NURSING RESEARCH:

DESIGN, STATISTICS AND COMPUTER ANALYSIS

NURSING RESEARCH:

DESIGN, STATISTICS AND COMPUTER ANALYSIS

CAROLYN FEHER WALTZ, Ph.D., R.N.

Professor
University of Maryland
School of Nursing
Baltimore, Maryland

R. BARKER BAUSELL, Ph.D.

Associate Professor
University of Maryland
School of Nursing
Baltimore, Maryland

 F. A. DAVIS COMPANY • **Philadelphia**

Library of Congress Cataloging in Publication Data

Waltz, Carolyn Feher.
  Nursing research: design, statistics and computer analysis
  Includes bibliographical references.
  1. Nursing—Research.   2. Nursing—Research—
Statistical methods. I. Bausell, R. Barker,
joint author. II. Title. [DNLM:
1. Nursing. 2. Research. 3. Computers.
WY20.5 W241n]
RT81.5.W37   610.73′072   80-18669
ISBN 0-8036-9040-1

PREFACE

This book is intended to serve as a comprehensive text for nurses who are involved in the design, analysis, and reporting of research. It is designed to present a pragmatic account of the process involved in designing and implementing research studies and to provide readers with the conceptual and operational basis for carrying out the process in their own settings.

Our own experiences in teaching research, statistics, and measurement to nurses and other health professionals, as well as in designing and implementing our own research studies guided the selection of topics and examples. This resulted in the inclusion of research content, strategies, and techniques with direct applicability for the investigation of nursing phenomena in a variety of settings. This book should have direct utility for those conducting research independently and collaboratively, and will aid consumers of research as well. Students in basic and advanced nursing research courses and graduate nurses with varying levels of preparation and experience in research will find it a valuable resource for expanding their repertoire of research knowledge as well as for guiding the conduct of research in educational, administrative, and clinical settings.

The authors do not assume that most readers have an extensive background in research design, statistics, or computer analysis. Rather, the discussions assume little or no background in research and consequently develop and explain in detail the concepts and principles that are operationally important to the content being presented. Computational procedures, although included, are de-emphasized and the focus is on the selection of an appropriate design, its implementation, and the utilization and interpretation of available computer programs for each of the statistical procedures presented. Many step-by-step examples are provided throughout the text. Attention is given to preparing a publishable report and opportunities for publishing nursing research results are examined. In addition, for the more sophisticated reader, care has been taken to include topics such as Bayesian analysis, criterion-referenced measurement, cross-lagged panel correlation analysis, and selected multivariate procedures that are currently underutilized in nursing research and are not found in existing nursing research textbooks, but have great potential for the investigation of nursing research questions and hypotheses.

References to additional sources are provided for readers who desire to further pursue the topics presented. References have been selected so that the material is readily available in most libraries and, whenever possible, comprehensive summaries of literature in an area or significant sources are cited rather than myriads of individual books and articles.

We are grateful to the Literary Executor of the late Sir Ronald A. Fisher, F.R.S., to Dr. Frank Yates, F.R.S., and to Longman Group Ltd., London, for permission to reprint Tables 1 and 2 of the Appendix from their book, *Statistical Tables for Biological, Agricultural and Medical Research* (6th edition, 1974).

CAROLYN FEHER WALTZ

R. BARKER BAUSELL

ACKNOWLEDGMENTS

I would like to express indebtedness for those sections of this book which I contributed (Protection of Human Subjects—Chapter 1; Hypothesis Testing—Chapter 2; Sampling—Chapter 3; Using the Computer for Data Analysis—Chapter 6; The Research Report—Chapter 7; Experimental Studies—Chapter 9; Selected Multivariate Procedures—Chapter 11) to my three research and statistical teachers: Drs. Joseph R. Jenkins, Jon Magoon, and James H. Crouse. Their personal attention and help will always be appreciated.

R. BARKER BAUSELL

CONTENTS

CHAPTER 1
INTRODUCTION

Nursing Research is a systematic, formal, rigorous, and precise process employed to gain solutions to problems and/or to discover and interpret new facts and relationships in the areas of clinical practice, nursing education, or nursing administration. When a study is undertaken to establish new knowledge or facts and develop theories or conceptual frameworks, it is often referred to as *basic* research. Research that attempts to find solutions to practical problems is termed *applied* research. Results of basic research are usually not immediately applicable to real world situations, while the new knowledge derived from applied research is generally used without much delay. Specific examples of basic and applied research are presented in Example 1-1.

EXAMPLE 1-1. Published Examples of Basic and Applied Research

Type: Basic.

Title: *Limiting intrusion — Social control of outsiders in a healing community: An illustration of qualitative comparative analysis.*

Source: Wilson, Nursing Research, vol. 26, no. 2, March – April, 1977, pp. 103 – 111.

Purpose: Explanatory propositions concerning the process of limiting intrusion were developed in the area of psychiatric care. Potential contributions of qualitative comparative analysis to nursing in general were suggested.

_____

Type: Applied.

Title: *Effect of Prepodyne as a perineal cleansing agent for clean catch specimens.*

EXAMPLE 1-1. *Continued*

Source: Moore and Bauer, Nursing Research, vol. 25, no. 4, July–August, 1976,
           pp. 259–261.

Purpose: Study was undertaken to determine a safe cleansing agent for collection of
           midstream urine specimens. Results suggested Prepodyne is a safe cleans-
           ing agent that shows a significant decrease in contamination levels
           which may give greater confidence to clinic diagnosis and reduce labora-
           tory costs.

Whether nursing research is basic or applied, it proceeds in the following
manner:

1. Identify the research problem.
   a. Survey the literature relating to the problem.
   b. Delimit the problem to be studied.
   c. State the purpose for the study in clear, specific terms.
2. Construct a research design.
   a. Formulate testable hypotheses.
   b. Define the variables.
   c. State underlying assumptions that govern the interpretation of results.
   d. Select subjects.
   e. Select or develop measures of outcomes.
   f. Specify data collection procedures.
   g. Select statistical procedures and computer programs for analyzing the
      data.
3. Execute the research design.
4. Evaluate the results and derive conclusions.

The focus of this book is the second step of the research process, constructing a
research design. The other steps of the process will be discussed only in terms
of their relationship to the research design.

THE RESEARCH PROBLEM

A *research design* is a plan that governs the conduct of a research endeavor.
The design employed in a particular study is a function of the research ques-
tion(s) to be answered. Questions for nursing research may generate from three
sources: (1) a theoretical or conceptual framework, (2) nursing practice experiences, and (3) the literature. When the researcher has identified a question or
topical area to be addressed by the study, a survey of the literature is indicated
in order to ascertain:

1. Some indication of the need for study in the area of interest, that is, justification for conducting the study.
2. Information regarding the activities of others in the same area.

3. Direction or focus for how to proceed with the proposed study.
4. A specific purpose for the study, for example, to describe, explain, or predict something relating to the problem's solution.

Specific strategies and techniques for conducting a literature search are presented in numerous sources[1, 13, 15] and, thus, will not be elaborated upon here. Borg[3] identifies two common errors to be avoided in conducting the literature search that have implications for the resulting research design: (1) conducting too cursory a review that overlooks previous studies containing ideas that might improve the proposed study design, and (2) focusing on research findings when reading research reports, thus missing valuable information on methods, measures, and the like. The review of the literature should be based on original articles, not on abstracts which can often be misleading.

Key sources for locating nursing literature include:

1. *Nursing Research, "Abstracts"*
   This was a regular component of the journal and appeared in each issue between 1959 and 1978. It represented a search of more than 200 nursing and health related periodicals.
2. *Cumulative Index to Nursing Literature*
   A quarterly publication with annual compilations since 1956, drawing from 54 periodicals in nursing and related fields. Published by Glendale Adventist Medical Center, Glendale, California.
3. *International Nursing Index to Periodical Literature*
   Published by the American Journal of Nursing Company, New York, New York, in cooperation with the National Library of Medicine in Bethesda, Maryland.
4. *Nursing Studies Index*
   An annotated guide to reported studies, research in progress, methods, and historical materials in more than 200 periodicals, books, and pamphlets. Published by J. B. Lippincott, Philadelphia, Pennsylvania.
5. Indexes to Nursing Periodicals
   Annual and cumulative indexes to nursing periodicals.
6. *Facts about Nursing*
   Published by the American Nurses' Association, Kansas City, Missouri. Includes data on numbers and distribution of nurses, employment conditions, numbers of students, graduations, withdrawals, and types of programs. A directory of major nursing organizations and statements of their purposes is also included.

To locate articles too recent to be included in the above sources, the tables of contents of nursing periodicals are useful.

Literature in fields related to nursing may be found using:

1. *National Library of Medicine Catalogue*
   Published monthly and contains listings of the holdings of the National Library of Medicine, Bethesda, Maryland.

2. *Index Medicus*
   Published monthly since 1960 by the National Library of Medicine. Contains guides to more than 5000 journals, including nursing journals.
3. *Excerpta Medica*
   An abstracting service published by Excerpta Medica, Elsevier North-Holland, New York, New York.
4. *Hospital Literature Index*
   A quarterly index of books, pamphlets, and articles from more than 300 periodicals including nursing journals. Published by the American Hospital Association, Chicago, Illinois.
5. *International Index*
   A quarterly guide to periodical literature in the social sciences and humanities. Published by H. W. Wilson Co., New York, New York.
6. *Research Grants Index*
   Published by the U.S. Government Printing Office, Washington, D.C.
7. *Psychological Abstracts*
   Abstracts materials from over 800 periodicals and 1200 other works per year.
8. *Dissertation Abstracts*
   Published monthly with annual listings since 1940. Contains abstracts of dissertations and monographs in microfilm at Ann Arbor, Michigan.
9. *Hospital Abstracts*
   Published since 1961 by H.M. Stationery Office, London, and prepared by Great Britain's Ministry of Health. Includes entries on nursing.
10. *Bibliography of Reproduction*
    Published since 1963 by Reproduction Research Information Service, Cambridge, England.
11. *Gale's Guide to the Use of Books and Libraries*
12. *McCormick's The New York Times Guide to Reference Materials*
13. *Medical Socioeconomic Research*
14. *Monthly Catalogue*
15. *Reader's Guide to Periodical Literature*
16. *Sociological Abstracts*
17. *Public Affairs Information Service*
18. *Education Index*
19. *Abstracts for Social Workers*
20. *International Pharmaceutical Abstracts*
21. *Poverty and Human Resources Abstracts*
22. *Resources in Education*
23. *Child Development Abstracts and Bibliographies*
24. *Bibliography of Suicide and Suicide Prevention*
25. *Quality Review Bulletin*, "Quality Assurance Rounds"

A number of *computerized information retrieval systems* are available to aid the researcher in conducting the literature search. These systems provide a quick, easy, efficient means for searching the literature to obtain a list of articles on a subject. Requests for a search are submitted through a computer terminal located in one's own library (most university libraries have access to one or more of these systems). This remote terminal taps directly into the main system where information is stored. A search analyst is available to help the researcher use the system. The researcher simply tells the search analyst what information is wanted and the analyst plans the search strategy and enters it into the terminal. In addition to being quicker than the traditional approach to conducting a literature search, these systems also provide more up-to-date information than the printed and published indexes discussed earlier.

Criteria for using these systems vary. Some systems are free, others have charges. A useful directory for obtaining this and other information about information retrieval systems is *Encyclopedia of Information Systems and Services*.[6]

Information retrieval systems that may be particularly useful in conducting nursing research are:

1. MEDLINE/MEDLARS
    Indexes over 2900 biomedical journals including all the journals indexed by *Index Medicus, International Nursing Index,* and *Index to Dental Literature.*
2. National Clearinghouse for Mental Health Information, National Institute of Mental Health
    Articles from more than 45,000 professional journals, books, conference proceedings, and other sources are abstracted. A bibliographic citation, the author's address, and abstract are retrievable by machine search techniques.
3. U.S. Commerce Department's National Technical Information Service
    Offers a computer-generated bibliographic search service of several hundred thousand Federally sponsored documents and abstracts published since 1964.
4. Smithsonian Science Information Exchange (SSIE)
    Contains more than 200,000 ongoing and recently compiled research projects in the life and physical sciences. Information can be retrieved in a variety of formats.
5. Psychological Abstracts Information Services (PAIS), including PATELL, PADAT, and PASAR
    Machine-readable tapes of PA records since 1967 are made available through a service called PATELL (PA Tape Edition Lease or Licensing). PADAT (PA Direct Access Terminal) allows researchers to conduct information searches on a computer terminal in their own facility. The method allows direct interaction with the PA data base. The output may be printed at the remote terminal location or printed on a high speed device at the main facility and mailed to the researcher.
    PASAR (PA Search and Retrieval) is accessible by mail. The individual submits a request form specifying information requirements following guidelines provided on the form. A computer printout of bibliographic

citations and full texts of abstracts is sent back to the requester by the main office.

6. Educational Resources Information Center (ERIC)
   A nationwide information network of the Department of Education, National Institute of Education, for abstracting and indexing education related reports. Computer searches are available.
7. Direct Access to Reference Information (DATRIX)
   Contains more than 150,000 dissertation abstracts that can be pinpointed by computer search. Reproduction by microfilm or hard copy is made possible by University Microfilms.
8. Health Education Information Retrieval System (HEIRS)
   Health education related reprints, book chapters, and other documents involving topics such as the philosophy of health care and health services planning are included.
9. NEXUS, American Association for Higher Education, Washington, D.C.
   A telephone information referral service that directs applicants to a clearinghouse agency or other service that meets their informational needs.

THE RESEARCH DESIGN

Depending upon the specific purpose for conducting the study, the researcher selects one of three types of research designs: descriptive, experimental, or correlational.

Descriptive Designs

Descriptive designs are employed when the researcher wishes to obtain information in areas in which little previous investigation has occurred and/or to construct a picture or account of events as they exist naturally. No attempt is made to introduce something new, or to in any manner modify or control the situation being studied. Specific examples of descriptive designs are presented in Example 1-2.

EXAMPLE 1-2. Published Examples of Descriptive Designs

Title: *Drug-drug interactions among residents in homes for the elderly: A pilot study.*

Source: Brown et al., Nursing Research, vol. 26, no. 1, January–February, 1977, pp. 47–52.

Purpose: The researchers contend that the clinically significant drug-drug interaction (D-DI), a subclass of adverse drug responses, is a neglected area of research. Studies in private community hospitals suggested clinically significant D-DIs occurred infrequently. The researchers speculated that the occurrence would be greater in homes for the elderly for a number of rea-

EXAMPLE 1-2. *Continued*

sons and thus set out to obtain information to support their supposition. The specific purposes they identified for their study were:
1. Describe the numbers and kinds of drug used for all residents in the institutions studied.
2. Describe the occurrence of the potential for clinically significant D-DIs.
3. Determine the distribution of certain drug factors among members of the study group (pp. 47 – 48).

Design: To meet their study purposes, the investigators:
1. Selected two settings as being representative of homes providing widely different services for the elderly in rural and urban settings.
2. Obtained a drug profile for each resident included in the study (n = 188).
3. Determined potential for clinically significant D-DIs by having physicians review the profiles.
4. Tabulated frequencies and discussed study results in terms of results obtained by others.

_ _

Title: *Needs of the grieving spouse in a hospital setting.*

Source: Hampe, Nursing Research, vol. 24, no. 2, March – April, 1975, pp. 113 – 119.

Purpose: The researcher sought to answer the following questions:
1. Can the spouse whose mate is terminally ill or has died identify his own needs?
2. What are these needs?
3. How are these needs affected by the death event of the mate?
4. Does the grieving spouse perceive that he, himself, has been helped by the nurses?
5. Which needs of the grieving spouse do nurses meet?
6. What nursing measures helped to meet these needs? (p. 114)

Design: The research questions were answered in the following manner:
1. Spouses whose mates had been determined by medical staff in a specific hospital center to be terminally ill were identified (n = 41).
2. Spouses were interviewed by the researcher to determine their needs and their perceptions of how they were met. Interviews were semi-structured and open ended and were tape recorded to facilitate data analysis.
3. Data were summarized by number and percent to determine and report answers to the study questions.

The bulk of the research in nursing to date has been descriptive in nature. In part, this has resulted from the value that such studies have as a mechanism for generating questions for future experimental study – an important concern for a profession, such as nursing, that is intent on developing theories and hypotheses to be tested. In addition, the accountability movement in nursing has stimulated educators, administrators, and practitioners to evaluate their respective programs. A descriptive study is usually the first step in a comprehensive evaluation because it allows the investigator to determine how the program is operating, that is, to find out what the facts are, so the investigator may then consider them in light of program objectives.

Experimental Designs

An experimental design is employed when the researcher seeks to determine whether or not a predicted or expected result occurs when a specified action is taken. Essential characteristics of a *true experimental design* are the utilization of a controlled situation and random assignment. When a controlled situation is established, certain factors are held constant, other factors are manipulated, and the results in the manipulated situation are evaluated and compared with those obtained in the controlled situation. Random sampling means that subjects are selected in such a way that every member of the population has an equal chance of being selected for inclusion in the study sample. The true experimental design is the most rigorous and precise approach to investigating nursing problems. The researcher uses the findings from a true experimental study to make inferences regarding the cause-effect relationships between factors. An example of a true experimental design is presented in Example 1-3.

EXAMPLE 1-3. Published Example of a True Experimental Design

Title: *Topical application of insulin in the treatment of decubitus ulcers: A pilot study.*

Source: Ort and Gerber, Nursing Research, vol. 25, no. 1, January–February, 1976, pp. 9–12.

Purpose: To evaluate the effects of topical application of insulin to promote healing of decubitus ulcers.

Design: To test the hypothesis that there will be a significantly greater increase in the rate of healing of decubitus ulcers in subjects who receive other forms of therapy evidenced by a decrease in the diameter of the ulcer, the researchers:
1. Randomly assigned subjects (n = 14) who developed decubitus ulcers to experimental and control groups.
2. Insulin therapy was provided subjects in the experimental group twice a day for five days.
3. Subjects in the control group received one of a variety of topical therapies other than insulin.
4. Subjects in both groups received routine supportive care (for example, turning and positioning).
5. Over a 15-day period, rate of healing of the ulcer, defined as the amount of decrease in diameter per day, was evaluated and compared for both groups.
6. Results supported the hypothesis, but generalizability was limited by the small size of the sample.

Quasi-experimental designs represent an attempt to approximate a true experimental design when certain essential characteristics of the true design cannot be attained. Campbell and Stanley[5] describe quasi-experimental designs as those in which the researcher can schedule data collection procedures even though the researcher is unable to (1) randomly sample, (2) manipulate factors, or (3) determine when or to whom the experimental treatment will be introduced. Quasi-experimental designs are less precise than true experimental designs and their results are more subject to disagreement. A researcher who employs a quasi-experimental approach must be very cognizant of the limitations of the specific quasi-experimental design selected. An example of a quasi-experimental design is presented in Example 1-4.

EXAMPLE 1-4. Published Example of a Quasi-Experimental Design

Title: *Nursing students' attitudes toward death.*

Source: Hopping, Nursing Research, vol. 26, no. 6, November–December, 1977, pp. 443–447.

Purpose: To determine changes in attitudes toward death and dying among baccalaureate nursing students associated with their participation in a clinical course focused on nursing care for the dying patient.

Design: A nonequivalent control group design (Campbell and Stanley, p. 47) was used to test three hypotheses (see article, p. 444). This quasi-experimental design was selected in lieu of an experimental one because the researchers were unable to randomly assign subjects to control and treatment groups. To implement the design, the researchers:
1. Designated an intact group of 20 students who elected to take the course as the experimental group.
2. Randomly selected a group of 20 students from those who were not in the course to serve as the control group.
3. Administered a questionnaire before and after the course to all students in the nursing program. Students were thus not aware of what data would be used (only data for the 40 subjects) or that two groups would be compared, and the researchers reasoned this fact might control for experimental bias in the results.
4. Compared resulting scores for the experimental group with those of the control group utilizing chi-square, t-tests, and an item analysis procedure.
5. Recognized the limitations in comparing two nonequivalent groups (that is, volunteers and nonvolunteers) and opted to consider their study as descriptive rather than experimental, viewing their statistical rejections of two null hypotheses as indicating differences between groups warranting further study.

The conduct of true experimental studies is a vital aspect of the continuing evolution of nursing theory and science. Nurses frequently, however, find themselves in situations in which they are unable to establish a controlled situation or in which all available subjects must receive the experimental program. It is in these instances that the value of quasi-experimental designs is realized and that they may make their contribution to the establishment of nursing practice based on validated theory and scientific investigation.

Correlational Designs

Correlational designs are employed when the researcher's interest is in exploring the relationships or commonalities among factors. In *regression* studies, a special case of correlational designs, the researcher attempts to explain or predict changes in one factor (the criterion factor) on the basis of changes in other factors (the predictor factors). An example of a correlational design is presented in Example 1-5.

> **EXAMPLE 1-5.** Published Example of a Correlational Design
>
> Title: *The student's perception of his creativity.*
>
> Source: Marriner, Nursing Research, vol. 26, no. 1, January–February, 1977, pp. 57–60.
>
> Purpose: To study the relationship of student's perceptions of his creativity with his educational major, hours completed toward graduation, grade point average, and rank among siblings (p. 58).
>
> Design: Subjects were 590 nursing and non-nursing students in one university. The criterion variable, students' perceptions of their creativity, was measured by asking students to rate their perceptions on a 1 (low) to 5 (high) scale. Predictor variables were educational major, hours completed toward graduation, grade point average, and sibling rank. Predictor variables were measured by having subjects respond to a questionnaire administered during a regular class period. Responses were summarized by number and percent. The relationship between the criterion variable and each of the predictor variables was assessed using an appropriate correlational statistical procedure.

Correlational designs derive their greatest utility from the flexibility they afford the researcher in investigating the complex relationships among the multiple factors that exist in nursing practice situations. In addition, when used for descriptive purposes, correlational studies provide more information than is usually obtained using other approaches to descriptive research. The reasons for this will become clearer when correlational designs are discussed in detail in a later chapter.

FACTORS AFFECTING SELECTION OF A RESEARCH DESIGN

Selection of the best design for a particular research problem requires a knowledge of the research area and a knowledge of different types of designs. Generally, several designs can be employed in studying a given research problem. However, alternative designs that are equally valid for investigating a problem are rarely equally efficient. Efficiency of alternative research designs may be defined in various ways. For example, efficiency may be defined in terms of the time required to collect data, cost of data collection, ratio of information to cost, and so forth.

Efficiency of a research design may be increased by the use of a larger number of subjects or by exercising additional controls during the conduct of the experiment. Similarly, efficiency may be enhanced if the most precise design or the one that allows for the more powerful statistical procedures to be used is employed. However, a design that is efficient in one research situation may not be in another. The researcher is thus forced to identify the best compromise that can be obtained within the constraints of the particular situation. For example, a researcher, because of the resources available, may find that the efficiency of the design can be increased by the use of a more complex experimental design that requires considerable time to plan and analyze, while in another situation, with fewer resources available, the same researcher may find the efficiency increased by using a simple design but a larger number of subjects. To determine the best design, the researcher should consider the following questions:

1. What kinds of data are required to study the research problem?
2. Is it possible to obtain subjects using a random sampling procedure?
3. How strictly controlled can the study be? Is it possible or desirable to include a control group? How important is it that the study be replicable?
4. What is the size of the problem to be studied? Is it significant enough to justify the time and effort needed to study it? Is there a large enough study population from which to obtain an adequate sample?
5. How much time are potential data sources willing to devote to data collection activities? How much effort is required to obtain the data needed to conduct the study? Are data available without too much trouble or cost?
6. What is the cost to subjects in terms of time, effort, and outcome if this study is conducted in a certain manner?
7. How much money is available for consultation time, computer time, instrument development?
8. What instruments are available? What instruments need to be developed? Who is available and willing to assume responsibility for their development and testing?
9. Will this be an individual or collaborative research effort? Who is available and willing to participate in the investigation of this problem? What are their strengths and weaknesses in the areas of research, statistics, and the content addressed?
10. Is sufficient time available to conduct the study?
11. Who is available to coordinate the research effort? What will be the nature and extent of this person's involvement in the tasks undertaken by

others (that is, consultative, active, administrative)? What are this individual's strengths and weaknesses in research, statistics, and the content area? Can this person serve as a resource to participants who are less sophisticated in these areas?

When the researcher has selected what is believed to be the best design for the study, it may be useful to evaluate the design using specific criteria that have been suggested by a number of authors.[9, 10, 17] Since these criteria are readily available they will not be enumerated here. The consensus is that a research design is adequate if it is relatively precise and efficient, affords the utilization of powerful statistical procedures, is economical for both researcher and subjects, produces valid and reliable results, allows an opportunity for comparison of study findings with the results of other investigations, and conforms to accepted practices and procedures used in the research area.

Whether or not a given research plan conforms to accepted practices and procedures used in the research area is currently one of the major factors affecting not only the selection of a research design but also the researcher's ability to implement it. This importance stems from the fact that the ethics of research efforts no longer rest solely with the individual researcher, but are subject to approval by institutional review boards who are charged with the protection of the rights of human subjects. Thus, subsequent to the researcher's own evaluation of the adequacy of the design, in most cases, the researcher will be required to submit the proposal to such an institutional review board for approval before the study can be conducted.

PROTECTION OF HUMAN SUBJECTS

Since nursing research almost always deals with human subjects, whether patients, well individuals, or other nurses, some provision must be made to insure that those individuals' rights, health, and safety are not violated. Only a few years ago, these provisions were very informal with the bulk of the responsibility lying with the professional integrity of the researcher, persons in charge of physical access to patients, and the willingness of the human subjects themselves to participate in any given study.

Unfortunately, as all health professionals now know, a few individuals in medical and behavioral research flagrantly violated the safety and rights of their subjects, sometimes with gruesome consequences. Perhaps due to humanitarian instincts, perhaps in response to the outrage generated by the fact that some of these studies were Federally funded, the Division of Health, Education, and Welfare (DHEW) in 1975 mandated that all institutions receiving funds from DHEW must provide formal assurance of compliance with DHEW regulations which specifically state that ". . . no activity involving human subjects to be supported by DHEW grants or contracts shall be undertaken unless an Institutional Review Board has reviewed and approved such activities. . . ."

One effect of this regulation has been to provide the impetus for those institutions that had not already established institutional review boards to do so (most had already done so). Another effect was to encourage those with review boards to use them more systematically and effectively. The summative result of the regulation was to force professionals to take a much closer look at *all* research (but especially clinical research involving patients) being conducted within the confines of their institutions, an effect which ultimately made the conduct of empirical research far more difficult from the researcher's perspective but hopefully safer from the patient's.

Most nursing research involves no experimental manipulation that could possibly be construed as placing a patient's life in jeopardy. Furthermore, very few studies even come close to violating their subjects' rights to privacy, simply because the very nature of empirical research precludes the need for it. (The purpose of research is to determine whether some effect or some relationship holds for *most* people; the identity of an individual participant is almost always irrelevant.) Why, then, the need for human subjects committees and review boards for research proposals?

One answer lies in such qualifiers as "most" and "very few," which imply that some studies do or may violate their subjects' rights. Most health care professionals subscribe to the belief that it is better to err on the patient's side than the researcher's. Even though patients may ultimately benefit from research results, it is reasoned that these benefits lie in the future and are tenuous at best. It is incumbent upon the researcher, therefore, to demonstrate that the potential benefits of the study far outweigh any potential danger to, or violation of privacy of, its subjects.

The actual subjects of a study, however, cannot be the researcher's only consideration in the conduct of research. The ANA's 1975 position paper entitled *Human Rights Guidelines for Nurses in Clinical and Other Research*,[2] for example, underscores the fact that informed consent applies not only to "subjects *per se* but also to any workers who are expected as part of their daily work to implement activities that potentially or actually carry risk for others or have uncertain outcomes." These guidelines further suggest that if nurses are expected to participate in clinical research as part of their jobs, then this participation should be spelled out as a condition of employment.

The document goes on to suggest that nurses, due to their professional responsibilities, must be vigilant of protecting the rights of individuals under their care "who by reason of their situation and/or illness are not able to protect themselves effectively from externally imposed threat or injury" and for this reason strongly suggests that nursing representation be present on all institutional review committees involving research in which nurses are likely to be involved whether directly or indirectly. In addition to these review committees, however, the guidelines specifically recommend that informed consent consist of (1) an explanation of the study procedures and purposes thereof, (2) a detailed description of any and all physical risk, discomfort, invasion of privacy, or threat to dignity entailed in the study, (3) an assurance that those procedures will be evoked to achieve anonymity, (4) an offer to discuss additional questions that the potential subject may have, (5) an assurance that quality of care will not be affected by failure to participate, and (6) an assurance that the subject may discontinue participation at any time he or she chooses.

The prospective researcher must be concerned with far more than simply protecting the rights of patients and staff, however, if the researcher expects to conduct research in a clinical setting. The researcher must satisfy at least one institutional review board, possibly more, within the institution in which the proposed research would be conducted. Usually, it is also necessary to obtain permission from the institution with which the researcher is affiliated, even though the data may not be collected within that institution. Applying for permission consists, in most cases, of the submission of a research protocol or proposal which is as formal, and in many cases as detailed, as the final report emanating from the finished research project. *Nursing Outlook* published an interesting article dealing with the institutional review process in a Boston area hospital.[8] In this particular institution, the division of nursing services set up a Nursing Research Review Committee which screens proposals and submits them to an ad hoc committee if approved, which in turn decides whether or not to submit the proposal to the overall Hospital Review Board. The author, who is also nursing research coordinator at this institution, concludes that it is impractical for nursing faculty to expect graduate students to be able to conduct clinical research as part of their curriculum because of the time constraints imposed by the review process. Although she vigorously defends her division's position in this regard, its implications for the profession are quite interesting, especially given the fact that such bureaucratic processes are being initiated and imposed by the profession upon itself.

Regardless of whether the character of this particular review process is considered laudable or not, the individual criteria used to judge proposals are quite reasonable and probably reflect current practices in most institutions. Generally, the members of the Nursing Research Review Committee ask themselves three genre of questions: (1) Is the project feasible given the facilities available, the time constraints, and so forth? (2) Does the proposal reflect good research practice and conception (for example, are purposes clearly stated, are procedures and instrumentation appropriate, are subjects' rights protected, are methods used to obtain informed consent clearly delineated and ethical, and will the study's results have potential utility and importance)? (3) How will the study fit into the overall treatment milieu (for example, will day-to-day routines be disrupted, will the study duplicate or interfere with other ongoing research, will the study conflict with institutional or departmental philosophy, objectives, or policy)?

Basically, these criteria reflect concerns common to all health agencies, both today and in the past. They should be of no less concern to researchers themselves. Is the study worth doing? Is it excessively disruptive of vital services being performed? Do the procedures constitute danger, embarrassment, or inconvenience to subjects already more vulnerable and fragile than the general population? The more seriously the researcher addresses these questions before a proposal is submitted, the more likely the proposal is to achieve acceptance. Also, the more the researcher knows about the idiosyncracies of a particular institution, the more likely is acceptance. (For example, patients and staff in a university affiliated hospital may be grossly overresearched; hence, an investigator might be wiser to submit the proposal to a less academically oriented facility.) Finally, the probability of a proposal being accepted is inversely proportionate to the amount of time and effort required of patients and staff; thus, time spent in planning ways to minimize such involvement is always an excellent investment.

In many ways, the effort invested in the preparation of a formal proposal for an institutional review board is well worthwhile. The process requires the researcher to think through and operationalize each step of the study. It requires the researcher to address difficult questions concerning minimal resources needed, protection of the rights of subjects, and so forth. Most practicing researchers, although sometimes decrying the excessive bureaucratization of the process, agree that the review performs a vital, helpful function and in many cases is necessary to protect the safety, health, and rights of human subjects.

REFERENCES

1. Abdellah, F. G. and Levine, E.: *Better Patient Care through Nursing Research*. Macmillan, New York, 1965.
2. American Nurses' Association: *Human Rights Guidelines For Nurses In Clinical and Other Research*, by J. Q. Benoliel and J. S. Berthold (ANA Publ. No. 0–46). American Nurses' Association, Kansas City, Missouri, 1975, p. 3.
3. Borg, W. R.: *Educational Research: An Introduction*. David McKay, New York, 1963, p. 67.
4. Brown, M. M., et al.: *Drug-drug interactions among residents in homes for the elderly: A pilot study*. Nurs. Res. 26:1, January–February, 1977, pp. 47–52.
5. Campbell, D. T. and Stanley, J.: *Experimental and Quasi-Experimental Designs for Research*. Rand McNally, Chicago, 1966.
6. *Encyclopedia of Information Systems and Services*, ed. 3. Gale Research Company, Detroit, Michigan, 1978.
7. Hampe, S. O.: *Needs of the grieving spouse in a hospital setting*. Nurs. Res. 24:2, March–April, 1975, pp. 113–119.
8. Hodgman, E. C.: *Student research in service agencies*. Nurs. Outlook 26:9, September, 1978, pp. 558–565.
9. Kirk, R. E.: *Experimental Design: Procedures for the Behavioral Sciences*. Brooks/Cole, California, 1968.
10. Lindquist, E. F.: *Design and Analysis of Experiments in Psychology and Education*. Houghton Mifflin, Boston, 1953.
11. Marringer, A.: *The student's perception of his creativity*. Nurs. Res. 26:1, January–February, 1977, pp. 57–60.
12. Moore, D. S. and Bauer, C. S: *Effect of Prepodyne as a perineal cleansing agent for clean catch specimens*. Nurs. Res. 25:4, July–August, 1976, pp. 259–261.
13. Notter, L. E.: *Essentials of Nursing Research*. Springer, New York, 1974.
14. Ort, S. and Gerber, R.: *Topical application of insulin in the treatment of decubitus ulcers: A pilot study*. Nurs. Res. 25:1, January–February, 1976, pp. 9–12.
15. Treece, E. W. and Treece, J. W.: *Elements of Research in Nursing*, ed. 2. C. V. Mosby, St. Louis, 1977.

16. Wilson, H. S.: *Limiting intrusion — Social control of outsiders in a healing community: An illustration of qualitative comparative analysis.* Nurs. Res. 26:2, March – April, 1977, pp. 103 – 111.
17. Winer, B. J.: *Statistical Principles in Experimental Design.* McGraw-Hill, New York, 1962.

CHAPTER 2
HYPOTHESIS TESTING

The purpose of all but purely descriptive research is to ascertain whether or not a relationship exists between variables. This relationship may take the form of seeing if one group of subjects performs better (or heals more quickly) than another as a result of an experimental treatment applied to one group but not the other, or it may simply involve seeing whether subjects who score highly on one measure also score highly on another.

Regardless of the nature of the relationship, the procedures used to establish its existence or nonexistence are conceptually identical. The first step involves clearly delineating the relationship to be examined prior to the conduct of the study. Once articulated, procedures are next worked out for collecting data to appropriately measure this relationship. The data are then collected and a decision is made regarding the existence or nonexistence of the posited relationship. Although conceptually simple, this basic process and its constituents comprise practically the entire subject matter of this book.

This chapter deals with the logic underlying the testing of the posited relationship and the subsequent decision-making process involved in deciding whether or not this relationship does actually exist.

THE HYPOTHESIS

As will be discussed in Chapter 8, all research studies are not concerned with examining the relationship(s) between variables. Most are, however, and it is these types of studies to which the concept of hypothesis testing is crucial.

The hypothesis is a formal statement of the purpose of a research study. It is, in fact, an operational definition of that purpose and as such has two necessary characteristics: it must delineate a relationship between variables and that rela-

17

tionship must be empirically testable through the collection of data. Implicit in these characteristics are the following conditions: only one relationship may be specified in a single hypothesis (although any given study may have several hypotheses); the hypothesis must be written before the study is conducted (to do otherwise would be like trying to bet on a horse race after the results are posted); only words describing an empirically testable relationship may be used in a hypothesis (phrases such as "the best method" or words such as "good," "harmful," and so forth have no place in a hypothesis).[2] Table 2-1 gives examples of acceptable and unacceptable hypotheses along with rationales for each.

Hypotheses are usually stated in the form of a declarative sentence as opposed to research problems which are often stated as questions. The chief distinction between the two formats usually resides in the greater specificity of the hypothesis. A research problem, for example, might be stated as the general question: "What is the nature of the relationship between age and blood pressure?" or "Is there a relationship between age and blood pressure?" A hypothesis, on the other hand, makes a clear statement regarding the explicit nature or posited relationship between the two variables: "There is no relationship between age and blood pressure" or "There is a relationship between age and blood pressure." Both of these statements delineate a testable relationship between two variables and as such fit the above definition of a hypothesis.

TABLE 2-1. Examples and Rationales of Acceptable and Unacceptable Hypotheses

---

Acceptable Hypotheses

1. There is no significant relationship between age and blood pressure.
2. An individual's blood pressure is a function of his age, weight, and daily exercise regimen.
3. There is no significant difference between students receiving and those not receiving instruction with respect to achievement scores.
4. The experimental group will achieve significantly greater attitudinal gains than the control group.

Unacceptable Hypotheses

1. There is no significant difference between age and blood pressure. (Age and blood pressure are measured with different metrics. To say there is no difference between the two is like saying there is no difference between apples and oranges.)
2. Administering instruction is the best way to increase students' achievement scores. (Research can only compare. To test the best possible method would necessitate the empirical comparison of all possible treatments.)
3. Group A is significantly better than groups B and C and group B is better than group C. (This hypothesis suffers from a dual fault. In the first place the dependent variable is not specified: better than what? Secondly, more than one relationship is presented. A hypothesis should be stated in such a way as to test only one relationship at a time.)
4. What is the nature of the relationship between an individual's blood pressure and his age, weight, and daily exercise regimen? (Hypotheses are stated as declarative sentences, not questions. A question cannot be tested; it cannot be accepted or rejected.)

It will be noted, however, that the first hypothesis is stated in negative terms as though the researcher expected to find no relationship between the two variables. This is really merely a convention and is called a *null hypothesis* and denoted as H_0. It does not mean that the researcher "believes" that there will be no relationship between age and blood pressure; the researcher's beliefs are irrelevant to the research process and null hypotheses are one means of emphasizing this fact. The null hypothesis simply states the relationship that will be tested. If a relationship is found, then H_0 will be considered probably *false*; if no relationship is found, H_0 will be considered probably *true*. (Many theoreticians prefer to talk in terms of failing to accept or reject the null hypothesis; the authors find it more convenient to consider hypotheses as probably true or probably false while recognizing the epistemological distinctions involved.)

A hypothesis that states the direction that a relationship is likely to take, or simply states that a relationship exists without dealing with directionality, is called a *research hypothesis* and denoted as H_1. In the above example, the statement "There is a relationship between age and blood pressure" is an example of a nondirectional research hypothesis. If the researcher had good reason to believe that older individuals possess higher blood pressures than younger individuals, then the direction of H_1 could be specified: "There is a positive relationship between age and blood pressure."

H_1 really differs from H_0 only in form. Functionally the two are simply different sides of the same coin: one gives the researcher's prediction or opinion, the other does not. When one is accepted as probably true, the other is automatically considered probably false.

HYPOTHESIS TESTING

Writing a hypothesis, although crucial, is only a small part of designing a research study. Far and away the greatest amount of work, skill, and thought goes into specifying the conditions under which the data will be collected and actually collecting that data. At this stage, these two extremely important steps will be saved for later chapters with the following discussion assuming that (1) a hypothesis has been written, (2) the conditions of the study have been specified, and (3) the data have been collected.

Once these tasks are accomplished, the next step in the process is to analyze the data in such a way that a decision can be made as to whether or not the relationship posited in the original hypothesis is present or absent. At first glance, this may seem like a ludicrously simple task. As an example, consider two groups of subjects, one having received preoperative instruction regarding what they could expect from their surgical experience, the other having received only the usual hospital routine. If these groups were to be compared with respect to the amount of postoperative medication they required, then all that would seemingly be necessary to test the null hypothesis would be to count up the number of times patients in each group requested medication and see if one group requested more than the other. Theoretically, it would seem that if the group that received the preoperative instruction requested exactly the same amount of medication as the group that did not receive said instruction, there would be no relationship between preoperative instruction and medication requests. Under such conditions, the null hypothesis would be considered to be probably true (that is, H_0 = "Patients receiving preoperative instruction do not differ from patients not receiving preoperative instruction with respect to the amount of medication requested following surgery").

With this particular outcome, such a conclusion would be difficult to refute. What, however, if the experimental group (that is, those subjects receiving preoperative instruction) had requested medication a total of 78 times and the control group's requests had totaled 79? Would the researcher be justified in arguing that the null hypothesis was probably false and that a relationship did indeed exist between the variables? Would a hospital administrator be justified in authorizing preoperative instruction for all patients on the basis of this minute difference between groups?

The probability is that after a little thought a reasonable administrator would conclude that the difference was too small to be sure that preoperative instruction had any real effect upon requests for medication. Such a decision would be correct because, in research dealing with different groups of people under different conditions, results are almost never identical across groups, people, and time. Given two or more groups, in fact, it is far more likely that in the final analysis these groups will differ *to some degree* than it is that they will not differ at all. Given this state of affairs, therefore, it should be obvious that some objective criterion should be available to ascertain whether or not a hypothesized relationship should be accepted as "real" or rejected as not real. Such a criterion does exist. It is called statistical significance and it is basic to all hypothesis testing.

STATISTICAL SIGNIFICANCE

Basically all that is involved in the concept of statistical significance is (1) the substitution of a statistical value for an observed relationship or difference and (2) the comparison of said statistical value to a distribution of other statistical values to ascertain how likely such a value (and hence the relationship it represents) would be to occur by chance alone. If the odds are on the side of the observed relationship not occurring by chance alone, then the null hypothesis is considered probably false (and H_1 probably true). If the odds seem to favor the relationship occurring by chance, then the null hypothesis is accepted as probably true.

Consider the following hypothetical example. Suppose the results shown in Table 2-2 had occurred when conducting the above mentioned study contrasting a group of patients receiving preoperative instruction (which could be called the experimental [E] group) with a group receiving none (the control [C] group) with respect to requests for medication following surgery. Patients receiving preoperative instruction *appeared* to request pain medications less frequently than control patients: the former registering 11 requests as opposed to 25 for the latter. The question becomes however: Since it is unlikely that the

TABLE 2-2. Hypothetical Postoperative Medication Requests of Patients Who Received and Patients Who Did Not Receive Preoperative Instruction

E (group receiving instruction)		C (group not receiving instruction)	
Patient	Number of medication requests	Patient	Number of medication requests
#1	3	#5	4
#2	2	#6	6
#3	1	#7	8
#4	5	#8	7
	11		25

two groups would have registered *identical* medication requests regardless of the experimental treatment (instruction), is the difference actually observed (that is, $25 - 11 = 14$) likely to have occurred by chance alone? If the answer is no, then the researcher can conclude that the observed difference (14) was due to the fact that one group received preoperative instruction and the other did not (if the study was conducted carefully) and that H_0 could be rejected as probably false. If the answer is yes, then the researcher would conclude that the instruction had no measurable effect and that H_0 was probably correct.

The actual decision of whether or not H_0 should be considered probably true or probably false is extremely easy to make. Conceptually, the process consists of two steps: (1) determining the level of error that can be tolerated in reaching the decision, and (2) determining how likely the actual results obtained were to have occurred by chance alone.

Level of Error

Usually nursing research follows the lead of psychological, educational, and behavioral research which by convention has decided that the maximum tolerable error for considering the null hypothesis probably false is 5 percent. Said another way, these researchers are willing to be wrong 5 times out of 100 when rejecting the null hypothesis, but no more than that. Implicit in this decision, of course, is the decision that if they are going to make an error they would prefer it to be on the side of not rejecting H_0 rather than rejecting it when it is "really" true.

This admittedly arbitrary level of tolerable error is called the *alpha level*, or sometimes simply the study's *level of significance*. It is not always set at 0.05. Sometimes it is set lower when researchers wish to be especially cautious about reporting false positive results, such as with clinical or applied research in which false positive errors could potentially be dangerous. In this vein, the next most popular level is undoubtedly 0.01 or 1 percent, which indicates that if the researcher concludes that a relationship exists in the data (and rejects H_0 as probably false), then the chances of being wrong are only 1 in 100. Some researchers have set even lower levels for themselves, such as 0.001.

In theory testing research, however, and in obviously exploratory work, the argument is occasionally made that higher significance levels (for example, 0.10 or a 1 in 10 chance of error) should be accepted using the rationale that no great harm would accrue from being wrong in rejecting H_0 and further that the researcher really does not wish to err on the side of reporting false negative findings (that is, by reporting that no relationship exists when in "reality" one does). Researchers simply must decide for themselves which alpha level to use, although the bulk of the academic community still seems to feel more comfortable with lower alphas (many journals, for example, will not publish results that have significance levels greater than 0.05).

Probability of Obtained Results Occurring by Chance

The second step in deciding whether or not H_0 should be rejected is to determine how likely the *actual results obtained were to have occurred by chance alone*. This value is then compared to the predetermined alpha level. If alpha had been set at 0.05, for example, and the observed relationship was found capable of occurring by chance alone more than 5 times out of 100 (for example, 0.06, 0.10, 0.50, and so forth), then H_0 would not be rejected. If the observed relationship would occur by chance alone less than the tolerable limit (for example, 0.049, 0.04, 0.002, and so forth), then H_0 would be rejected as probably false.

The actual significance level of the obtained relationship is determined in practice by (1) choosing an appropriate statistic to represent said relationship, (2) computing the statistic (which is really nothing more than translating the relationship in such a way that it can be represented by the statistic), and (3) comparing the statistic to its particular distribution to see how likely it (and hence the relationship it represents) was to occur by chance alone. This entire procedure is an extremely simple process when data are analyzed via the computer because steps two and three are accomplished for the researcher automatically. Since you will thus never be forced to sit down and work through the concepts underlining statistical significance, it might be instructive to demonstrate how the significance level of the hypothetical results in Table 2-2 could be obtained without the use of computers, statistics, or statistical tables. Although no one ever computes statistical significance by the methods discussed, working through the process should enhance your understanding of the conceptual basis behind hypothesis testing.

Returning to the hypothetical data in Table 2-2, the question of exactly what statistical significance means, hence exactly what "obtained by chance alone" means, can be rephrased as "given the eight medication requests observed in the study (that is, 3, 2, 1, 5, 4, 6, 8, and 7), what is the probability that a difference as large as 14 (25 − 11) would occur by chance alone?" One way to answer this question would be to write the eight numbers on slips of paper, mix them thoroughly in a hat, and draw two groups of four numbers from the hat without looking. Each group of four numbers could then be totaled and the difference between these totals could be considered a "chance" occurrence since they obviously occurred by chance alone.

If, for example, the first randomly drawn group had consisted of the numbers 3, 2, 4, and 6 and the second group of 1, 5, 7, and 8, then the difference between these groups would be $21 - 15$ or 6. This number could, therefore, serve as the researcher's definition of a relationship that occurred by chance alone. The researcher could then theoretically compare the difference actually obtained (14) in the study to this chance difference and conclude that H_0 should be rejected, since the difference that occurred following instruction was greater than the difference that occurred by chance.

An obvious problem with this strategy lies in the fact that very few people would be willing to accept one chance occurrence (that is, drawing two groups of four numbers from a hat) as an absolute definition of "chance." What, they might ask, if it just so happened that two comparably homogeneous groups of numbers were drawn by accident? Anything could happen on a single drawing.

The researcher could counter these arguments, of course, by conducting many more drawings and recording the results. The researcher would thus construct a sampling distribution of thousands of chance differences between groups to which the obtained difference could be compared. If 95 percent or more of the chance differences were smaller than the obtained difference of 14, then the researcher could safely conclude that the difference between the experimental and control groups was not random and thus reject H_0.

Although the significance level of any experiment could be determined in this manner, very few researchers would have the patience to construct a unique sampling distribution for each study they completed. Actually a much more direct method of constructing a sampling distribution exists. The total number of combinations of two groups of four numbers each can easily be calculated mathematically. Starting with the eight numbers listed in Table 2-2, therefore, it is possible to construct 70 different combinations, of which having the numbers 3, 2, 1, and 5 in the experimental group and 4, 6, 8, and 7 in the control is only one. Table 2-3 shows a few of these combinations.

The researcher could then compute differences between these 70 unique combinations of four numbers and construct a frequency distribution of the differences between the two groups. (Note that although there are 70 different

TABLE 2-3. Examples of Possible Combinations for the Two Groups of Four Numbers in Table 2-2

(1)		(2)		(3)		(4)		(5)		(6)		.... (70)
E	C	E	C	E	C	E	C	E	C	E	C	
1	5	1	4	1	2	1	2	2	1	5	1	
2	6	2	6	3	4	3	4	3	4	6	2	
3	7	3	7	6	5	6	5	6	5	7	3	
4	8	5	8	7	8	8	7	7	8	8	4	
10	26	11	25	17	19	18	18	18	18	26	10	
16		14*		2		0		0		16		

*The configuration that actually occurred.

TABLE 2-4. Frequency Distribution of Differences Between the Two Groups in Table 2-2

Differences between E and C totals	Total number of unique combinations that can produce these differences
16	2
14	2
12	4
10	6
8	10
6	10
4	14
2	14
0	8
	70

combinations of four numbers possible, there are not 70 unique differences between groups.) This distribution is presented in Table 2-4.

This particular frequency distribution represents all the possible chance differences that could occur between the two groups of four numbers and the possible ways in which each difference can occur. Once constructed, all the researcher need do to determine how likely the observed difference of 14 was to occur by chance alone is to determine how many ways a difference of 14 *or greater* could occur and divide that figure by the total number of unique combinations of two groups of four numbers each. Referring to the distribution, it is found that there are two ways by which the difference of 14 could have occurred by chance *and* two ways in which an even greater difference (16) could have occurred. This means that a difference as great as 14 could have occurred by chance a total of 4 times out of 70, thus the probability that the observed 14 did occur by chance alone is 4 divided by 70 or 0.057. If the level of significance or alpha level of this study had been set at 0.05, which is likely, then the null hypothesis could not be rejected because the researcher would be wrong 5.7 out of 100 times rather than the permissible 5 out of 100. The results were very close to being statistically significant, but did not "quite make it," thus the null hypothesis would have to be accepted as probably true.

Directionality

The above discussion assumed that the researcher did not wish to specify the direction of the hypothesized relationship *before* conducting the study, although obviously the researcher hoped that any obtained difference would favor the experimental group. This is certainly the most common practice in research, although another option exists.

As presented, the researcher tested the following H_1: "Patients receiving preoperative instruction differ significantly from patients not receiving preoperative instruction with respect to number of postoperative medication requests." Given this hypothesis, a difference of 14 favoring the control group would receive the same treatment as the observed difference of 14 favoring the experimental group. A very different situation would exist, however, if the researcher had posited a direction to the relationship.

Suppose the following H_1 had been tested: "Patients receiving preoperative instruction register significantly fewer postoperative medication requests than patients not receiving preoperative instruction." In this situation, unlike the previous one, a difference of 14 favoring the control group *would not* receive the same treatment as the observed difference of 14 favoring the experimental group. The reason for this should be obvious. H_1 posited a significant (that is, an alpha of 0.05 or less) difference between the groups *favoring* the experimental group, hence any difference favoring the control group would be considered supportive of H_0, not H_1. In other words, no matter how great a difference observed in favor of the control group, H_1 would be automatically rejected as probably false.

Given the directional H_1 positing a difference favoring the experimental group therefore, a question arises concerning how to redefine differences occurring by chance and consequently how to determine the probability of a difference as large as 14 *favoring the experimental group* occurring by chance. Obviously, Table 2-4 can no longer be used because no distinctions were made between the direction of the difference between E and C. Referring to that distribution indicates, for example, that from the total of 70 unique combinations of groups of four numbers, two could be expected to produce differences as large as 16 and two produce differences as large as 14. In actuality, only one combination was capable of producing a difference of 16 favoring the experimental group (that is, E = 1, 2, 3, and 4; C = 5, 6, 7, and 8), the other difference of 16 favored the control group (that is, E = 5, 6, 7, and 8; C = 1, 2, 3, and 4) as indicated in Table 2-3. The same held for differences of 14; only one unique combination of the 70 possible favored the experimental group, the other consisted of a mirror image favoring the control group. To ascertain the probability of a 14 favoring E when such a direction had been hypothesized a priori, therefore, the researcher would count only the single difference of 16 and the single difference of 14 favoring the experimental group, and would ignore the 16 and 14 differences favoring the control group. Thus, instead of dividing 4 (two differences of 16 and two of 14) by 70, the researcher would divide 2 by 70 and obtain 0.0285 instead of 0.057, thereby rejecting H_0 as probably false and accepting H_1 as probably true. (Table 2-5 illustrates the frequency distribution of the differences between the 70 pairs of groups of four from a directional perspective.)

In other words, if everything else is equal, the same difference is half as likely to occur by chance in a directional hypothesis as in a nondirectional one *if that difference occurs in the proper direction.* A re-examination of Table 2-5 should indicate the propriety of this convention.

As was discussed earlier, no one actually uses so cumbersome a procedure for ascertaining the significance level of an obtained set of data. All researchers translate their observed relationship into a statistic and then compare that to a distribution of statistics. Most such distributions contain provisions for both

TABLE 2-5. Frequency Distribution of Differences Between the Two Groups in
Table 2-2 Showing Directionality

Differences between E and C totals *	Total number of unique combinations that can produce these differences
+16	1
+14	1
+12	2
+10	3
+8	5
+6	5
+4	7
+2	7
0	8
−2	7
−4	7
−6	5
−8	5
−10	3
−12	2
−14	1
−16	1
	70

*A + difference indicates E superiority; a − favors C.

directional and nondirectional hypotheses (usually calling the former one-tailed, the latter two-tailed tests). When a particular distribution does not contain such a provision, the researcher using a directional hypothesis must compensate by comparing the statistic to the critical value of an alpha twice the one chosen to test the hypothesis (that is, 0.10 for 0.05; 0.02 for 0.01). Computer programs, such as SPSS, that automatically compare the obtained statistic to a distribution usually allow the researcher to specify a directional or a nondirectional test.

Most researchers employ a nondirectional test in their studies and many journals require a very strong theoretical rationale before they will accept a directional test. The reason for this practice is not entirely clear, but may reside in the fact that, to be appropriate, a directional test must be specified in *advance* of conducting a study and there is no easy way for anyone, including journal editors, to be sure that a researcher did indeed hypothesize the direction of a relationship in advance. There is no question that it is exactly twice as easy to attain "significance" by using a directional test once the direction of a relationship is known, hence in effect changing actual hypotheses in midstream. There is also no question that some researchers have been guilty of this practice, although perhaps they would have been less likely to do so if they understood the implications of such a strategy.

There is, however, no good reason why a researcher should not use directional hypotheses if the researcher (1) is really just interested in a relationship manifesting itself in one direction and is willing to "throw away" results in the other direction no matter how impressive, (2) has some theoretical or empirical rationale (over and above a simple "hunch") for specifying said direction, and (3) specifies the direction *before* collecting the data. If these three criteria can be met there is absolutely nothing "wrong" with using a directional or one-tailed hypothesis, because in reality H_0 is just as difficult to reject and the probability of error (that is, of H_0 "really" being true) is still equal to the alpha level.

POWER

There are only two possible decisions that can be made when testing a null hypothesis: the researcher can reject it as probably false or accept it as probably true. In each case, the decision can either be right or wrong, although unfortunately the researcher can never be sure which. As discussed in the previous section, however, it is possible to estimate how likely the decision to reject H_0 was to be incorrect by simply computing the significance level of the relationship. The likelihood of this genre of error is also sometimes called the probability of Type I error, which of course implies the existence of a Type II error as well.

Type II error occurs only when the researcher *fails* to reject H_0. In this case Type I error is completely irrelevant, but obviously error could be present just as easily in failing to find a significant relationship as in finding one. Just as obviously, the researcher will never know for sure whether the decision to accept H_0 as probably true is right or wrong, but again the likelihood (or probability) of making such an error can be estimated although the process is a bit more complex.

At first glance, these two sources of error may appear to be independent of one another since only one genre need be considered for any one study (Type I error is irrelevant when failing to reject H_0; Type II irrelevant when succeeding in rejecting H_0), the two concepts are very closely related. The reason for this is probably best illustrated through the concept of power and its relationship to statistical significance.

Power is defined as the probability of rejecting the null hypothesis when it should be rejected (that is, when in "reality" it is false) and is really nothing more than $1 -$ Type II error. Since statistical significance determines whether or not the null hypothesis is rejected, the same parameters that influence statistical significance also influence power (and hence Type II error). Power then, like statistical significance, is a function of the alpha set by the researcher prior to the study (the more stringent the alpha, the lower the power), the homogeneity of the subjects (the more homogeneous the criterion scores within groups, the greater the power), the difference between the groups with respect to the dependent variable (the greater the difference between groups, the greater the power), and the relative size of the sample (the more subjects participating in a study, the greater the power).

The reasons that these four parameters are related to power are relatively straightforward. The relationship of the alpha level to power is probably the most obvious. The more stringently statistical significance is defined, the more difficult will be the rejection of H_0. For example, it is far less likely to achieve significance at 0.01 than 0.05, and even less likely to achieve it at 0.001. Thus, the alpha level set by the researcher prior to the study definitely influences the likelihood of achieving statistical significance and hence power.

A re-examination of Tables 2-4 and 2-5 indicates the relationship between the relative difference between groups with respect to medication requests and the achievement of statistical significance: the largest differences between groups are the ones least likely to occur by chance alone (for example, differences of two and four are seven times as likely to occur by chance as differences of 14 and 16).

The connection between the homogeneity of the patients comprising the sample and power is not quite as obvious, although the concept should be much clearer after reading Chapter 9. At present, suffice it to say that there are techniques for decreasing *within group* variability.

A similar relationship holds with the relative size of the sample. In the hypothetical data presented in Tables 2-3 to 2-5, the largest possible discrepancy between any two randomly constructed groups was 16, which could occur only if all the low numbers (for example, 1, 2, 3, and 4) happened by chance to fall into one group and all the high numbers in the other group. Although unlikely, such an occurrence is possible, as are approximations such as the one that actually occurred in which three of the four smallest numbers occurred in the experimental group. As unlikely as these extreme differences would be to occur by chance alone with four patients per group, they would be even less likely to occur if 10 or more patients were present in each group. The corollary of this phenomenon is that *the more subjects contained in two or more groups the smaller the difference (and hence the smaller the relationship) necessary to reject H_0.*

These, then, are the four parameters directly related to the ease with which statistical significance is obtained. All good researchers do everything they possibly can to maximize power (hence minimizing Type II error) in order to reject the null hypothesis. At first glance, this statement may seem antithetical to the concept of research being an objective and dispassionate search for truth, but in reality it is not. In almost all cases, studies are conducted because the researcher *believes* that a relationship does in fact exist. In other words, although the null hypothesis may be the formal statement of the object of the study, the real purpose is to use every *legitimate* means to attempt to reject H_0 at the lowest alpha possible. To do this is to come to as close an approximation to the "truth" as anyone possibly can, and that is the real purpose of research.

The reason for this lies in the repeated assertion that no one ever knows what the truth is, although researchers are in the enviable position of being able to estimate how close their results were to being correct. Now certainly if the researcher fails to reject H_0, the probability of Type II error in the study can be estimated by computing the study's power and subtracting it from 1 (Type II error = 1 − power). The reality of the situation is, however, that this value will be considerably greater than the alpha at which the same study's null hypothesis would be rejected (which would probably be no greater than 0.05). The reason for this is simply that it can sometimes be quite difficult to achieve a power much greater than 0.80 when the alpha level is set at 0.05 or below, especially if the sample size is limited. This means that should the researcher fail to reject the null hypothesis, the probability of being wrong (Type II error) would be 0.20 or more, considerably greater than the Type I error of 0.05 should the researcher succeed in rejecting the null hypothesis at that level.

For this reason, experienced researchers tend to manipulate all the parameters available to them to increase the power of their studies, hence increasing the probability of obtaining significance as well as of lending credence to those results that fail to achieve same. To do otherwise would be economically unsound, both with respect to time and money. It makes very little sense to conduct a study that has a low probability of success, especially when the means by which that probability can be computed are so clearly defined. Journal editors are therefore most reluctant to publish studies that do not achieve statistical significance unless they are assured that the power of the study was reasonably high; hence the computation of power for those studies that fail to reject H_0 is almost essential for any serious researcher. For those readers interested in the computational procedures involved in the process as well as a more detailed discussion of the concept, Cohen[1] presents a thorough, easy to follow development.

SUMMARY

This chapter has attempted to present the logic of hypothesis testing on a primarily intuitive level. Hypotheses were defined as formal statements of the purposes of research studies and their acceptance or rejection was discussed in terms of a nonmathematical, nonstatistical approach that has little practical utility other than its explanatory power. The types of error that can be made both when H_0 is rejected (Type I) and when it is not rejected (Type II) were presented along with the related concepts of statistical significance and statistical power. Parameters related to these concepts were discussed along with a recommendation for computing the power in those cases in which statistical significance is not achieved.

REFERENCES

1. Cohen, J.: *Statistical Power Analysis for the Behavioral Sciences*. Academic Press, New York, 1969.
2. Kerlinger, F. N.: *Foundations of Behavioral Research*. Holt, Rinehart and Winston, New York, 1973.

CHAPTER 3
SAMPLING

Since almost all nursing research involves the use of people, whether patients or nurses themselves, a crucial decision that must be made early in any research project is which people shall be selected to participate (or more accurately, which shall be *asked* to participate). The first step in making this decision must be dictated by the research question, which delineates not only what facts or relationships are to be studied but also *to whom* these facts or relationships are relevant.

A researcher never states, for example, the purpose of the study as generally as "to ascertain attitudes toward increasing the availability of contraceptives to adolescents." An interested reader would immediately ask "attitudes of whom?" forcing the definition of a group of people in whose attitudes the researcher is interested. This group could include everyone in the world, everyone in the United States, everyone of voting age in South Dakota, all the registered nurses in the country, or all the public health nurses in the South. Regardless of how the group is defined, it becomes the focus of the study and is referred to as the research *population*.

A problem should be immediately apparent. How could anyone hope to interview (or question) everyone in the world or even all the public health nurses in the South? If these tasks are clearly impossible, then how could one possibly determine either group's opinions regarding contraceptive availability? The answer is that (1) some manageable number of the group or population of interest must be studied rather than the entire population and (2) the results obtained from this subset, called a *sample*, must be used to represent the results that would have been obtained had it been feasible to have studied the entire population. This process is referred to as generalizing the results of a study from a sample to the population from which it was drawn and is a concept crucial to all research.

The chief problem with including only a sample of subjects (Ss) from a larger population in a study is that the sample will most definitely differ in some ways from that population, since the latter contains many people not present in the former. If the two entities differ substantively enough, then generalization is not possible and the entire study may be wasted. The extent to which the sample is likely to be representative of the population from which it was drawn is dependent upon two things: the way in which its membership was selected and its relative size with respect to the population.

A sample must be selected in as unbiased a manner as possible. If a researcher simply decides to interview acquaintances, a convenient captive audience, or the first 100 people met in the hospital lobby, there is every reason to expect that sample to be unrepresentative of the larger population that the researcher aspires to study. Even if the researcher conscientiously selects "representative" Ss, or Ss from representative institutions or settings, bias is still likely to be present simply because enough is not known about the many ways people can differ to match a sample and a population with respect to all possible relevant characteristics. If a truly representative method for selecting sample Ss cannot be found, then the only real option left to the researcher is to make the sample very large, large to the point that even if some unknown bias does exist its effect will be vitiated by the fact that the sample size approaches that of the population. Obviously, this alternative will usually be impractical for the very reason that sample selection was necessitated in the first place (that is, the impossibility of studying an entire population, or even a large portion of it), thus necessitating the use of a selection procedure that controls for all known and unknown sources of bias.

At first glance, this may appear to be a very tall order indeed. In reality, however, it is not at all difficult. Basically, all that such a procedure must entail is to give every person eligible to participate in a study (that is, in the population) an *equal* chance to so participate. If this one condition can be met, then Ss with all possible combinations of characteristics have a chance to be represented in the sample, hence the researcher need not worry about identifying possible sources of bias and controlling for them.

RANDOM SAMPLING

Ironically, researchers are able to achieve this truly impressive feat by admitting the extent of their ignorance with regard to the attributes that are and are not relevant to the study. This admission comes in the form of leaving sample selection totally to random chance, which again is defined as giving every person in the population an equal chance of being selected. It can be accomplished in several ways.

If the population is sufficiently manageable in size, then a researcher could conceivably place everyone's name (that is, everyone eligible to participate in the study) in a hat, mix them up, and draw as many names as needed for the sample. If a reasonable number of names were to be drawn in this way, then the sample should be very similar to the entire population of names in the hat. Obviously if only one or two Ss were selected in this manner,

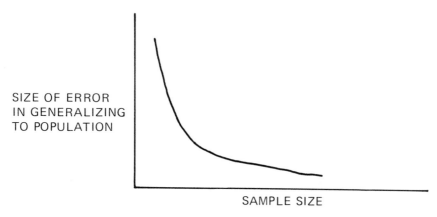

SIZE OF ERROR
IN GENERALIZING
TO POPULATION

SAMPLE SIZE

FIGURE 3-1. Relationship between sample size and representativeness. As can be seen from this graph, discrepancy between the sample and the population is not linear. Actually the discrepancy is a function of the square root of the sample size, hence a sample of 100 is not four times as accurate as a sample of 25 but only twice as precise.

no real confidence could be placed in the sample's representativeness. Everything else being equal, the larger a sample the more representative it will be (Fig 3-1).

A less cumbersome procedure than drawing names out of a hat might entail the assigning of a number to each member of the population and randomly selecting a number rather than a name. If, for example, all the public health nurses in the country who met a given criterion were to serve as the population for a study, a list would have to be secured and each nurse on that list assigned a number starting with 1 for the first name and proceeding to, say, 10,431 for the last (assuming that the list contained 10,431 names). The number of people that the researcher estimates are needed for the study would then be decided upon and that many random numbers between 1 and 10,431 would be generated through the use of a table of random numbers (Fig. 3-2) or via a computer. The individual names corresponding to the numbers selected would then serve as the sample to be studied.

To illustrate on an extremely small scale, assume that a researcher wished to randomly select three members from the following group of 10 nurses to serve as study Ss. The first step would involve defining the population, which in this case simply entails being cognizant of its membership:

> B. Ward
> B. Smith
> M. Jones
> L. Smith
> D. Walker
> J. Bowman
> K. Turner
> S. Suter
> K. Rogers
> L. Samison

```
48593640884753748593627364856372647856485993546311273641736
48571234950687463526176364766282938475621101983740048575631
38495869209485739283901834785783772818398475869573810384919
29301928374657829183746576273847617010192837475009283746587
03948578283949580019293847565839291093849857384758473821700

12839347593018736457890094857367118938374857475837585738283
12374857684939209485869084736271728374859009228374575763610
20394857888273948716737074858574732819293048575758493928181
03948576647483728273847058784758676847378475837283746758588
89398403984509839848586118498592029384095802840981093850983
```

FIGURE 3-2. Using a table of random numbers. The above list of five digit random numbers is illustrative of what tables of random numbers often look like, although the list will typically continue for many pages. To use such a list, the researcher may start at any point in the list (at the beginning, middle, end, second line, and so forth) and choose as many numbers as needed to fulfill his requirements. If the researcher decided to begin at the beginning of the second row of five digit numbers above, for example, the first random number would be 11208, the second 22039, and so on. Should only three digit numbers be needed, then the researcher could use the top three numbers of each row (for example, 112, 220, 833 in the second column). Numbers that are larger than the total number of Ss in the population are ignored.

Although tables of random numbers such as this can be very helpful for selecting relatively small samples, their use can be rather tedious for extremely large studies. In such cases, a researcher would be well advised to allow the computer or minicomputer to select the needed random numbers. This is easily accomplished by simply informing an appropriate program of the largest and smallest number assigned to the population and how many random digits are required. The requisite sample is then printed out automatically.

The second step is to number these ten Ss in any order that is convenient (for example, the order in which records are filed, the order in which their names appear on a computer printout, and so forth):

> 1. B. Ward
> 2. B. Smith
> 3. M. Jones
> 4. L. Smith
> 5. D. Walker
> 6. J. Bowman
> 7. K. Turner
> 8. S. Suter
> 9. K. Rogers
> 10. L. Samison

Finally three random numbers between 1 and 10 are generated. Suppose in the present case they were 4, 5, and 9, which means that L. Smith, D. Walker, and K. Rogers would be identified as Ss comprising the study's sample.

Although random selection of Ss can be a time consuming process when a population of substantial size is involved, there is usually no viable alternative. The most difficult part is almost always obtaining a list of the membership of any given population (generating even large groups of random numbers is not difficult given the use of ready made computer and minicomputer programs), but if the researcher wishes to make the case that the sample is similar to a much larger group, then the membership of that group must be known or else no credence can be placed in the contention. It is simply not possible to randomly select Ss from a population if its membership is not known (or not ascertainable, see section on Cluster Samples below) because of the impossibility of insuring that every member of the population had an equal chance of being selected.

This is not to say that there are no alternatives at all to random sampling. If the exact incidence of a variable in a population is known, for example, and if that variable is highly related to the variable(s) under study, then it is possible to statistically extrapolate from a slightly biased (that is, not randomly selected) sample via regression techniques (see Chapter 10) to estimate what the incidence of the variable under study is *likely* to be in the population. It is very rare, however, that all these conditions can be met and even when they are the margin of error is often so great that the researcher would have been better advised to have chosen a less ambitious target population and to have randomly sampled from it.

If, in the final analysis, the membership of a population (and characteristics of that membership) is not known to a researcher, then that population has no relevance to any study conducted by the researcher regardless of the researcher's objectives or aspirations. Suppose, for example, that a nurse researcher wished to ascertain the degree of compliance of cardiac patients to diet and exercise regimens prescribed following hospitalization for major infarctions. Suppose further that a decision was made to randomly select one half of the qualifying patients admitted to the cardiac ward of a convenient hospital. (This might be accomplished by flipping a coin at the entry of each new patient or using a table of random numbers.) Now even though this nurse might be interested in generalizing the results to all patients suffering major infarctions as defined in the study, all such patients were not the population from which the sample was randomly selected, hence strictly speaking the results can only be generalized to the population of patients admitted *to the floor of Hospital X during the time span of the study.* Furthermore, if the researcher were required to obtain patient consent to participate in the study, then the population would be further limited to patients admitted to *the floor of Hospital X during the time span of the study who volunteered for a research project.* Fortunately, as will be discussed in Chapter 9, extenuating circumstances often exist that help make a study more general than the strict logic sampling theory permits, especially for correlational and experimental research. Purely descriptive studies, however, which are only interested in measuring the incidence of a variable or phenomenon in society, are usually constrained to this logic unless compelling exceptions can be advanced.

As hard line as this position may appear, it is easily defensible. How could the results of the above study be veridically generalized beyond the specific hospital in question unless a great deal of detailed information were known about other institutions? How, for example, could the researcher be sure that the hospital did not employ more (or fewer) persuasive techniques to insure compliance? How could the researcher be sure that patients from Hospital X were not systematically different from those in other hospitals (for example, were perhaps older, less educated, more seriously ill, and so forth)? A corollary of these questions, of course, is that the more that is known about the fit between the *actual* population serving a study and the desired target population, the more faith a researcher and the research consumer can have that the obtained results may be applicable to both. The harsh reality is that true random samples are relatively rare in nursing as in other behavioral research, hence results are usually simply intuitively and broadly generalized to people and settings "similar to the ones studied." Both researchers and readers of research reports, however, should constantly be vigilant to the actual population serving a study. As already suggested, studies relying upon volunteers can really only be generalized to volunteers; studies relying upon specially accessible subsets of a larger group can only be generalized to those subsets. (For example, if the ANA membership list were the basis of a random selection of nurses within a state, then the resulting study would be generalizable only to ANA members within that state, not to non-ANA members and not to ANA members outside the state.) Again, however, sight should not be lost of the fact that the researcher must do the best that conditions permit in a world not created for the practice of research; thus, if the sample to which a researcher can generalize is relatively restricted, the study may still be worth conducting and considering. This is especially true if researchers are objective enough to make a conscientious and thorough search for possible biases within a sample or restricted population. If a study is sufficiently thought provoking then other researchers can see if the results replicate with other Ss in other settings. If they do, then their overall generalizability is vastly expanded.

Random Sampling versus Random Assignment

The present chapter is concerned with methods of selecting Ss for participation in a study, not in what occurs to them once selected. In experimental research (see Chapter 9) Ss once selected are randomly assigned to two or more groups in which they receive different treatment at the hands of the experimenter. Procedures used to effect this situation can entail random sampling. For example, if the experimenter wishes to contrast two groups, an experimental and a control, each could be randomly selected from the same population, in which case random sampling would be involved. This strategy is very rare, however, usually a sample is first selected and then the group membership of Ss is determined by random assignment. What often results, therefore, is random assignment of a sample to groups in a situation in which the sample itself was *not* randomly chosen. Although such a procedure augurs well for the experimental versus control contrast, it does nothing to increase the generalization of the study's results to the population from which the sample was drawn. Random sampling should therefore be considered a separate concept from random assignment of Ss *within* a research study: the former referring to how Ss were selected for participation in the study as a whole; the latter to how Ss were selected for participation in different groups *within* the study.

STRATIFIED RANDOM SAMPLES

The reader may have inferred by now that the authors lean heavily toward random selection of Ss as the primary mechanism for insuring generalizability of research results. This is certainly the case, but some mention should be made of other types of sampling procedures, both random and otherwise.

As stated above, everything else being equal the larger the sample the more faith that can be had in its representativeness. The use of very large samples has some very obvious and distinct disadvantages as well, however, chief of which is their expense, both in money and time.

If the researcher has the luxury of knowing not only a population's membership, but also possesses accurate estimates of certain relevant population characteristics (that is, relevant to the objectives of the study), then the study's sample size can be drastically reduced without losing any degree of generalizability by employing a procedure known as *stratified random sampling.* The procedure is able to accomplish this truly impressive feat by the process of choosing one or more attributes that are related to, but not identical with, the chief object of study and *forcing* the sample to have the same proportion of Ss containing those attributes as the population as a whole.

Pollsters of public opinion, for example, are masters of these techniques. Wishing to predict how the voting public of the United States will respond to a certain issue, they are able to drastically reduce their sample size and still make astonishingly accurate predictions by, among other things, (1) identifying voter characteristics that are related to responses on certain issues (for example, geographic region, party registration, age, sex, and so forth), (2) ascertaining the exact incidences of these characteristics in the population as a whole (for example, perhaps 50 percent of all registered voters are Democrats, 40 percent are Republicans and 10 percent are Independents), and then (3) randomly selecting proportionate numbers from these subgroups (for example, exactly 50 percent of the sample would be randomly selected from individuals registered as Democrats, 40 percent from Republican roles, and so forth). This procedure still fits the definition of random selection *within* any given category or level, but insures a more representative sample. (If simple random sampling had been employed, for example, the resulting sample might have only been 47 percent Democrats, which is close, but not as close as could be achieved via stratifying techniques.) The extent to which stratifying procedures can result in a reduction in sample size and retain a given level of representativeness is directly dependent upon the strength of the relationship between the stratifying variable(s) and the variable constituting the focus of the study. (If no relationship exists at all, then stratification constitutes absolutely no advantage over simple random selection.) A corollary of this fact is that stratified random sampling is really feasible only if the researcher knows a good deal about the relationship between the variables.

CLUSTER SAMPLING

Another type of random sampling often used by professional pollsters involves randomly selecting superordinate units and then, from those selected, randomly selecting ever smaller units.

An example might entail the problem of interviewing a representative sample of American clinical specialists. The selection and subsequent interviewing of a simple random sample from such a large population would be horrendously costly. In the first place, all clinical specialists in the country would have to be listed in order to give each an equal chance of being selected; secondly, the final sample would contain individuals from every nook and cranny in the United States, hence necessitating the interviewers' logging a great deal of travel time to obtain relatively little data.

These disadvantages could be reduced by first randomly selecting a given number of states to participate in the study, then randomly selecting several hospitals in each state, and finally, randomly selecting several clinical specialists within each hospital to interview. Besides saving a great deal of time, effort, and money, this method should result in a reasonably representative sample.

OTHER TYPES OF SAMPLING

Some research texts make distinctions between *convenience* sampling (picking whomever is available), *purposeful* sampling (picking Ss believed by the researcher to be representative), and so forth. All these techniques have one thing in common: every member of the population from which they are drawn does not have an equal chance of being selected and hence no real protection against bias is available. Perhaps the only real option that a researcher has who cannot randomly select is to limit the scope of the study to a much smaller unit (for example, one hospital) and study as many Ss therein as possible. This at least affords the possibility of drawing some reasonable conclusions regarding that unit with the attendant possibility of tenuously generalizing to other, similar units.

CHAPTER 4

MEASUREMENT*

Measurement is the process of assigning numbers to objects using a rule. It is presumed that the rule assigns the numbers to represent the amounts of a specific attribute possessed by the objects being measured. For example, a tape measure is a measurement rule that allows one to represent an individual's height; thus, using a tape measure to quantify individuals' heights is one type of measurement. A test is a measurement rule consisting at a minimum of (1) a set of items, for example, statements to be verified or completed, or questions to be answered, (2) a set of directions telling the examinee how to respond to the items, and (3) a scoring procedure for converting the collection of item responses for each examinee to a number. The application (that is, administration and scoring) of a test to one or more examinees is a type of measurement and is in fact not very different from using a tape measure to quantify height.[13]

The *rules* used for assigning numbers to objects to represent the amounts of a specific attribute possessed by them may be classified in several ways. The most frequently encountered system for categorizing measurement rules is that of Stevens.[23] He classified rules into four hierarchical categories in terms of the amount and kind of information retrievable from the numbers they assign to objects. Stevens' four categories, nominal, ordinal, interval, and ratio, are defined and illustrated in Table 4-1. *Nominal* level measurement allows one to tell which objects are in the same category and which are in different categories. *Ordinal* level measurement allows one to not only tell which objects occupy the same or different categories, but also allows the researcher to order the objects according to the amount of the measured attribute they possess. At the *interval* level, one can not only categorize and rank objects, but can also order

---

*A portion of the material in this chapter is adapted from Staropoli and Waltz,[22] pp. 111 to 140 and 166 to 196, with permission.

the objects by the magnitude of their numerals and by the relative sizes of the differences between pairs of objects. *Ratio* level measures provide all the information inherent in interval level plus information concerning the absolute amount of the measured characteristic possessed by an object. That is, each number represents the quantity of the attribute possessed by the object which is possible only when the scale has a natural zero point that represents complete absence of the attribute in question. It should be noted that a set of categories is exhaustive if every object to be classified belongs to at least one category. Cate-

TABLE 4-1. Stevens' Levels of Measurement

Level	Rule	Example	Salient characteristics
Nominal	Numbers assigned represent an object's membership in one of a set of mutually exclusive and exhaustive categories that cannot be ordered.	In responding, check 1 if you are an RN and 2 if you are not. —1. RN —2. Not RN	Allows researcher to tell which objects are in the same category and which ones are in different categories. No statements may be made regarding the amount of the attribute possessed.
Ordinal	Numbers assigned represent an object's membership in one of a set of mutually exclusive and exhaustive categories that can be ordered.	Rank the nurses working on Ward B from most competent to least competent. Assign the number 1 to the most competent, 2 to the next most competent, and so forth.	Researcher can identify membership in categories and can also order the objects according to the amount of the attribute possessed.
Interval	Numbers assigned represent membership in one of a set of mutually exclusive and exhaustive categories that can be ordered and that are equally spaced.	A patient's oral temperature at 12 noon on three consecutive days was: Day 1, 104° Day 2, 101° Day 3, 99°	Membership can be identified, objects can be ordered, and in addition, the researcher can order the relative sizes of the differences existing between pairs of objects, that is, statements such as: the patient's temperature on Day 1 was 5° higher than on Day 3, or the drop in temperature between Day 1 and Day 2 was greater than the drop in temperature between Day 2 and Day 3.

TABLE 4-1. *Continued*

Level	Rule	Example	Salient characteristics
Ratio	Numbers assigned represent membership in mutually exclusive and exhaustive categories that can be ordered and are equally spaced. In addition, the scale has an absolute zero point.	The heights of three children are obtained using a tape measure: Sarah = 60″ Barker = 50″ Perry = 30″	The researcher can identify membership and order objects according to amount and relative sizes of the differences between pairs. In addition, the researcher can speak of one object being n times more than another, that is, statements may be made such as: Sarah is two times taller than Perry.

gories are mutually exclusive if each object belongs to no more than one category. If categories differ in quality rather than quantity they are unorderable. Categories that differ quantitatively are orderable on the basis of amount.

A great deal of controversy exists regarding levels of measurement and the proper statistical treatment of the resulting scores. Researchers usually take one of two bipolar views of measurement rules. The *fundamentalists* believe (1) there are distinct types of measurement scales into which all possible measures of attributes can be classified, (2) each measure has some real characteristics that permit its proper classification, and (3) once a measurement is classified, the classification specifies the types of statistical analysis that can be employed with the measure. The *pragmatists,* on the other hand, contend that the classification systems established by most measurement rules are not as clear-cut and readily serviceable as the fundamentalists would like to believe and consequently much confusion and disagreement arises among researchers, and time and effort is wasted in merely attempting to assign a level of measurement to a variable.

At the operational level in the Stevens System, much controversy exists over the differentiation between ordinal and interval levels of measurement. Some argue that test scores, for example, represent an ordinal level of measurement because they simply order examinees according to the amount of the measured attribute they possess, while others insist test scores do more than rank order examinees and that one can in fact speak to the amount of an attribute possessed (that is, treat them as interval). Nunnally[15] presents a cogent argument for minimizing the emphasis on rules of measurement that is worthy of the reader's attention. In the pragmatists' view, then, the techniques applied to any set of numbers should be determined by the nature of the research question one is trying to answer and not by the level of measurement attained. If a statistical procedure provides a meaningful answer to the question, it should be employed regardless of the level of measurement.

Since the nurse needs to be aware of the fundamentalist view and the implications for the research resulting from such efforts, the statistical procedures presented in this book will take into account levels of measurement. However, it should be made perfectly clear that the authors believe that the statistical treatment of any set of numbers or scores should be determined by the nature of the question one is trying to answer and not by the level of measurement. If the question makes sense, then the best statistical technique available for finding the answer should be used.

TYPES OF MEASURES

The mystique surrounding the topic of measurement stems in large part from the esoteric terms employed by those in the field. Whether selecting from available instruments or developing new devices or methods, the work of the researcher will be facilitated by a familiarity with the jargon used in relation to measurement.

Tests and other measuring devices can be classified by (1) what they seek to measure, (2) the manner in which they are constructed and interpreted, (3) the type of subject performance they seek to measure, and (4) who constructs them.

What is Measured

In nursing research, four types of measurement devices are of interest: those that seek to measure cognition, affect, psychomotor skills, and physical functioning.

COGNITIVE MEASURES

Cognitive measures are tests of subjects' knowledge or achievement in a specific content area. Indicators of cognitive behavior include:

1. Achievement tests (objective and essay) that measure the extent to which cognitive objectives have been attained.
2. Self-evaluation measures designed to determine subjects' perceptions of the extent to which cognitive objectives have been attained.
3. Rating scales and checklists for judging the qualities of products produced in conjunction with or as a result of an experience.
4. Sentence completion exercises designed to categorize the types of responses and to enumerate their frequencies relative to specific criteria.
5. Interviews to determine the frequencies and levels of satisfactory responses to formal and informal questions raised in a face-to-face setting.
6. Peer utilization surveys to ascertain the frequency of selection or assignment to leadership or resource roles.

7. Questionnaires employed to determine the frequency of responses to items in an objective format or number of responses to categorized dimensions developed from the content analysis of responses to open-ended questions.

8. Anecdotal records and critical incidents to ascertain the frequency of behaviors judged to be highly desirable or undesirable.

9. Reviews of records, reports, and other written materials (for example, articles, autobiographical data, awards, citations, honors) to determine the numbers and types of accomplishments of subjects.

In terms of numbers alone, cognitive measures are the most important types of methods. Although they encompass more than paper and pencil tests per se, written tests are by far the most widely used, especially multiple choice tests because they are the most objective of the various types available, the most reliable, and because they have the greatest utility, that is, they can be used to test all types of knowledge even those formerly felt to be testable only by essay.

A *multiple choice item* consists of (1) a stem, which is an introductory question or incomplete statement and (2) responses, which are the suggested answers. The responses for a multiple choice item consist of two elements: (1) the answer, that is, the correct response, and (2) distractors, misleads, or foils, which are the incorrect responses. The term options or alternatives refers to both the distractors and the correct answer. Usually no more than three or four options are used for any given item. Whether or not the items are actually being constructed by the researcher, the following aspects should be considered before employing a multiple choice test:

1. Does the writer have a thorough mastery of the subject matter being tested? Does the writer know not only the facts but implications as well, that is, fallacies and popular misconceptions?

2. Is there a well developed set of objectives that directed the test's construction?

3. Does the writer understand the psychologic and educational characteristics of the individuals for whom the test is intended? This is important in determining the difficulty level as well as distractors.

4. Is the writer aware of various interpretations of word meanings, precise in word usage, and organized in verbal expression?

5. Is the writer familiar with the types and varieties of test items, particularly their possibilities and limitations?

6. Does the writer convey the belief that some kinds of subjects are more difficult than others and that item writing is not a unitary skill?

7. Does the writer avoid lifting items verbatim from text? Such items are usually inadequate. A sentence presented out of context frequently loses much of its meaning and is likely to be ambiguous. Sentences that can be readily extracted from context without conceptual loss are likely to measure trivia, that is, such items frequently measure only memory for fact rather than understandings, generalizations, or principles.

Table 4-2 presents examples of well written multiple choice items. Before employing a multiple choice test, the researcher should ascertain that:

1. Items are expressed as clearly as possible and, whenever possible, words with precise meanings are chosen.
2. Complex or awkward word arrangements are avoided as are nonfunctional words. Nonfunctional words are those that do not contribute to the basis for choosing a given response.
3. All qualifiers needed to provide a reasonable basis for responding are included, that is, to whom and for what purpose.
4. Unessential specificity in the item stem or response is avoided.
5. The level of difficulty of the item is adapted to the level of subjects and is in concert with the purpose for the measurement.
6. Irrelevant clues to the correct response are avoided. Irrelevant clues include pat verbal associations, grammatical constructions, correct response consistently stated more precisely and at greater length than the distractors, systematic formal differences between the answer and distractors (that is, common elements in the stem and response, including interrelated items in the statement or response of one question that give a clue to another question).
7. The content of questions has been exposed to expert editorial scrutiny.
8. Specific determiners (all, none, certainly, never, always) are avoided as is stereotyped phraseology.

TABLE 4-2. Desirable Characteristics of Multiple Choice Items

Desirable characteristic	Example*	Comment
Permits a correct answer.	The basic service unit in the administration of public health is: a. the Federal government. b. the state health department. c. the local health department. d. the public health nurse.	Items that require or permit a correct answer are those that eliminate the need for the respondent to make a judgment regarding the correctness of the response, i.e., matters of fact provide a suitable basis for such items.
Requires the respondent to select the best answer from among several answers.	The primary responsibility of the instructor in health services is: a. to provide an emotional and social environment that adds a wholesome and healthful tone to the child's school day. b. to provide emergency or first aid care when a child becomes ill or injured in school. c. to provide up-to-date material about health as part of the curriculum plan. d. to screen for abnormalities and sickness and to record the findings.	For many of the important questions that need to be asked, it is impossible to state an absolutely correct answer within the reasonable limits on a multiple choice item. Even if space limitations were not a factor, two experts would probably not agree on the precise wording of the best answer. The use of this type of item, which has one best answer, permits the item writer to ask more significant questions and frees the writer from the responsibility of stating a correct answer so precisely that all au-

TABLE 4-2. Continued

Desirable characteristic	Example*	Comment
		thorities would agree that the particular wording used was the best possible wording.
Based on matter of opinion.	Advocates of the specialized approach to school nursing point out that: a. the health of the child cannot be separated from that of the family and community as a whole. b. specialized nursing of the child cannot be separated from that of the family and community as a whole. c. a specialized program offers greater diversity and challenge to the well-prepared community health nurse. d. specialized nursing in the school allows the nurse to function without the disadvantages of a dual channel of administrative responsibility.	The responses to this question represent generalizations on the basis of literature written by the advocates of the specialized approach to school nursing. No authoritative sanction for one particular generalization is likely to be available, yet respondents familiar with this literature would probably agree on a best answer to this item.
Based on a novel question.	The problem of air pollution is most likely to be reduced in the future by which of the following: a. urban population will wear air purifying equipment. b. cities will be enclosed to facilitate air purification. c. development of processes that will not produce air pollutants. d. use of nonpollutant producing fuels.	Requiring the respondent to predict what would happen under certain circumstances is a good way of measuring understanding of the principle involved.
Requires selective recall.	The U.S. Public Health Service was reorganized in 1966 to: a. include the UNICEF program. b. include the Agency of International Development. c. combine the Voluntary Agency Services with the official ones. d. provide leadership in control of disease and environmental hazards and in development of man-power.	Unless this item had been made the specific object of instruction, it will function to assess the learner's ability to recall a variety of information about the Public Health Service, to select that which is relevant, and to base a generalization upon it.
Descriptive responses.	The child's socialization may be defined as: a. a behavioral process in which the child's behavior conforms to the social practices of family and extra family groups.	Inexperienced item writers tend to seek items having very short responses. This can seriously limit the significance and scope of the achievements measured. In an item measuring the ability

TABLE 4-2. *Continued*

Desirable characteristic	Example*	Comment
	b. a process of developing an effective set of performances characteristic of self-control. c. the genetically determined or hereditary mechanisms that determine the individual's physical traits. d. all of the above.	to define an important term, it is usually better to place the term to be defined in the item stem and to use definitions or identifications as the responses. The same principle should be applied to other items, i.e., one-word responses need not be avoided altogether but they should seldom be prominent in any measure.
Combines two elements to give four responses.	A school community safety program should be concerned with: a. teaching children how to avoid accidents. b. teaching adults and children to eliminate physical hazards that endanger them. c. eliminating physical hazards that endanger children and teaching them to avoid accidents. d. teaching children and adults to avoid accidents and eliminating physical hazards that endanger them.	A difficulty with four-option multiple choice items is that of securing four good alternatives. One solution to this problem is to combine questions with two alternatives each to give the necessary four alternatives.
Combines a question with an explanation.	When was the World Health Organization created and why? a. 1945, to prevent the spread of disease from one continent to another. b. 1948, to achieve international cooperation for better health throughout the world. c. 1945, to structure health privileges of all nations. d. 1948, to provide for a liberated population and aid in the relief from suffering.	This is a variation of the item type in which essentially two or more alternatives are combined to give four alternatives.
Uses an introductory sentence.	When a group is working as a health team, overlapping of activities may occur. What is essential if this is to be prevented? a. auxiliaries will work within a fairly circumscribed field. b. the public health nurse will assume responsibility for all phases of the nursing team's activities. c. the functions of all personnel will be defined. d. maximum skills of each team member will be utilized.	The use of a separate sentence frequently adds to the clarity of the item stem if it is necessary to present background information as well as to ask the question itself. Combining these two elements into a single question-sentence probably would make it too complex.

TABLE 4-2. *Continued*

Desirable characteristic	Example*	Comment
Includes a necessary qualification.	Generally speaking, the environmental health program personnel in urban centers are: a. persons with professional training in civil or sanitary engineering. b. sanitary inspectors or nonengineering personnel with indoctrination and orientation provided by the health department. c. public health engineers whose training embraces the public health aspects of both sanitary engineering and santary inspection. d. all of the above.	If this question asked only about environmental health program personnel in general without qualifying urban personnel, it would be difficult for the respondent to give a firm answer to the question given the existing differences between the environmental health programs in other than urban areas, i.e., county, state, Federal.
Uses the options, none of these, and/or all of these appropriately.	A necessary requirement for receiving funds under the Comprehensive Health Planning Act of 1966 is that: a. state boards of health must have at least 10% lay representation. b. the council responsible for developing a comprehensive health plan for the state must have 50% consumer participation. c. health and welfare councils, whether or not actively involved in health planning on the state level, must have at least 25% lay representation. d. none of the above.	Whenever each of the responses can be judged unequivocally as correct or incorrect in response to the question posed in the item stem, it is appropriate to use none of the above as a response. It would be appropriate to use all of the above in a similar situation where more than one perfectly correct answer is possible.
Uses true statements as distractors.	The general purpose of a parent education program is: a. to teach parents information they need to know throughout their children's changing developmental stages. b. to help parents reinforce their understanding and strengths in regard to themselves and their children. c. to develop attitudes of healthy family life in parents of young children. d. to cover a wider range of subject matter, format, and method than is possible on an individual basis.	It is not necessary for the incorrect options to a test item to be themselves incorrect statements. They simply need to be incorrect answers to the stem question. Judgments concerning the relevance of knowledge may be as important as judgments concerning its truth. This is particularly useful as a technique for testing achievement, which is sometimes thought to be testable only using essay measures.

TABLE 4-2. *Continued*

Desirable characteristic	Example*	Comment
Uses sterotypes in distractors.	The particular process of interaction between the organism and its environment that results in a specifiable change in both is referred to as: a. homeostasis. b. human behavior. c. operant behavior. d. developmental dynamism.	Phrases such as operant behavior and homeostasis, which a respondent may have heard without understanding, provide excellent distractors at an elementary level of discrimination.
Uses heterogeneous responses.	The index of economic welfare is: a. square feet of housing space. b. per capita national income. c. rate of growth of industrialization. d. morbidity and mortality rates.	The responses to this item vary widely. Because of their wide differences, only an introductory knowledge of indices of economic welfare is required for a successful response.
Uses homogeneous responses (harder item).	Funds for occupational health programs were allocated to state and local health departments as a result of: a. Social Security Act. b. Clean Air Act. c. Community Health Centers Act. d. Occupational Health Act.	The homogeneity of the responses in this item requires a considerably high level of knowledge of public health acts and hence makes the item difficult in comparison to an item utilizing heterogeneous options.
Presents multiple clues (easier item).	The amount estimated to eliminate poverty in our country is said to be which of the following: a. 2% of the gross national product and $\frac{1}{5}$ of the cost for national defense. b. 3% of the gross national product and $\frac{1}{6}$ of the cost for national defense. c. 4% of the gross national product and $\frac{1}{4}$ of the cost for national defense. d. 5% of the gross national product and $\frac{1}{3}$ of the cost for national defense.	The use of the values of two variables fitting the specification in the item stem makes it a fairly easy question. That is, the examinee need only know one of the values or know one in each of the three distractors to respond successfully.

From Staropoli and Waltz,[22] with permission.
*Some of these items are from Borlick et al.,[2] with permission.

AFFECTIVE MEASURES

Affective measures seek to determine interests, values, and attitudes. *Interests* are conceptualized as preferences for particular activities. Examples of statements relating to interests are:

I would rather provide nursing care to children than to adults.
I like to work with student nurses as they give care to patients.
I would enjoy having one day a week to devote to research in patient care.
I prefer teaching responsibilities to administrative responsibilities.

Values concern preferences for "life goals" and "ways of life" in contrast to interests, which concern preferences for particular activities. Examples of statements relating to values are:

I consider it important to have people respect nursing as a profession.
A nurse's duty to the patient comes before duty to the community.
Service to others is more important to me than personal ambition.

Attitudes concern feelings about particular social objects, that is, physical objects, types of people, particular persons, and social institutions. Examples of statements relating to attitudes are:

Nursing as a profession is a constructive force in determining health policy today.
All continuing education programs should be open to participants free of charge.
Certification should be contingent on a nurse's participation in continuing education activities.

The feature that distinguishes attitudes from interests and values is that attitudes always concern a particular target or object. In contrast, interests and values concern numerous activities — specific activities in measures of interest and very broad categories of activities in measures of values.

It is extremely difficult to preserve the conceptual differences between interests, values, and attitudes when actually constructing measures of affect. Thus, for the purposes of rendering them measureable, they are all subsumed under the rubric of *acquired behavioral dispositions*[3] and are defined as tendencies to respond in a consistent manner to a certain category of stimuli. For example, when subjects are asked to evaluate a continuing education experience in nursing, one is interested in measuring their tendency to consistently respond favorably or unfavorably to a set of questions about the course (the stimuli).

The most direct approach to the determination of affect is to ask individuals directly what their attitudes, interests, or values are. For example, subjects are given a list of favorable and unfavorable statements regarding the antagonistic patient and asked to agree or disagree with each. Such self-report inventories are called attitude scales. *Self-report inventories* are designed to yield measures of adjustment, appreciation, attitudes, interests, temperament, and the like from which inferences can be made concerning the possession of psychologic traits (for example, defensiveness, rigidity, aggression, cooperativeness, and anxiety). Other indicators of affective behaviors are:

1. Sentence completion exercises designed to obtain ratings of the psychologic appropriateness of an individual's responses relative to specific criteria.

2. Interviews.
3. Questionnaires.
4. Semantic differential, Q sort, and other self-concept perception devices.
5. Physiologic measures.
6. Projective techniques, for example, role playing, picture interpretation.
7. Observational techniques and behavioral tests including measures of congruence between what is reported and how an individual actually behaves in a specific situation.
8. Anecdotal records and critical incidents.

From the empirical evidence that exists concerning the validity of different approaches, it appears that self-report offers the most valid approach currently available.[15] For this reason, at present, most measures of affect are based on self-report and usually employ one of two types of scales: a summated rating scale or semantic differential scale.

A *scale* is a measuring device comprised of:

1. A stem, which is a statement relating to attitudes or an attitudinal object to be rated by the respondent.
2. A series of scale steps.
3. Anchors that define the scale steps.

Table 4-3 presents an example of the components of a scale.

There are different types of anchors that can be employed: numbers, percentages, degrees of agreement-disagreement, adjectives, actual behavior, and products (for example, samples of nursing care plans to be rated 1 to 6). Usually numerical anchors are preferred because:

1. If the meaning of each step on the scale is specified at the beginning of the rating form, as is usually the case, numbers provide an effective means of coordinating those definitions with the rating scales.
2. Numbers on scales constantly remind subjects of the meanings of scale steps.
3. Numbers facilitate the analysis of data, for example, placing ratings on cards for computer analysis.[15]

TABLE 4-3. Example of the Components of a Scale

Component	Example
	Indicate your degree of agreement with the following statement:
Stem	Antagonistic behavior on the part of a patient indicates a need on the patient's part for additional attention and time from the nurse.
Scale steps	1 / 2 / 3 / 4 / 5 / 6
Anchors	Completely disagree Completely agree

From Staropoli and Waltz,[22] with permission.

Summated Rating Scales

A summated rating scale contains a set of scales all of which are considered approximately equal in attitude or value loading. The subject responds with varying degrees of intensity on a scale ranging between extremes such as agree/disagree, like/dislike, or accept/reject. The scores for all scales in the set are summed or summed and averaged to yield an individual's attitude score. An example of a summated rating scale is given in Table 4-4. These scales are easy to construct, usually reliable, and flexible in that they can be adapted to the measurement of many different kinds of attitudes. The reliability of summated scales depends directly on the number of items. If there are only a few (for example, six) items on the scale, the reliability can be increased by increasing the number of scale steps for each item. If, on the other hand, there are many (for example, 20) items on the scale, fewer scale steps for individual scales are required for a high degree of reliability. In most instances, 10 to 15 items using five or six steps are sufficient. Individual scales on summated atti-

TABLE 4-4. Example of a Summated Rating Scale

Indicate your degree of agreement with each of the following statements:

a. Antagonistic behavior on the part of the patient indicates a need for additional attention and time from the nurse.

   1   /   2   /   3   /   4   /   5   /   6

   Completely   Completely
   agree   disagree

b. Antagonistic behavior is used by patients to obtain more than their usual share of the nurses' time and attention.

   1   /   2   /   3   /   4   /   5   /   6

   Completely   Completely
   agree   disagree

c. The nurse should spend more time with antagonistic patients in an attempt to allay their fears.

   1   /   2   /   3   /   4   /   5   /   6

   Completely   Completely
   agree   disagree

d. The nurse should place limits on the time and attention given to antagonistic patients to avoid reinforcing their undesirable behavior.

   1   /   2   /   3   /   4   /   5   /   6

   Completely   Completely
   agree   disagree

From Staropoli and Waltz,[22] with permission.

tude scales tend to correlate substantially with each other because they obviously relate to the same thing. That is, it is easy for the constructor to intuit items that will correlate highly with one another and for the subject to see the common core of meaning in the items.[15]

The researcher needs to take into account several principles when employing a summated rating scale:

1. All the statements in the item pool should concern a particular attitudinal object.
2. Since it is usually easy to obtain a homogeneous scale for the measurement of attitudes, seldom are more than 40 items required for the item pool.
3. Since the purpose for each item on a summated scale is to obtain reliable variance with respect to the attitude, most of the items should be either moderately positive or moderately negative, that is, there is no place for neutral statements in summated scales. Statements that are very extreme in either direction tend to create less variance than statements that are less extreme.
4. The pool of items should be evenly divided between positive and negative statements.
5. In the development of summated scales, it is very important that reliability and validity information be obtained under circumstances very similar to those in which the final scale will be employed (that is, similar subjects, same administration procedures, same instructions, and so forth).
6. Numerous weighting schemes have been proposed for the scoring of the items on summated scales. It is usually not necessary to apply weights to summated items because (a) it is difficult to defend any particular method for weighting responses over the method of simply using the unweighted sum, and (b) weighted and unweighted summated scores usually correlate highly.[15]

For a guide to the construction of summated attitude scales, the reader is referred to Nunnally,[15] Edwards,[6] or Shaw and Wright.[19]

Semantic Differential Scales

Semantic differential scales employ direct ratings of concepts with scales anchored on the extremes by bipolar adjectives. This is a method developed by Osgood, Suci, and Tannenbaum[16] for measuring the meaning of concepts. The semantic differential scale has three elements: (1) the concept to be evaluated in terms of its semantic or attitudinal properties, (2) the polar adjective pair anchoring the scale, and (3) a series of scale positions that for practical purposes usually contains not fewer than five or more than nine steps, with seven steps as the optimal number identified by Osgood. Table 4-5 presents an example of a semantic differential scale.

In Table 4-5, the respondent is instructed to rate the concept "antagonistic

TABLE 4-5. Example of a Semantic Differential Scale

Antagonistic Patient

| 1 | / | 2 | / | 3 | / | 4 | / | 5 | / | 6 |

Ineffective   Effective

| 1 | / | 2 | / | 3 | / | 4 | / | 5 | / | 6 |

Foolish   Wise

| 1 | / | 2 | / | 3 | / | 4 | / | 5 | / | 6 |

Weak   Strong

| 1 | / | 2 | / | 3 | / | 4 | / | 5 | / | 6 |

Useless   Useful

| 1 | / | 2 | / | 3 | / | 4 | / | 5 | / | 6 |

Bad   Good

From Staropoli and Waltz,[22] with permission.

patient" according to how the respondent perceives it or feels it at the moment by placing an X somewhere along each of the six-point scales anchored by polar adjectives pairs. The resulting scale responses can then be converted to numerical quantities and treated statistically.

Nunnally[15] explains that the logic underlying the semantic differential stems from the recognition that in spoken and written language, characteristics of ideas and real things are communicated largely by adjectives. If it is reasonable on this basis to assume that much of "meaning" can be and usually is communicated by adjectives, it is also reasonable to assume that adjectives can be used to measure various facets of meaning. It is useful to distinguish among three overlapping facets of meaning investigated by the semantic differential, that is, denotation, connotation, and association. *Denotation* concerns a description of an object's physical properties. For example, an orange is denoted as a round yellowish fruit. The denotative aspects of meaning are those that direct a person to a specific object to the exclusion of all other objects. *Connotation* refers to what implications the object has for the particular person. After denoting the orange, the person might say "I like them very much," which would represent a connotation or sentiment for that individual. *Associations* consist of other objects that are brought to mind when an individual sees or hears about a particular object. Associations to an orange would be fruit, seed, and apple. The semantic differential mainly measures connotative aspects of meaning, particularly the evaluative connotations of objects. For that purpose it is one of the most valid measures of meaning available.

Numerous factor analytic studies of semantic differential scales have suggested that there are three major factors of meaning involved. The most frequently found factor is *evaluation*, which is defined by pairs of adjectives, such as:

good — bad   honest — dishonest
fair — unfair   successful — unsuccessful
positive — negative   valuable — worthless

The second strongest factor is *potency*. Some of the pairs of adjectives that load on this factor are:

strong — weak   severe — lenient
large — small   hard — soft

The third factor is *activity*. Examples of pairs of adjectives relating to this factor are:

active — passive   tense — relaxed
quick — slow   sharp — dull

Typically, it is found that scales for measuring potency and activity also correlate with the factor of evaluation, which is by far the strongest factor statistically.[15]

Before using a semantic differential scale, the researcher should ascertain:

1. The meaning of the scales does not depend on the concept being rated. For example, whereas "chubby" may be positively evaluative when applied to babies, it may not be positively evaluative when applied to adults. This interaction of scales with concepts, when it occurs, places a limit on the extent to which factors in semantic differential scales can be employed as general yardsticks regardless of the concepts in a particular study. Less scale concept interaction is likely to occur when all the concepts in a particular study are selected from the same domain of interest.
2. The concepts to be rated should be relevant to the research problem and sensitive to differences or similarities among the participants.
3. When the scores are summed over a number of scales, the logic of constructing semantic differential measures is the same as for the construction of summated scales, that is, a homogeneous group of scales that meets the requirements of reliability is sought, and is not usually difficult to attain.
4. It is usually good to employ numbers to designate steps on semantic differential scales. The meanings of numbers should be carefully defined and illustrated in the instructions to the inventory.
5. Although in many studies it has been the practice to reverse the polarity of scales to prevent subjects from being influenced from scale to scale by ratings made on previous scales, the weight of the argument is for keeping scales pertaining to any factor all pointing in the same direction (for ex-

ample, making the "good" pole of all evaluative scales either on the left or the right).

6. In addition to summing scores over groups of scales, in many studies it is also instructive to compare concepts on individual scales.[15]

Additional information regarding the construction of semantic differential scales can be obtained from Osgood, Suci, and Tannenbaum,[16] Snider and Osgood,[20] and Nunnally.[15]

PSYCHOMOTOR MEASURES

Psychomotor measures seek to assess subjects' skill, that is, their ability to perform specific tasks, carry out specific procedures, techniques, and the like. An important consideration in the measurement of psychomotor objectives involves the manner in which the skills and materials or objects to be manipulated or coordinated are specified. That is, criteria for the successful manipulation or coordination of an object must be clearly and unambiguously stated at the time when objectives are made explicit. Task analysis procedures are often used to accomplish this. Additional content on the specifics of task analysis procedures is available in Gagne.[7]

Given the existence of explicit criteria upon which to base the measurement of psychomotor activities, the most viable approach at this time is the observation method combined with a performance checklist or rating scale. The observation method always involves some interaction between respondent and observer in which the observer has an opportunity to watch the respondent function. Although in some cases free and unstructured observation is desirable for the purposes of measuring psychomotor skills, it is necessary that the researcher prepare an observation guide to structure the observations and train the observer in its use. This guide facilitates the researcher's maximization of the likelihood that the crucial activities with which the study is concerned will be considered and hence increases the reliability and validity of the method.

No matter how structured the observation or how well trained or competent the observers, sound observation techniques require more than one observer. This provides an estimate of the accuracy or reliability of the observations and provides a basis for determining the degree of confidence to be placed in the data.

Three factors must be considered in the discussion of observation techniques: (1) interaction between observer and respondent, (2) whether or not the respondent knows he is being observed, and (3) whether or not the respondent knows when he will be observed. Observation is difficult because watching a situation often changes it so that the observer is no longer certain of what he is observing. This implies that a basic criterion for evaluating studies in which observation is used is the extent to which the situation observed was natural. Whether or not observation is known or unknown to the respondent raises ethical questions regarding subjects' rights which will not be dealt with here. The important point is that observations of subjects' psychomotor skills should be accomplished with as little effect on the natural situation in which the skills are normally performed as possible. Suggestions as to how this might be accomplished can be found in Webb and associates.[25]

Observation techniques may be direct or indirect. In *direct* observation the observer evaluates psychomotor performances by simply watching the participant perform. A limitation of this method stems from the fact that it is both time consuming and expensive. It is, however, an excellent technique for the assessment of behavior in conjunction with clinical performance in nursing. One of its strengths results from the fact that if the researcher wishes to learn how a subject functions under the pressure of supervision, there is no substitute for direct observation that is known and scheduled.

Indirect methods of observation include motion picture, television, videotaping, and other devices for recording subjects' activities. The value of indirect techniques results from the opportunities they afford for the subject to become involved in the evaluation of his performance as the recording is viewed jointly by observer and subject. Indirect observations are limited in that they are not sensitive to the tone, mood, or affect of a situation. In addition, important observational data may be missed because of logistic difficulties and/or selectivity on the part of the individual operating the equipment.

Both direct and indirect observations should be structured by a guide for conducting the observations that is constructed on the basis of the important behaviors to be observed. A rating scale format is usually utilized for such a guide.

PHYSIOLOGIC MEASURES

Physiologic measures seek to quantify the level of functioning of living beings. Indicators of physiologic functioning include:

1. Blood pressure readings.
2. Temperature readings.
3. Respiratory measures.
4. Metabolic readings.
5. Diabetic and other screening devices.
6. Readings from cardiac and other life-monitoring instruments.
7. EKG and EEG readings.
8. Results of blood tests and analyses.
9. Measures of height and weight.

Physiologic measures are among the most precise methods one can employ, yield data measured at the interval or ratio level of measurement, allow a wide range of statistical procedures to be employed in their analysis, and tend to produce results that demonstrate a high degree of reliability and validity. Thus, the advantages of employing physiologic measures in nursing research are:

1. They yield data that are more precise and objective than those obtained when other types of measures are employed.

2. The collection, tabulation, and analysis of data are more efficient in that results are expressed in numerical form and need no conversion prior to analysis. Similarly when data are in numerical form, the researcher can readily compare the results with those obtained in other studies. This is important in secondary and meta research (discussed in Chapter 11) in which the goal is the linking of data from different studies to provide the basis for the accumulation of a body of scientific knowledge.

3. They yield a higher level of measurement, thus facilitating the utilization of more powerful statistical procedures and promoting the researcher's obtaining the maximum amount of information from the data.

4. They permit the researcher to exercise greater control over the study. For example, checks can be performed to assess the tenability of statistical assumptions as well as to test the reliability of the data which depend on mathematical models requiring numerical data such as the normal curve of error. Similarly, a higher degree of control over the behavior of the study variables is available.

How Measures Are Constructed and Interpreted

Two distinctions to be considered here are (1) whether a measure is norm-referenced or criterion-referenced and (2) whether a device is subjective or objective.

When a *norm-referenced measure* is employed, a subject's performance or physical functioning is evaluated relative to the performance of others in some well defined comparison or norm group. The National League for Nursing Achievement Test Battery is an example of a norm-referenced test in that the scores of subjects taking the test are compared with scores obtained by other students taking the test in other parts of the country, that is, compared to national norms. Similarly, the results of the application of physiologic measures (for example, blood pressure readings) are often interpreted on the basis of norms (usually ranges of values) considered normal for some well defined comparison group.

In measurement, the term *norms* refers to statistical information that describes the distribution of scores of a well defined population or representative sample of subjects on a particular test and provides information re a subject's performance as represented by that subject's test scores in relation to the norm population on that test.[14] National norms are those based on the test performances of a well defined national sample of subjects. Interpretation of National League for Nursing (NLN) Achievement Tests are based on national norms. Thus, in this case, one is chiefly interested in determining how nursing students in a particular nursing program achieve when compared with nursing students exposed to a wide variety of nursing programs. Local norms are developed by teachers, counselors, administrators, practitioners, and the like for the purpose of comparing how subjects in their school, agency, or district, all of whom receive essentially the same treatment (that is, are in the same educational program, receive care in the same hospital, or reside in the same community health census tract), compare with each other. For a more detailed discussion of the various types of norms, the reader is referred to Angoff[1] and Martuza.[14]

The task of the test constructor when a norm-referenced approach is used is to construct test items that measure a specific characteristic and maximally discriminate among subjects possessing differing amounts of that characteristic, for example, if the characteristic to be measured is knowledge of human sexuality content, then test items are constructed to sort those individuals who really know the content from those who know less. The goal is to spread scores out along the scale, that is, to have a few high scores, most scores in the middle, and a few scores at the low end.

How well subjects' performances compare with the performances of others is irrelevant when a *criterion-referenced measure* is employed. The sole purpose of a criterion-referenced device is to determine whether or not a subject has acquired a predetermined set of target behaviors. The task of the test constructor in this case is to (1) specify the important target behaviors precisely and (2) construct a test or measure that discriminates between those subjects who have and those who have not acquired the target behaviors.

Objective instruments contain items that allow subjects little if any latitude in constructing their responses and that spell out criteria for scoring so clearly that scores can be assigned by individuals who know nothing of the content or similarly by mechanical means. Multiple choice questions and physiologic measures are examples of the most objective devices that can be employed.

Subjective tests allow the respondent considerable latitude in constructing responses. In addition, the probability that different scorers may apply different criteria is greater. Examples of subjective instruments are essay tests, term papers, and case studies.

Types of Examinee Performance

A researcher may seek to measure an individual's typical performance or an individual's maximum performance. If the interest is in assessing subjects as they produce their highest quality work, then a *maximum performance* measure is appropriate. Such measures are indices of cognitive behavior that generally measure a set of skills a subject possesses but differ among themselves in the specificity of their focus and the use to which scores are put. Maximum performance measures of particular interest include aptitude measures, achievement measures, and diagnostic measures.

Aptitude tests tend to focus on various general aspects of human ability (for example, mechanical or artistic aptitude). They are often used as predictors of performance in special fields.

Achievement measures are tests of particular skills and knowledge, and are more specific than aptitude tests. They usually sample a wide range of skills and are constructed by researchers for their own use. Commercially produced achievement measures also are available in many different content areas.

Diagnostic tests usually are even more specific in their focus than achievement measures, although this need not always be the case. They focus on specific skills and often employ multiple measures of a particular skill. Their intent is to pinpoint specific weaknesses that might not be apparent otherwise. Once specific deficiencies are identified and remediation has taken place, one might predict that achievement assumed to be dependent on these more specific skills will improve.

If information about subjects' typical behaviors (that is, what they usually do or would do) is of interest, it is appropriate to utilize a *typical performance* measure. These are measures of affective behavior and usually attempt to have respondents describe the way they typically perceive themselves or their behavior. Typical performance measures usually ask the subject for scaled responses, forced choice responses, or criterion-keyed responses. Table 4-6 presents examples of each of these types of responses.

TABLE 4-6. Sample Responses of Typical Performance Measures

Scaled Response

In a scaled response situation, the respondent indicates on a scale what the rating or answer is to the question posed.

Example:

Did this course provide information that will be meaningful to you in your clinical work?

Please rate.

not at all	very little	somewhat	enough	very much
1	2	3	4	5

Forced Choice Response

With a forced choice response item, the respondent is asked to choose between two or three different alternatives, all of which may be appealing responses. The point is that one particular response is most appealing to the subject.

Example:

A program of ongoing evaluation of patient care does not exist in the agency with which you are affiliated. You are aware of a need to evaluate the various approaches to patient care management. You would prefer to have this need met by:

1. Referring the task to someone else.
2. Supporting the activities of the professional nursing organizations that are seeking to stimulate interest and involvement in evaluation of patient care.
3. Supporting a policy change in the agency responsible for care.
4. Acting as a resource person to staff by providing them with knowledge and materials to enable them to develop such a program.
5. Becoming a member of a committee of practitioners who are developing and testing a pilot program of evaluation in conjunction with the patients to whom they deliver care.
6. Initiating the idea of such a program by providing care to a small group of clients and sharing with staff your evaluation of the various approaches you use.

Criterion-Keyed Response

Criterion-keyed responses depend on information previously obtained about how certain groups answered the items. If a present respondent's score looks like those from

TABLE 4-6. *Continued*

members of a certain predefined group, then the respondent is classified as a member of that group. Criterion keying assumes that the criterion for membership in a particular group is having a set of responses on the measurement instrument that look like those from the predefined group.

Example:

Minnesota Multiphasic Personality Inventory (MMPI) was originally used with hospitalized psychiatric patients and normals (i.e., nonhospitalized respondents) to construct a criterion-keyed set of questions that had some value as predictors of mental stability, i.e., if a particular item was responded to differently by the two groups, it was included in the test.

From Staropoli and Waltz,[22] with permission.

Who Constructs Measures

Standardized measures are developed by specialists for wide use. Their content is set, the directions for administering the test (often including time limits) are clearly described, and the scoring procedure to be used is completely prescribed. Norms information concerning test scores is generally available.

Informal instruments are typically constructed by researchers for their own use. They are not content-constrained, that is, the researcher is free to define the content as well as administration procedures and scoring. Norms may be available for local groups but usually are not available for any group.

The type of measures employed in a given study will have important implications for what can be done with and on the basis of the resulting information. Thus, the researcher must clarify at the outset the type of measurement that will yield data appropriate for the types of research questions or hypotheses the researcher seeks to answer.

RELIABILITY AND VALIDITY OF MEASURES

Two important characteristics of every measuring device or technique are reliability and validity. *Reliability* refers to the consistency with which a measurement rule assigns scores to a group of examinees. Factors that may affect the degree of consistency obtained for a given measure are (1) the manner in which the measure is scored, (2) characteristics of the measure itself, (3) the physical and emotional state of the individual at measurement time, and (4) properties of the situation in which the measure is administered (for example, the amount of noise, the lighting conditions, temperature of the room).

In general, a measurement instrument is valid if it does what it is intended to do. More specifically, after the instrument has been constructed, the next step is to find out whether or not it is useful for the purposes for which it was constructed. This step is usually referred to as determining the *validity* of the instrument. Strictly speaking then, one validates not the measuring instrument but rather some use to which the instrument is put. For example, a test designed to select participants who would benefit from a particular workshop experience must be valid for that purpose but would not necessarily be valid for other purposes such as measuring how well participants master objectives at the completion of the learning experience.

Both validity and reliability are matters of degree rather than all or none properties. Measures should be assessed each time they are used to see if they are behaving as planned. New evidence may suggest modifications of an existing measure or the development of a new and better approach to measuring the attribute in question.

TABLE 4-7. Procedures for Estimating the Reliability of Subjectively Scored Measures

	Interrater reliability	Intrarater reliability
Definition	Refers to the agreement among two or more raters in assigning scores to the objects or responses being judged.	Refers to the consistency with which one test rater assigns scores to a single set of test item responses on two occasions.
Procedure	1. Two or more competent raters score the responses to a set of subjective test items. 2. If only two raters are used, the Pearson correlation coefficient (r) may be used to measure the degree of agreement among them. If more than two raters are used, coefficient alpha may be used with the column headings representing the judges and the row headings representing the objects being rated.	1. A large number of persons respond to one subjective item. 2. Scores are assigned to the items on some fixed scale. Answers are not recorded on the respondents' answer sheets. 3. Approximately two weeks later, response sheets are shuffled and rescored using the same procedure used on the first occasion. 4. The Pearson correlation coefficient (r) between the two scorings is determined as a measure of agreement.
Interpretation	A coefficient of 0 means complete lack of agreement; a coefficient of 1.00 indicates complete agreement. Note: Agreement does not mean that the same scores were assigned by all raters; it means that the relative ordering of scores assigned by rater 1 matches the relative order assigned by rater 2, and so forth.	A zero value for the correlation coefficient is interpreted as inconsistency; a value of 1.00 is interpreted as complete consistency.
Utility	Raters are often trained to a high degree of agreement in scoring subjective measures using the interrater reliability measure to determine when the raters are using essentially the same criteria for scoring the responses.	This technique is useful in determining the extent to which an individual applies the same criteria to rating responses on different occasions and should be used for this purpose by those who use subjective-type measures. This technique enables one to determine to some extent the degree to which ratings are influenced by temporal factors.

From Staropoli and Waltz,[22] with permission.

Reliability is a necessary prerequisite for validity, that is, if an instrument does not assign scores consistently it cannot be useful for the purposes for which it is intended. Tables 4-7 and 4-8 compare and contrast the general types of reliability and outline the usual procedure carried out in estimating each type. Table 4-9 compares and contrasts the general types of validity and discusses the usual procedure for determining each type.

TABLE 4-8. Procedures for Estimating the Reliability of Measures

	Test-retest reliability	*Parallel-form reliability*	*Internal consistency*
Definition	Consistency of performance a measure elicits from one group of subjects on two separate occasions.	Consistency of performance alternate forms of a test elicit from one group of subjects on one testing occasion. Two tests are considered parallel if (1) they have been constructed using the same objectives and procedures, (2) have approximately equal means, (3) have equal correlations with any third variable, and (4) have equal standard deviations.	Consistency of performance of a group of individuals across the items on a single test.
Procedure	To estimate the 2-week test-retest reliability for a particular test, the researcher would: 1. Administer the test under standardized conditions to a single group of examinees representative of the group for which the measure was designed. 2. Two weeks later, re-administer the same test under the same conditions to the same group of subjects. 3. Determine the extent to which the two sets of scores are correlated. The correlation coefficient (r) is taken as the estimate of reliability.	To estimate parallel-form reliability, the researcher would: 1. Administer two alternate forms of a test to one representative group on the same test occasion or on two separate test occasions. 2. Determine the extent to which the two sets of scores are correlated utilizing the Pearson correlation coefficient as an estimate of reliability. If both forms are administered on the same testing occasion, the coefficient reflects form equivalence only. If they are administered on two occasions, stability as well as form equivalence is reflected.	To estimate the internal consistency of a test, the researcher would: 1. Administer the measure under standardized conditions to a representative group on one occasion. 2. Determine the value of the alpha coefficient.

TABLE 4-8. Continued

	Test-retest reliability	Parallel-form reliability	Internal consistency
Interpretation	This coefficient reflects the extent to which the measure rank orders the performances of the subjects the same on the two separate measurement occasions. For this reason, it is often referred to as the coefficient of stability. The closer the correlation is to 1.00, the more stable the measuring device is presumed to be.	Values above 0.80 are usually taken as evidence that the forms may be used interchangeably.	The alpha coefficient measures the extent to which performance on any one item in the test is a good indicator of performance on any other item in the same test.
Utility	This procedure is appropriate for determining the quality of instruments designed to measure characteristics known to be relatively stable over the period under investigation. Since achievement tests measure characteristics that tend to change rapidly, this procedure is not appropriate for estimating the reliability of measures of this type.	Whenever two forms of an instrument can be generated, this is the preferred method for assessing reliability.	Alpha is the preferred measure of internal consistency because (1) it has a single value for any given set of test data and (2) it is equal in value to the mean of the distribution of all possible split-half coefficients associated with a particular set of test data.

Adapted from Martuza,[13] with permission.
From Staropoli and Waltz,[22] with permission.

The determination of the reliability and validity of a specific device or method is faciliated when multiple measures of the same thing are employed, that is, more than one type of instrumentation is used to answer a given research question. Similarly, the reliability and validity of the overall study results and the utility of the findings increase when the researcher employs multiple measures of each research question.

Specific Procedures for Estimating Reliability and Validity

The specific procedures utilized for determining the types of reliability and validity outlined in Tables 4-7 to 4-9 will differ depending upon whether the measure is norm-referenced or criterion-referenced. Procedures discussed for norm-referenced reliability and validity are also applicable to any non-normed,

TABLE 4-9. Procedures for Estimating the Validity of Measures

	Content	Construct	Criterion-related
Important: When intent is to	Determine how an individual performs at present in a universe of situations that the test situation is claimed to represent.[21]	Infer the degree to which the individual possesses some hypothetical trait or quality presumed to be reflected in the test performance.[21]	Forecast an individual's future standing or estimate present standing on some variable of particular significance that is different from the test.[21]
Greatest utility for	Cognitive measures, e.g., achievement testing in which subject performance on a small set of items in one test serves as lone indicator of how well content is mastered.	Affective measures e.g., measures of creativity and anxiety in which believed individual differences in test performance reflect individual differences in the trait about which the inference is being made.	Measures used to predict present or future performance, e.g., clinical performance test at end of a clinical course used to predict students' ability to perform in the clinical setting.
Procedure	Review of objectives and test items by a panel of experts.	Comparison of student scores on test with scores of individuals known to have high and low amounts of trait being measured.	Correlation of test scores with present or future performance on a second measure of the same thing.

*From Staropoli and Waltz,[22] with permission.

informal instrument whose purpose is to measure a specific characteristic and maximally discriminate among subjects possessing differing amounts of that characteristic.

NORM-REFERENCED RELIABILITY

Given an understanding of correlation and prediction (see Chapter 10), the procedures for test-retest reliability and parallel-form reliability estimations are straightforward. They will not be given further attention here.

Alpha is the preferred measure of internal consistency. It measures the extent to which performance on any one item in an instrument is a good indicator of performance on any other item in the same instrument. The formula for determining the alpha coefficient is:

$$\text{(Formula 4-1)} \qquad \text{alpha} = \left(\frac{K}{K-1}\right)\left[1 - \left(\frac{\Sigma \text{ VAR ITEMS}}{\text{VAR TEST}}\right)\right]$$

where:

K = number of items in the test.

Σ VAR ITEMS = sum of the individual item variances.

VAR TEST = variance of the distribution of test scores.

TABLE 4-10. Hypothetical Test Scores on a Five-Item Achievement Test Administered to Four Students

Student	Item 1	2	3	4	5	6	Total test score
A	5	3	3	2	2	6	21
B	3	2	5	3	2	5	20
C	2	2	5	3	3	9	24
D	0	3	2	2	0	5	12
E	5	0	0	0	3	5	13
Total	15	10	15	10	10	30	90
Mean	3	2	3	2	2	6	18
Variance	3.6	1.2	3.6	1.2	1.2	2.4	22

Suppose a six-item test were given to five participants in a continuing education learning experience to assess their knowledge of interviewing principles and the scores shown in Table 4-10 were obtained. Alpha as an indicator of reliability for this test is calculated in the following manner:

1. $K = 6$, since there are six items.
2. VAR TEST, the variance for the test score distribution, calculated in the usual manner is:
$$SS\ (X) = (31 - 23)^2 + (19 - 23)^2 + (23 - 23)^2 + (22 - 23)^2 + (20 - 23)^2$$
$$= 90$$
$$= 90/5$$
$$= 18$$
3. VAR ITEM, the variance for each item on the test, is calculated in the same manner:
$$SS\ (ITEM\ 1) = (5 - 3)^2 + (3 - 3)^2 + (2 - 3)^2 + (0 - 3)^2 + (5 - 3)^2$$
$$= 18$$
$$= 18/5$$
$$= 3.6$$
4. Substituting in the formula for alpha:
$$Alpha = \left(\frac{6}{5}\right) \left[1 - \left(\frac{13.2}{22}\right)\right]$$
$$= \left(\frac{6}{5}\right) [1 - 0.6]$$
$$= (1.2)\ (0.4)$$
$$= 0.48$$

The resulting alpha value indicates that the test has only a moderate internal consistency. As a result, performance on any one item is only a fair predictor of performance on any other item. A high alpha value is usually taken as evidence that the test as a whole is measuring just one attribute, for example, achievement of interviewing principles.

Several considerations need to be made when alpha is employed as a measure of reliability:

1. It is affected by the length of the test. The longer the test (the more items contained on the test), the higher the value of the alpha coefficient (the higher the reliability estimate).
2. It is necessary to assume, when using alpha, that conditions were such that all subjects had ample time to complete all items on the test. Administering a test under speeded conditions (that is, conditions that make it impossible for most of the subjects to attempt all of the items) spuriously raises the value of the alpha coefficient obtained. If less than 85 percent of the subjects respond to all the items on a test, the test is considered a speeded one and alpha should not be used as an estimate of reliability.
3. As with all reliability measures, an alpha value obtained in one situation is not generalizable to other situations. Alpha should be calculated each time a measure is used.
4. The size of the alpha coefficient obtained in any situation is directly related to the total test variance. The greater the value of the total test variance, the greater the value of the alpha coefficient obtained.
5. Alpha measures are not appropriate for utilization as measures of internal consistency in a criterion-referenced framework. Within a criterion-referenced context, a skewed test score distribution (see Chapter 8) usually results and this type of distribution generally has little variance.
6. Alpha is the preferred estimator of reliability in a norm-referenced measurement framework. Norm-referenced tests are constructed to maximize total test score variance.[13]

CRITERION-REFERENCED RELIABILITY

Estimating the reliability of criterion-referenced measures has been and remains a thorny problem. This problem can be examined by considering the implications that the utilization of a criterion-referenced framework has with respect to reliability and how this differs from the estimation of reliability when the norm-referenced framework is used.

Norm-referenced measures are used to ascertain an individual's performance in relationship to the performance of the other individuals on the same measuring device. Criterion-referenced measures, on the other hand, are used to ascertain an individual's status with respect to some criterion, that is, performance standard. An important distinction between the two types of measurement is that in the case of criterion-referenced measures, the interest is in knowing what the individual can do, not how he stands in comparison to others as in the norm-referenced approach. In general, a norm-referenced measure is employed when a degree of selectivity is required by the situation. For example, there are only limited openings in a continuing education learning experience and the continuing educator is anxious to identify the best potential participants. In situations in which the interest is in whether an individual possesses a particular competence and there are no constraints regarding how many individuals can possess that skill, criterion-referenced measures are appropriate.

Norm-referenced measures are designed to spread people out, that is, to maximize the variability of the scores on the measure. With criterion-referenced measures, variability is irrelevant, that is, the meaning of the scores flows directly from the connection between the instrument and the criterion. Variability is not an essential characteristic of a criterion-referenced measure. The issue of variability is not only at the core of the differences between norm- and criterion-referenced measures, but it is also the crux of the problems in estimating the reliability of criterion-referenced instruments. This is because the reliability procedures for norm-referenced measures are based on the desirability of variability among scores.

It is obvious that a criterion-referenced measure should be internally consistent. If the argument is to be made that the items are tied to a criterion, then the items should be quite similar in terms of what they are measuring. The problem, however, is that procedures for determining internal consistency (for example, alpha), because they are dependent on score variability, are not appropriate for criterion-referenced measures and it is not clear what should replace them.

Other aspects of reliability are equally problematic. Stability might be important for a criterion-referenced measure but a test-retest correlation coefficient, dependent on its own variability, is not necessarily the way to assess it. It is all right if a criterion-referenced measure has a high inter-item correlation or test-retest correlation. The point is not that these indices cannot be used to support the consistency of the measures. A criterion-referenced measure could be highly consistent and yet indices dependent on variability (that is, alpha, r) might not reflect that consistency.

The literature on criterion-referenced reliability is fraught with disagreement among experts regarding appropriate measures for determining criterion-referenced reliability. Carter[5] suggested administering a single form to two comparable groups and then comparing the percent that met criterion in one group with the percent that met criterion in the other group. He also suggested determining the percent of respondents who achieved criterion on parallel tests. Livingston[12] suggested a procedure for determining the squared deviations of the individual's score from a performance standard or cutting score. This procedure was similar to that utilized in the norm-referenced case but, rather than determining the individual's distance from the mean of the group, the individual's score distance from the performance standards (that is, mastery level) formed the basis for Livingston's procedure. Hambleton and Novick[8] suggested that the primary purpose for criterion-referenced testing in objective-based instructional programs is to classify respondents into mastery states or categories on each of the objectives included in the test. They argued that the concern in criterion-referenced measurement should not be with how far a respondent deviates from a fixed standard, but rather the problem is one of deciding whether a respondent's true performance level is above or below some cutting score. Their approach, based on Bayesian statistics, concerns itself with the proportion of times the same decision is made regarding an individual's true mastery with two parallel instruments.

Swaminathan, Hambleton, and Algina[24] extended the earlier work of Hambleton and Novick[8] and suggested a technique for estimating the reliability of criterion-referenced measures that is rapidly gaining the favor of experts in the field. Reliability is defined by them in terms of the consistency of decisions made about mastery states over repeated administrations of the same instrument. More specifically, reliability is defined as a measure of agreement over and above that which can be expected by chance alone between the decisions made about respondent's mastery states in repeated administrations for each objective measured by the criterion-referenced instrument. If an instrument consists of items measuring several objectives, then it is necessary to determine the reliability for each subtest (that is, group of items) measuring a particular objective. A criterion-referenced test will, therefore, have as many reliabilities as there are objectives included in the instrument. The statistic used to reflect consistency in this approach is Cohen's Coefficient K.

(Formula 4-2) $K = (P_o - P_e)/(1 - P_e)$

where:
   K = agreement over and above chance between the decisions made about mastery states in repeated administrations of the measure.
   P_o = observed proportion of agreement.
   P_e = expected proportion of agreement.

P_o, the observed proportion of agreement, is determined by finding the proportion of respondents who achieved mastery on both administrations of the measure and the proportion of the respondents who achieved nonmastery on both administrations, and calculating the sum of these two values. P_e, the expected proportion of agreement, is determined by multiplying the proportion of respondents who achieved mastery on the first administration by the proportion of respondents who obtained mastery on the second administration and adding the resulting value to the product of the proportion of respondents who were nonmasters on the first and second administrations. The following example may clarify the procedure.

A workshop objective is that, at the completion of the learning experience, participants be able to write at least eight principles of interviewing that are relevant to their work with the dying patient. An achievement test is then constructed to measure this objective and its reliability estimated using the following procedure. A sample of 100 who participated in the workshop is identified and then given the test on two separate occasions. The results of these two testings are summarized in Table 4-11.

Mastery is determined by whether or not an individual correctly lists a minimum of six principles. The values in the table are interpreted in the following manner: the value 0.80 in the upper left-hand cell indicates that 80 percent of the respondents who achieved mastery at the time of the first administration also achieved mastery at the time of the second administration; the value 0.05

TABLE 4-11. Results of Achievement Test Administered to 100 Subjects on Two Separate Occasions

| | Administration 2 | | Marginal proportion |
Administration 1	Master	Nonmaster	
Master	0.80	0.05	0.85
Nonmaster	0.10	0.05	0.15
Marginal proportion	0.90	0.10	1.00

in the upper right-hand cell indicates that 5 percent of the respondents who achieved mastery on the first administration did not achieve mastery at the time of the second administration. The values in the two lower cells are interpreted in a similar manner. These values are obtained by counting the number of respondents in each cell and then dividing this number by the total number of respondents to obtain a proportion. Utilizing the values in Table 4-11, K is then calculated in the following manner:

$$P_o = 0.80 + 0.05 \qquad\qquad P_e = (0.85)\,(0.90) + (0.10)\,(0.15)$$
$$= 0.85 \qquad\qquad\qquad\quad = 0.77 + 0.02$$
$$= 0.79$$

$$K = \frac{0.85 - 0.79}{1 - 0.79}$$
$$= \frac{0.06}{0.21}$$
$$= 0.285$$

which reflects only 29 percent agreement over and above that attributed to chance.

The K value of 0.285 indicates only moderate agreement between the decisions made on the two administrations of the test. The upper limit of K is +1 and may occur only when the marginal proportions for different administrations are equal. If any respondent is classified differently on repeated administrations, the value of K will be less than 1. The lower limit of K is −1. A negative value indicates extreme decision-making inconsistency and hence indicates unreliability of the measure.

The coefficient of agreement, K, and hence the reliability of the criterion-referenced measure is dependent on factors that affect the decision process. Factors that affect decision making include the method of assigning respondents to mastery states, selection of the cutting score, test length, and heterogeneity of the respondent group. Decision-making consistency then is a measure of the reliability of the entire decision-making process. The instrument or test provides only one input into the decision-making process and all the other factors that affect the process must be considered when an attempt is made to generalize reliability data to a new decision-making situation.

It should be noted that K is very much situation-specific and, therefore, information such as cutting scores and respondent ability as measured by the instrument should be reported along with the reliability index. The authors recommend that K be utilized to determine the reliability of criterion-referenced measures.

It is important that the researcher who uses criterion-referenced measures be aware of the issues that relate to the determination of reliability for these measures and keep up to date with new procedures as they are developed. The *Journal of Educational Measurement*, published quarterly by the National Council on Measurement in Education, is an excellent source for keeping current in this area.

NORM-REFERENCED VALIDITY

Different types of measures are often used for different aims. *Validity* refers to the degree to which a measure is capable of achieving the purposes for which it was developed. Thus, the kind of validity information to be gathered depends on the aim(s) of the measure rather than on the type of measure. If an instrument is used for more than one purpose, it is necessary to investigate more than one type of validity.

Content Validity

This type of validity is important for instruments designed to measure cognition. The process for the most part is subjective. The determination of whether or not a particular instrument has an acceptable degree of content validity for use in a given situation can only be determined by having individuals who are knowledgeable about that particular content make judgments concerning the adequacy of the instrument in measuring that content in a representative manner.

Content validity is closely related to the manner in which an instrument is developed. When a representative sample of content is to be measured, the researcher should construct an exhaustive set of items to measure each objective and then use a random sampling procedure to select a subset of items from this larger set to use for the instrument.

The researcher should give the list of behavioral objectives and a separate list of the items constructed to specifically test the objectives to at least two specialists in the area of content addressed by the objectives and ask them to link each objective with its respective item(s). In addition, the judges should be asked to assess the relevancy of the items to the content addressed by the objectives and to indicate if they believe the items are a representative sample of the content behaviors of interest.

In the case of criterion-referenced measures, a few attempts have been made to quantify the judgment of content specialists by using an index of interjudge agreement as the measure of item content validity.[10, 17, 18] Unfortunately, most of these techniques are cumbersome or have limitations that lessen their utility, or both. An approach worth noting because of its practicality is one described by Hambleton and coworkers.[9] It involves supplying the objectives and items to two content specialists and having them independently rate the relevance of each item to the objective(s) using a four-point rating scale (for example, 1 — not relevant, 2 — somewhat relevant, 3 — quite relevant, and 4 — very relevant). The *index of content validity* (CVI) is then simply defined as the proportion of items given a rating of 3 or 4 by both raters involved. For example, suppose the relevance of each of four items on an instrument to a particular objective is independently rated by two experts using the four-point scale and the results are those displayed in Table 4-12. Thus, using these data:

$$CVI = \text{proportion of items given a rating of 3 or 4 by both raters}$$
$$CVI = 3/4$$
$$= 0.75$$

If all items are given ratings of 3 or 4 by both raters, inter-rater agreement would be perfect and the value of the CVI would be 1.00. If half of the items are jointly classified as 1 or 2 while the others are jointly classified as 3 or 4, the CVI would be 0.50 indicating an unacceptable level of content validity.

Limitations of the approach are:

1. The CVI may be inflated by chance.
2. The value of CVI in a given situation is a function of the number of rating categories and the manner in which categories are combined.

Thus, this approach has practical merit in quantifying content validity if used as outlined above and interpreted with care. Content validity judgments require subject matter expertise and are different from the judgments made in determining face validity. *Face validity* refers to the appearance of the instrument to the layman, that is, if upon cursory inspection an instrument appears to measure what the test constructor claims it measures, it is said to have face validity.

TABLE 4-12. Results of Relevance Rating of Four Items by Two Raters Using a Four-Point Rating Scale

Rater 2	Rater 1		Total
	1 or 2	3 or 4	
1 or 2	1	0	1
3 or 4	0	3	3
Total	1	3	4

Construct Validity

This type of validity is especially important for measures of affect. It is evaluated by determining the degree to which certain explanatory concepts or constructs account for performance on the measure. Studies of construct validity involve essentially three steps: (1) the researcher asks what hypotheses can be stated regarding the behavior of persons with high and low scores on this measure, (2) the researcher gathers data to test these hypotheses, and (3) in light of these findings, the researcher makes an inference as to whether the rationale underlying the instrument's construction is adequate to explain the data collected. If the rationale fails to account for the data, the researcher should revise the measure, reformulate the rationale, or reject the rationale altogether. Fresh evidence would then be required to demonstrate construct validity for the revised measure.[21]

Three specific procedures for determining construct validity are (1) the contrasted groups approach, (2) the experimental manipulation approach, and (3) the multitrait-multimethod approach.[14]

Contrasted Groups Approach. This approach requires that the researcher identify two groups of individuals: one known to be extremely high and the other extremely low in the characteristic being measured by the instrument. For example, in estimating the validity of an instrument that purports to measure anxiety, the researcher would identify a group of individuals who are known to be extremely anxious and a group of individuals who are known to have a low degree of anxiety. The researcher would then administer the instrument to both groups and examine the differences in the scores obtained by each. If the instrument is sensitive to individual differences in anxiety, then the mean performance of these two groups should differ significantly. Whether or not a difference in the two group means is significant is determined using an appropriate statistical test (for example, the t-test, or an analysis of variance test).

If a significant difference is found between the means of the two groups, the researcher can say that some evidence was obtained to support the claim that the instrument has construct validity, that is, that the instrument measures anxiety. It should be noted that evidence is not absolute proof that the test measures anxiety. Since the two groups differ in many ways, the mean difference in test scores may be due to group noncomparability on some other variable that was not measured.

If the data collected indicate there is no significant difference between the means of the two groups' test scores, it may be concluded that (1) the test is unreliable, (2) the test is reliable but not a valid measure of anxiety, or (3) the test constructor's conception of the construct anxiety is faulty and needs to be reformulated. That is, there is no basis for claiming that the test is sensitive to individual differences on the hypothesized anxiety continuum.

Experimental Manipulation Approach. The theory or rationale underlying the construction of the measure is used to predict how a group of individuals will perform on the instrument under a variety of experimentally induced conditions. The individuals are then placed in these conditions and measured using the instrument in question. If the individuals as a group behave as predicted on the test, one can offer this as evidence for construct validity. If the individuals behave in a manner inconsistent with the prediction, then the same alternatives exist as those mentioned in the discussion of the contrasted groups approach with the additional possibility that the experimental design might not have provided an adequate test of the hypothesis in question.[14]

Multitrait-Multimethod Approach. This approach is based on two premises: (1) that different measures of the same construct should correlate highly with each other and (2) that measures of different constructs should have a low correlation with each other. The first is referred to as the *convergent validity principle* and the second the *discriminant validity principle.*[4]

Two types of variance are of concern when this approach is employed: (1) variability in a set of scores resulting from individual differences in the trait being measured, that is, *trait variance,* and (2) variability resulting from individual differences in subjects' ability to respond appropriately to the particular type of measure used, that is, *method variance.* The size of the correlation between two measures is a function of both trait and method variances. For example, a high correlation between two scores on two self-report measures of clinical performance may be explained by individual differences in clinical performance or it may be more a function of using the same approach to instrumentation (that is, self-report). The separation of trait variance from method variance is an inherent aspect of the multitrait-multimethod approach and accounts for one of its advantages over other approaches to the determination of validity.

When this technique is employed, the researcher's attention is focused not only on the size of the correlations, but the patterns of the relationships between correlations as well. Suppose the researcher had two instruments designed to measure confidence in medical-surgical nursing skills, two instruments designed to measure incorporation of learnings into nursing practice, and two instruments designed to measure empathy. Furthermore, one measure of each construct utilizes a semantic differential scale and the second measure of each construct utilizes an adjective checklist. Each of these six instruments is administered to all subjects during the same point in time. Then the reliability of each form is determined utilizing a measure of internal consistency

		METHOD 1 (SEMANTIC DIFFERENTIAL)			METHOD 2 (ADJECTIVE CHECKLIST)		
		CONFIDENCE	INC.	EMPATHY	CONFIDENCE	INC.	EMPATHY
SEMANTIC DIFFERENTIAL	CONFIDENCE	.90					
	INCORPORATION		.88				
	EMPATHY			.81			
ADJECTIVE CHECKLIST	CONFIDENCE				.80		
	INCORPORATION					.91	
	EMPATHY						.79

FIGURE 4-1. Reliability diagonals in constructing a multitrait-multimethod matrix. (From Staropoli and Waltz,[22] with permission.)

		METHOD 1 (SEMANTIC DIFFERENTIAL)			METHOD 2 (ADJECTIVE CHECKLIST)		
		CONFIDENCE	INC.	EMPATHY	CONFIDENCE	INC.	EMPATHY
SEMANTIC DIFFERENTIAL	CONFIDENCE	.90					
	INCORPORATION		.88				
	EMPATHY			.81			
ADJECTIVE CHECKLIST	CONFIDENCE	.61			.80		
	INCORPORATION		.63			.91	
	EMPATHY			.60			.79

FIGURE 4-2. Validity diagonal in constructing a multitrait-multimethod matrix. (From Staropoli and Waltz,[22] with permission.)

(alpha) and the correlation (r) between each pair of forms is computed. Validity is then assessed by constructing a multitrait-multimethod matrix and entering the resulting correlations in the following manner.

First, the researcher enters the reliability estimate for each form as shown in Figure 4-1. The sets of three reliability estimates in the upper left and lower right blocks of Figure 4-1 are the *reliability diagonals*. If these estimates are sufficiently high, the researcher proceeds to the next step, if not, the procedure terminates because reliability is a prerequisite for validity. The values of the reliability estimates in Figure 4-1 range from 0.79 to 0.91 indicating reasonably high reliability and thus the analysis may continue.

Next, to assess *convergent validity*, the correlations between the two measures of each construct measured using different approaches is entered in the lower left block of the matrix as shown in Figure 4-2. The *validity diagonal* in Figure 4-2 indicates that the relationships between the two measures of the same trait using different instrumentation range from 0.60 to 0.63, high enough to provide evidence of convergent validity.

Correlations between measures of different constructs employing a semantic differential scale are entered in the upper block of Figure 4-3 and the correlations between measures of different constructs using an adjective checklist are

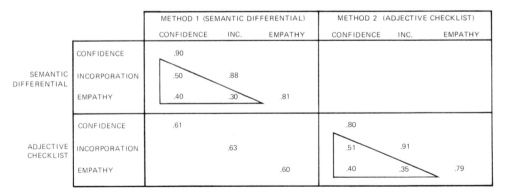

FIGURE 4-3. Heterotrait-monomethod triangles in constructing a multitrait-multimethod matrix. (From Staropoli and Waltz,[22] with permission.)

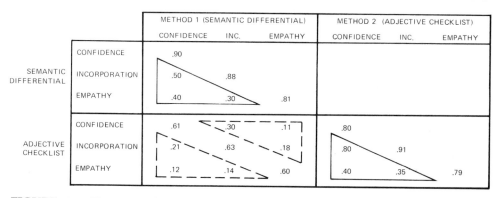

FIGURE 4-4. Heterotrait-heteromethod triangles in constructing a multitrait-multi-method matrix. (From Staropoli and Waltz,[22] with permission.)

entered in the lower right block of the matrix. These coefficients are indicators of the relationship between measures of different constructs that use the same method of measurement. Hence, these values are a function of the relationships existing between the three constructs and the utilization of a common instrumentation. The values in this *heterotrait-monomethod* triangle should be lower than the values in the validity diagonal if variability is more the result of trait variance than method variance. In Figure 4-3, triangle values are in fact lower than the values in the validity diagonal and thus provide evidence for *construct validity*.

The remaining correlations between measures of different constructs measured by different methods are entered in the triangles in the lower block in the left of the matrix as shown in Figure 4-4. The values in these *heterotrait-heteromethod* triangles should be lower than the values in the validity diagonal and the corresponding values in the heterotrait-monomethod triangles. In Figure 4-4 this pattern is observed and hence provides evidence of *discriminant validity*.

In summary, if the information in Figure 4-4 resulted from an actual study, it would provide evidence for reliability, convergent validity, construct validity, and discriminant validity. Hence, whenever the necessary conditions can be met, the multitrait-multimethod approach to instrument validation produces more data with more efficiency than most other techniques available.

CRITERION-RELATED VALIDITY

Criterion-related validity is important when the researcher wishes to infer from a measure an individual's probable standing on some other variable called a criterion. *Predictive validity* indicates the extent to which an individual's future level on the criterion can be predicted from a knowledge of prior test performance. *Concurrent validity* refers to the extent to which a measure may be used to estimate an individual's present standing on the criterion. The distinction between these two types of criterion-related validity is important. Predictive validity involves a time interval during which something may happen (for example, people gain experience or are subjected to some type of learning experience).[21]

In each of the questions below, the researcher wants to know the extent to which performance on a criterion variable can be estimated using information about another variable, hence they are questions of criterion-related validity.

1. Are scores on a confidence in nursing practice measure at the completion of a continuing education learning experience good predictors of participants' incorporation of learnings into ongoing nursing practice?
2. Is performance on an achievement test of learnings a good predictor of performance in a patient care situation?

In both cases, the researcher wants to know the extent to which performance on an important criterion variable (that is, incorporation of learnings into nursing practice and performance in a patient care situation) can be estimated using information on a less costly, more easily obtained measure (that is, confidence scores, achievement test scores). Criterion-related validity is assessed by measuring the performance of the target population or a representative sample of that population on both the predictor and criterion variables and then determining the linear correlation, that is, Pearson r, as a measure of the quality of the predictor for estimating performance on that particular criterion in that target population. It should be noted that the utility of most criterion-related validity coefficients is limited by the fact that salient characteristics in most populations are dynamic and changing. Similarly, the value of the results of criterion-related validity studies is a function of the representativeness of the sample and the choice of a criterion measure. Criterion measures must be valid and, more importantly, must be reliable and meaningful. Many important nursing variables are difficult to define and measure. Too often a criterion is determined by convenience. For example, when the criterion of interest is not readily available, it is tempting to use some substitute criterion rather than to wait until the desired criterion is available. This is a potential hazard in nursing because of the long time frequently required to collect information (for example, the incorporation of learning into practice may involve years of data collection). However, the relevance of the criterion used may not typically bear the same relevance to the predictors as the desired criterion. This possibility must be given careful consideration, and expediency should not be allowed to rule the conduct of the study.

CRITERION-REFERENCED VALIDITY

Most of the procedures discussed for estimating the validity of norm-referenced measures are based on correlations and thus on variability. As with reliability, the results of these procedures when applied to criterion-referenced measures are useful if they are positive but not necessarily cause for alarm if they are unfavorable. Criterion-referenced measures are valid primarily in terms of the adequacy with which they represent the criterion. Therefore, content validity approaches are the most appropriate estimators of validity for criterion-referenced measures. That is, a careful judgment made by experts, based on the test's apparent relevance to the behavior legitimately inferable from those delimited by the criterion, is the general procedure for validating criterion-referenced measures. The reader is referred to the previous discussion of content validity.

This is not to imply that other strategies for determining validity (for example, construct validity) cannot also be utilized to gain additional evidence for the validity of a criterion-referenced instrument. For example, the researcher may be interested in estimating the validity of a criterion-referenced measure (for example, administered at the completion of a program) as a predictor of some more distant criterion (for example, occurring a year or years later). If positive intercorrelations are found among several predictors of the same criterion, this would add to the researcher's confidence regarding whether or not a given predictor is meeting its stated purpose.

Item Analysis Procedures

Item analysis is a procedure used to increase the reliability and validity of a measuring device by separately evaluating each item to determine whether or not that item discriminates in the same manner that the overall measure is intended to discriminate.[11]

NORM-REFERENCED PROCEDURES

Three item analysis procedures have utility when a norm-referenced approach to measurement is employed: (1) item p level, (2) discrimination index, and (3) item response chart.

Item p level

The p level or difficulty level of an item is the proportion of correct responses to that item. To determine the p level, one simply counts the number of subjects selecting the correct or desired response to a particular item and divides this number by the total number of subjects in the group.

Example: A 10-item achievement test is given to 40 participants in a continuing education program. Upon scoring, it is determined that 20 subjects selected the correct response to item 1, the remaining subjects did not. The p level for this item is 20/40 or 0.50.

The limits for p are 0 to 1.00. The closer the value of p is to 1.00, the easier the item, the closer p is to zero, the more difficult the item. In norm-referenced measures, p levels between 0.30 and 0.70 are desirable, because extremely easy or extremely difficult items have very little power to discriminate or differentiate among subjects.[13]

Discrimination Indices

D is a measure of an item's discriminatory power. If performance on an item is a good predictor of performance on the overall measure, the item is a good discriminator. To obtain D, scores for all subjects on the overall measure are ranked from high to low. Then ranked scores are divided into two groups, one group comprised of the highest 25 percent and the second comprised of the lowest 25 percent. The remaining (middle) scores are set aside. For each item, the proportion of persons in the top 25 percent who answered the item correctly is determined. This value is labeled P_u. Next, the proportion of persons in the lowest 25 percent who answered the item correctly is determined and designated P_l. D is determined by subtracting P_l from P_u. D ranges from -1.00 to $+1.00$. A positive D value indicates the item is discriminating like the total test. A negative D value suggests that people who get low scores on the total measure tend to get the item correct while those who score high on the total measure tend to select incorrect responses to this item. Negative D values usually indicate that the item is in need of improvement. It may be that the item is misinterpreted by the more knowledgeable subject or that the item provides a clue to the less knowledgeable subject that enables a correct guess at the answer. D values greater than $+0.20$ are desirable in a norm-referenced context.

Item Response Charts

One question answered by item response charts is: given a particular measure, will subjects in the top 25 percent of the score distribution also tend to get a particular item correct and subjects in the bottom 25 percent of the distribution tend to miss the same item? If so, such an item has favorable discriminating power and contributes to the overall reliability and validity of the measure. To answer this question, it is first necessary to rank order the subjects and identify the highest and lowest 25 percent as in the discussion of D. A fourfold table is then constructed based on two pairs of categories. The first pair is simply right/wrong for a specific item; the second pair is the category high/low scorers (Fig. 4-5). The chi-square value of the resulting proportions is calculated using the formula in Chapter 10. If chi-square is significant, it can be concluded that a difference exists in the proportion of high and low scoring subjects who gave correct responses. Items that meet this criterion should be retained, those that do not should be discarded.

Inspection of the total response pattern in an item response chart is useful for identifying malfunctioning or nonfunctioning distractors. The p lev-

	WRONG	RIGHT
HIGH	0	50
LOW	10	40

FIGURE 4-5. Item response chart for norm-referenced procedure.

el and D index for the item in Figure 4-5 are 0.90 and +0.20, respectively. Thus, the item is easy and discrimination is positive but not strong. Examination of the response chart indicates that the item does not discriminate well. The incorrect option was selected by only 10 percent of the subjects. It would, therefore, be prudent to examine the item to determine if these results are due to some item defect and to revise the item accordingly. Potential problems might be that the correct option contains a clue that is used by many of the lower group in responding or that the incorrect option is grammatically inconsistent with the stem and thus clues subjects not to select it. If the item appeared sound as constructed, it would be useful to analyze the content and instructional procedures to which this item relates for the purpose of determining why the item's discriminating power is marginal.

CRITERION-REFERENCED PROCEDURES

In a criterion-referenced measurement framework, the concern is with items that discriminate between subjects who have achieved a particular task or objective and those who have not.

Discrimination Indices

A criterion-referenced discrimination index is a measure of the item's ability to discriminate between (1) subjects who have acquired the target behavior and those who have not and (2) subjects who have been exposed to a relevant treatment and those who have not. Two such indices have been developed for this purpose, D', a modified version of D, and the pretest-posttest procedure.

D' is the proportion of subjects who get a particular item correct and meet criterion on the measure as a whole minus the proportion of subjects who get the item correct and fail to meet the criterion on the overall measure. It is assumed that all items on the measure relate to a single objective or collection of highly related objectives. The value of D' ranges from −1.00 to +1.00 and is interpreted in the same manner as D in the norm-referenced approach.

The pretest/posttest difference index (PPDI) is the proportion of subjects getting the item correct on the posttest minus the proportion of subjects getting the item correct on the pretest. A negative value or a value near zero indicates that the item is either insensitive to the treatment or faulty. The same kind of information can be obtained by comparing one group of subjects after they receive the treatment with a comparable control group, that is, a group not exposed to the treatment.

Item Response Charts

Additional information may be obtained from the PPDI results if, for each item, the type of fourfold table shown in Figure 4-6 is constructed. The distribution of subjects in the cells of Figure 4-6 provides information regarding the objec-

POST-TEST

		CORRECT	INCORRECT
PRETEST	INCORRECT	(A)	(B)
	CORRECT	(C)	(D)

FIGURE 4-6. Item response chart for criterion-referenced procedure.

tive upon which the item is based, the effectiveness of the treatment relative to the objective, or the quality of the item itself. For example, a relatively large proportion of subjects in cell c may indicate either that the item contains a specific determiner, thus cluing a large number of subjects to the correct answer, or that the objective the item is designed to measure is not treatment specific (that is, subjects acquired the target behavior prior to the treatment). A relatively large proportion in cell b may indicate that the objective is unattainable by most subjects, that the objective is attainable but the treatment is ineffective, or that the item is faulty. A relatively large proportion of subjects in cell d would suggest that the treatment was detrimental to performance on the item and must be reconsidered.

SUMMARY

Measurement is the process of assigning numbers to objects using a rule. The rule is presumed to assign numbers to represent the amount of a specific attribute possessed by the subjects measured.[13] The most frequently encountered system for categorizing measurement rules is that of Stevens[23] who classified rules into four hierarchical categories, nominal, ordinal, interval, and ratio, in terms of the amount and kind of information retrievable from the numbers they assign. A great deal of controversy exists regarding the importance of levels of measurement. The nurse needs to be aware of both the fundamental and pragmatic viewpoints and the implications each has for the research resulting from their efforts.

Tests and other measuring devices can be classified by (1) what they seek to measure (cognitive, affective, psychomotor skills, physiologic functioning), (2) the manner in which they are constructed and interpreted (norm-referenced versus criterion-referenced, objective versus subjective), (3) the type of subject performance they seek to measure (maximum versus typical performance), and (4) who constructs them (standardized versus informal). The type of measures employed in a given study will have important implications for what can be done with and on the basis of the resulting information. Thus, the researcher must clarify at the outset the type of measurement that will yield data appropriate for the kinds of research questions or hypotheses the researcher seeks to answer.

Two important characteristics of every measuring device or technique are reliability and validity. Reliability refers to the consistency with which a measurement rule assigns scores to a group of subjects. An instrument is valid if it does what it is intended to do. Both reliability and validity are matters of degree rather than all or none properties. The researcher should assess the measures each time they are used to determine if they are behaving as planned. New evidence may suggest modifications of an existing measure or the development of a new and better approach to measuring the attribute in question.

Specific procedures for estimating the reliability of norm-referenced measures include test-retest, parallel form, and alpha. Determination of Cohen's Coefficient K is the preferred procedure for estimating reliability in the criterion-referenced case.

Approaches to validity when a norm-referenced measure is utilized include (1) content validity index, (2) contrasted groups approach, (3) experimental manipulation, (4) multitrait-multimethod matrix technique, and (5) correlation and regression procedures. Criterion-referenced measures are valid primarily in terms of the adequacy with which they represent the criterion. Therefore, content validity approaches are the most appropriate estimators of validity in this case.

Item analysis procedures are used to increase the reliability and validity of measuring devices by separately evaluating each item to determine whether or not that item discriminates in the same manner that the overall measure is intended to discriminate. Norm-referenced item analysis procedures include (1) item p level, (2) discrimination indices, and (3) item response charts. Modifications of the same three procedures exist for use with criterion-referenced devices.

REFERENCES

1. Angoff, W. H.: *Scales, norms, and equivalent scores.* In R. L. Thorndike (ed.): *Educational Measurement*, ed. 2. American Council on Education, Washington, D.C., 1971.
2. Borlick, M., et al.: *Nursing Examination Review Book, vol. 9, Community Health Nursing*, ed. 2. Medical Examination Publishing Co., New York, 1974.

3. Campbell, D. T.: *Social attitudes and other acquired behavioral dispositions.* In Koch, S. (ed.): *Psychology: A Study of a Science, vol. 6.* McGraw-Hill, New York, 1963.
4. Campbell, D. T. and Fiske, D. W.: *Convergent and Discriminant Validity by Multitrait-Multimethod Matrix.* Psychol. Bull. 56:81, 1959.
5. Carter, R. P.: *Special problems in measuring change with psychometric devices.* In *Evaluative Research: Strategies and Methods.* American Institute for Research, Pittsburgh, 1970.
6. Edwards, A.: *Techniques of Attitude Scale Construction.* Appleton-Century-Crofts, New York, 1957.
7. Gagne, R. M.: *The acquisition of knowledge.* Psychol. Rev. 69:355, 1962.
8. Hambleton, R. and Novick, M.: *Toward an integration of theory and method for criterion-referenced tests.* Journal of Educational Measurement 10:159, 1973.
9. Hambleton, R. K., et al.: *Criterion-Referenced Testing and Measurement: Review of Technical Issues and Developments.* An invited symposium presented at the Annual Meeting of the American Educational Research Association (mimeo.), Washington, D.C., 1975.
10. Hemphill, J. and Westie, C. M.: *The measurement of group dimensions.* J. Psychol. 29:325, 1959.
11. Isaacs, S. and Michael, W. B.: *Handbook in Research and Evaluation.* Edits Publishers, San Diego, California, 1975.
12. Livingston, S. A.: *Criterion referenced application of classical test theory.* Journal of Educational Measurement 9:13, 1972.
13. Martuza, V. R., et al.: *EDF 660 Tests and Measurements Course Manual,* revision 4. University of Delaware College of Education, 1975 (unpublished).
14. Martuza, V. R.: *Applying Norm-Referenced and Criterion-Referenced Measurement in Education.* Allyn and Bacon, Boston, 1977.
15. Nunnally, J. C.: *Psychometric Theory.* McGraw-Hill, New York, 1967.
16. Osgood, C. E., Suci, G. J., and Tannenbaum, P. H.: *The Measurement of Meaning.* University of Illinois Press, Chicago, 1957.
17. Rovinelli, R. and Hambleton, R. K.: *Some Procedures for the Validation of Criterion-Referenced Test Items. Final Report.* Bureau of School and Cultural Research, New York State Education Department, Albany, 1973.
18. Rovinelli, R. and Hambleton, R. K.: *On the Use of Content Specialists in the Assessment of Criterion-Referenced Test Item Validity. Laboratory of Psychometrics and Evaluative Research Report No. 24.* University of Massachusetts, Amherst, Mass., 1976.
19. Shaw, R. E. and Wright, J. M.: *Scales for the Measurement of Attitudes.* McGraw-Hill, New York, 1967.
20. Snider, J. G. and Osgood, C. E. (eds.): *Semantic Differential Technique.* Aldine, Chicago, 1969.
21. *Standards for Educational and Psychological Tests.* American Psychological Association, Washington, D.C., 1966.
22. Staropoli, C. and Waltz, C.: *Developing and Evaluating Educational Programs for Health Care Providers.* F. A. Davis, Philadelphia, 1978.
23. Stevens, S. S.: *On the theory of scales of measurement.* Science 103:677, 1946.
24. Swaminathan, H., Hambleton, R., and Algina, J.: *Reliability of criterion-referenced tests: A decision-theoretic formation.* Journal of Educational Measurement 2:263, 1974.
25. Webb, E. E., et al.: *Unobtrusive Measures: Nonreactive Research in the Social Sciences.* Rand McNally, Chicago, 1966.

CHAPTER 5
INSTRUMENTATION

Instrumentation is the process of selecting or developing devices and methods appropriate for measuring the variables identified in relation to a research problem. A device or method will be effective only as it relates specifically to the study purposes and elicits data that allow the researcher to answer the research questions or test the research hypotheses. A number of sources are available to researchers who prefer to select an existing tool or method rather than develop their own. The more significant resources include:

1. Buros, O. (ed.): *The Sixth Mental Measurements Yearbook.* Gryphon Press, New Jersey, 1965.
2. Buros, O. (ed.): *Tests in Print.* Gryphon Press, New Jersey, 1961.
3. *Journal of Educational Measurement.*
4. *Educational and Psychological Measurement.*
5. *Review of Educational Research.*
6. *Psychological Abstracts.*
7. *Educational Index.*
8. ERIC (Educational Resources Information Center), Washington, D.C.
9. Thorndike, R. L. and Hagen, E.: *Measurement and Evaluation in Psychology and Education,* John Wiley and Sons, New York, 1969.
10. Webb, E. J., et al.: *Unobstrusive Measures: Nonreactive Research in the Social Sciences.* Rand McNally, Chicago, 1966.
11. Educational Testing Service, *Microfiche File,* Princeton, New Jersey, A comprehensive file of measures and instruments reported by researchers in the literature.
12. Shaw, M. and Wright, J.: *Scales for the Measurement of Attitudes.* McGraw-Hill, New York, 1967.
13. Oppenheim, A.: *Questionnaire Design and Attitude Measurement.* Basic Books, New York, 1966.

14. Ward, M. J. and Lindeman, C: *Instruments for Measuring Nursing Practice and Other Health Care Variables, vols. 1 and 2.* Western Interstate Commission for Higher Education, Colorado, 1978.

15. Ward, M. J. and Fetler, M: *Instruments for Use in Nursing Education Research.* Western Interstate Commission for Higher Education, Colorado, 1979.

Whether the researcher develops a method or selects an existing one, there are a number of general considerations that should be applied regarding instrumentation:

1. A rationale must serve as the basis for determining the nature and specific content of the device or method. The rationale may derive from a theoretical framework, empirical evidence obtained in earlier studies, or a combination of both.
2. All information elicited by the device should be directly related to the study and must be necessary to test the hypotheses or answer the research questions. To ensure that all data gathered by a particular method will be useful to the researcher: (a) an objective should be specified for each item included, and (b) the manner in which the information obtained by each item will be used in the analysis should be clearly stated prior to employing the device or method.
3. The device or method should be practically designed. It should not be too long or too comprehensive to be completed by respondents within a reasonable amount of time. The arrangement or sequence of items should appear logical to the subject and should contribute to gaining and maintaining the subject's interest. Directions for taking or using the device or method should be simply and clearly stated so they are easily understood by the respondent.
4. If the instrument is to be used as the researcher intends, guidelines should exist for whomever administers the device that clearly specify the exact extent and limitations of that role. In addition, the instrument should be as easy as possible to administer.
5. The instrument should be free of bias. For example, the instrument should not contain clues that may lead subjects to respond in a manner they deem desirable on the part of the researcher.
6. A pretest of the instrument should be undertaken by the researcher using subjects similar to those who will be included in the study in order to estimate the reliability and validity of the device or method.

PRETESTING THE INSTRUMENT

A pretest is a trial run of the instrument or method that is to be used in collecting data for answering the research questions or testing the research hypotheses. The purposes of the pretest are to provide the researcher with information regarding the method's reliability and validity, and to reveal problems relating to its content, administration, and scoring. If these purposes are to be met, the method must be pretested on subjects who meet the criteria for inclusion in the study sample, but who will not participate in the study per se. Similarly, the pretest conditions should approximate as nearly as possible the conditions expected to exist during the conduct of the study.

During the conduct of the pretest, the researcher should be attentive to the reactions, comments, and nonverbal communications of the subjects that might give clues to problems with the method. Similarly, the researcher's own observations and concerns that may suggest needed improvements should be recorded. For example, the researcher should note any difficulties in locating subjects, problems of maintaining interest, questions raised by respondents and the researcher's responses to them, adequacy of the time allowed for administering the method, adequacy of the space provided for recording responses, length, and the like.

After the pretest data have been collected, the researcher should ask subjects to identify difficulties they encountered in completing the instrument, suggestions they may have for improving the method, and possible discrepancies between the researcher's intent in asking questions and how the subjects understood and responded to the questions. In addition, the researcher should tabulate and compile the data, including the preparation of tables and graphs, so that the researcher may note any difficulties encountered in preparing the data for analysis. Appropriate item analysis procedures and procedures for estimating the method's reliability and validity should be employed using the pretest data.

On the basis of the information obtained from the pretest, including the resulting evidence for the method's reliability and validity, the researcher should decide either that the method may be used as is for the collection of data for the study and proceed, or that the method needs modifications before it can be employed. If the researcher determines that the method needs modifications for improvement, these should be made and the method pretested again prior to conducting the study.

METHODS OF INSTRUMENTATION

In designing a nursing research study, the investigator needs to select or develop methods and techniques for collecting data necessary for answering the research questions or testing the research hypotheses. Unfortunately, too many otherwise well planned and executed designs have failed because researchers did not give adequate attention to the employment of appropriate and correct methods for the collection of data *specific* to their research concerns.

A number of methods may be utilized for the collection of data. An overview of basic techniques that the authors have found especially pertinent in nursing research is presented in Table 5-1. The intent in presenting this information is twofold: (1) to expand the nursing researcher's repertoire of measurement approaches and (2) to stimulate the researcher to consider essential characteristics and requirements of specific approaches before the study in order to avoid

TABLE 5-1. Selected Methods for Collection of Data in Nursing Research

Method	Essential characteristics	Aspects to consider before using and/or constructing

Anecdotal notes	1. A recorded description of the behavior and activities of the subject during a particular performance of short duration.
	2. The note is usually written informally without modifying expressions and contains only data that clarify the image of the event.
		1. A systematic approach should be developed for the collection of anecdotal notes.
		  a. Critical behaviors should be identified.
		  b. Number of notes to be selected for each subject predetermined.
		2. Researcher and subject may consider the notes together, thus they are effective for formative evaluation.
		3. Notes are especially useful for recording longitudinal data re subject's progress in developing competency.

Content analysis	1. This method involves the systematic analysis of the text of written material in order to document, describe, and quantify a specific phenomenon.
	2. A checklist is frequently employed as a vehicle for recording how many times a particular type of response occurs.
	3. The intent is generally to produce a descriptive statement concerning an attitude, word or concept frequency, a change, or a social condition, e.g., a search of professional periodicals to determine changes over the last 20 years re nurses' attitudes toward research.
		1. Content analysis may provide information not only in regard to the topics under study, but may also provide insight into the communication vehicle itself, and professional and/or societal changes.
		2. The method may be excessively time consuming unless the researcher employs a random sampling procedure for obtaining data.
		3. Care must be taken to ensure the selection of documents that are representative of the topic under study. To allow for the quantification of data and avoid bias:
		  a. A systematic classifying scheme must be determined prior to the collection of data.
		  b. Categories in the scheme should be relatively unambigous and mutually exclusive.
		  c. Independent, unbiased experts' shared reviews and reactions to the scheme should be sought before it is employed.

TABLE 5-1. *Continued*

Method	Essential characteristics	Aspects to consider before using and/or constructing
Critical incident technique	1. A critical incident is "one that makes a significant difference in the outcome of an activity. It may be the positive factors that contribute toward the success of the behavior or it may be the negative factors that interfere with the completion of the assignment."[3] 2. Critical incidents should be selected because they are relevant to the behavioral objective being evaluated.	1. This technique is an effective mechanism for enabling the researcher to assess the subject's behaviors in relation to their impact on the outcome of an action.
Decision-making exercises	1. A description of a nursing action that involves a nursing decision is provided the subject, usually in one of three ways: a. The situation is described to the point at which a decision must be made and then the subject is asked to make a decision and provide the rationale for the choice. b. The situation is described, including the decision, and then the subject is asked to state agreement or disagreement with the decision and to state why. c. The situation and decisions are described, and the subject is asked if the information provided is sufficient for a decision; if not, the subject indicates what information is needed.	1. These exercises allow one to assess subject's performance at the higher levels of the learning taxonomies and are especially valuable for this reason.
Delphi technique	1. The Delphi method[5, 6] is generally employed for quantifying expert judgments, determining priorities, or making long range forecasts. It proceeds in the following manner:	1. The greatest merit of the technique stems from its adaptability to a variety of research situations. Other advantages are that: a. Experts need not attend a meeting, be intimidated

TABLE 5-1. *Continued*

Method	Essential characteristics	Aspects to consider before using and/or constructing
	a. A panel of experts on the topic of interest is asked to complete a questionnaire designed to elicit opinions, estimates, or future predictions re the topic. b. Responses are collected, summarized, and returned to the experts. c. Using the combined information of all the experts, each member of the panel again predicts, comments, and responds to the new information in another questionnaire. d. This process is repeated until the resulting data are a consensus of the opinions, predictions, or beliefs of all the experts.	or influenced by other experts, and may remain anonymous. b. The method affords a procedure for condensing the opinions of many experts into a few precise and clearly defined statements. 2. Disadvantages are that: a. The procedure is costly and time consuming for the researcher (e.g., postage, tabulating results, printing a variety of questionnaires). b. The time requirement for the collection of data is dependent on the speedy response of each expert, i.e., subsequent questionnaires cannot be distributed until the responses from the preceding one are received and tabulated. c. Results represent opinions of experts and may or may not be consistent with reality. 3. When the procedure is employed, it is paramount that the researcher: a. Carefully select the panel so that a variety of personalities, interests, etc., are represented to avoid biases as a result of panel membership. b. Assess the reliability and and validity of the questionnaires as each set of data is returned.
Interviews	1. Reliability is increased if a well defined format is employed, e.g., objective ques-	1. An interview is a desirable method when it is necessary to probe for complete data or

TABLE 5-1. *Continued*

Method	Essential characteristics	Aspects to consider before using and/or constructing
	tionnaire format that allows clarification and elaboration within narrow limits. 2. Interviews should be factually oriented, aimed at specific information, and relatively brief.	to obtain relatively in-depth information. 2. This method is costly, time consuming, and often inconvenient.
Multimedia	1. Using media in research increases the variety of senses used by the subject and thus adds more depth in a measurement situation and increases the scope of evaluation. 2. Media are usually used in combination with other methods, e.g., observation, simulation, process recording etc.	1. Films provide for visual and auditory stimulation and are particularly useful in critical incident and decision-making testing. 2. Videotapes have the same use as films, but in addition have a start-stop capacity that allows the researcher and subject to jointly appraise and critically analyze subject's performance. Hence they are very useful in evaluative research. 3. Tape recordings add an auditory dimension and are especially useful for assessing sounds, e.g., heart, lung, or subject's competency in interpreting or analyzing interviews. 4. Slides and pictures provide visual imagery and are useful in attitude testing (e.g., if the subject is asked to interpret the meaning of a scene depicted) or in assessing subject's ability to interpret or critically analyze steps in a process.
Multiple choice tests	1. A multiple choice item includes: a. *Stem* — introductory question or incomplete statement. b. *Responses* — suggested answers 1) *Answer* — correct response.	1. Does the writer have a thorough mastery of the subject matter being tested? Does the writer know not only the facts, but implications as well, i.e., fallacies and popular misconceptions? 2. Is there a well developed set of educational objectives that

TABLE 5-1. *Continued*

Method	Essential characteristics	Aspects to consider before using and/or constructing
	2) *Distractors* (misleads, foils) — incorrect response. 2. Multiple choice questions are constructed: a. Using an available cognitive taxonomy, e.g., Bloom's Taxonomy of the Cognitive Domain.[1, 13] b. According to principles of good item writing.	directs the test's construction? 3. Does the writer understand the psychologic and educational characteristics of the individuals for whom the test is intended? This is important in determining the difficulty level as well as distractors. 4. Is the writer aware of various interpretations of word meanings, precise in word usage, and organized in verbal expression? 5. Is the writer familiar with the types and varieties of test items, particularly their possibilities and limitations? 6. Does the writer convey the belief that some kinds of subjects are more difficult than others and that item writing is not a unitary skill? 7. Does the writer avoid lifting items verbatim from text? Such items are usually inadequate. A sentence presented out of context frequently loses much of its meaning and is likely to be ambiguous. Sentences that can be readily extracted from context without conceptual loss are likely to measure trivia, i.e., such items frequently measure only memory for fact rather than understandings, generalizations, or principles.
Nursing audit	1. The audit is a protocol for ascertaining quality nursing care based on the use of the patient's chart as the source of data.	1. Subject's recordings of patient may be analyzed over a period of time or may represent one particular interval.

TABLE 5-1. *Continued*

Method	Essential Characteristics	Aspects to consider before using and/or constructing
	2. The criteria employed relate to the appropriateness and comprehensiveness of significant facts, the accuracy of data collection and interpretation, and the consistency with which reported plans and actions are congruent with assessment data.[11]	
Nursing care studies	1. A problem-solving activity whereby the subject undertakes the comprehensive assessment of a particular patient's problems leading to planning, implementing, and evaluating nursing care measures.[12]	1. In selecting this method, one must be certain that the nature of the problem to be addressed and the number of variables with which the subject must deal are within the subject's educational level, i.e., behavioral objectives must be clearly stated.
Observation	Observations may be: a. Direct—observer evaluates the subject by simply watching the subject perform. b. Indirect—observer uses devices for recording subject's activities, e.g., motion picture, television, videotaping. 2. The observation should be structured by a guide for conducting the observations that is constructed on the basis of the important behaviors to be observed (i.e., the objectives).	1. Direct observation a. Is time consuming and expensive. b. Allows one to learn how a subject functions under the pressure of supervision. 2. Indirect observation a. Affords opportunity for a subject to become involved in the evaluation of performance. b. Is not sensitive to tone, mood, or affect of the situation. c. Is subject to selective perception problems.
Physiologic techniques	1. Physiologic techniques are those methods that employ existing instruments or tools for collecting information regarding subjects' physical status. Examples of physiologic techniques frequently employed in clinical nursing research are:	1. Physiologic techniques are often used in conjunction with other techniques such as checklists, observations, rating scales, media, and records. 2. Physiologic techniques, if employed correctly, are among the most reliable

TABLE 5-1. *Continued*

Method	Essential characteristics	Aspects to consider before using and/or constructing
	a. Electrocardiogram. b. Electroencephalogram. c. Thermometers. d. Urinalyses. e. X-ray equipment. f. Sphygmomanometers. g. Thermography. h. Variety of electronic monitoring devices, e.g., in sleep research for determination of REM.	and valid methods available. Thus, the nurse who employs physiologic techniques should have a familiar background and understanding of physiology and anatomy, and be thoroughly familiar with the theoretical basis for the instrument, the correct procedure for its utilization, possible contraindications for its use, and interpretations that may be made on the basis of its results.

Problem oriented records	1. A systematic record keeping centered around the patient's health problems.[14]
	2. Consists of four major components;
	  a. Data base—all appropriate information about the patient for assessing patient's condition.
	  b. Problem list—list of the conditions, systems, or circumstances identified from the data base that have implications for the patient's health. Each problem is numbered.
	  c. Initial plans—diagnostic and therapeutic orders for each problem listed. Plans are keyed to each problem.
	  d. Progress notes
	    1) Narrative note, an expository comment relative to each problem.
	    2) Flow sheets, graphic forms to record repetitive and serial data.
	    3) Discharge summary, followup organized around each problem.
		1. Requires subject to integrate all aspects of a patient's care.
		2. Reports more than events relative to the patient, i.e., also conveys rationales of practitioners so there is a better understanding of therapeutic actions.
		3. Format is compatible with the nursing process as the methodology of nursing.
		4. In assessing the subject using this method, one needs to consider not only the substance of what is included, but also the subject's skill in communicating the message.

TABLE 5-1. Continued

Method	Essential characteristics	Aspects to consider before using and/or constructing
Process recording	1. A verbatim, serial reproduction of the verbal and nonverbal communication between two individuals for the purpose of assessing interactions on a continuum, leading toward mutual understanding and interpersonal relationships.[12] 2. The process recording has four main components: a. Client communication. b. Nurse communication. c. Nurse's interpretation of client's communication. d. Implications of the communications for nursing actions. 3. The report should be written immediately after the interaction occurs, while the event is vivid in the recorder's mind.	1. This technique is amenable to any interaction of the subject with another individual: a. Subject-client. b. Subject-health team member. c. Subject-subject. 2. The procedure is time consuming. 3. Behavioral objectives must be explicitly defined so that the subject focuses on them in recording the interaction. 4. This approach is best when used in conjunction with individual conferences.
Q sort	1. The conceptual basis for the Q sort method is small sampling theory. The study population consists of traits, characteristics, and attitudes for a small number of subjects. The intent is to evaluate performance for each subject and then determine the relationship between subjects' responses.[2] 2. The technique was devised for scaling or ranking items. a. The items to be ranked, usually 50 or more, are placed on cards. b. The subject(s) is asked to sort a predetermined number of items into a specified number of piles, usually 9–11, according to the study purpose.	1. The major advantages of the Q sort are that: a. It is relatively inexpensive and adaptable to a variety of research situations and theoretical perspectives. b. Resulting data are complete and relatively simple to handle and analyze. c. It demonstrates reliability for studying self concept, attitudes, and behavior. 2. Major disadvantages stem from the fact that: a. It is time consuming to administer. b. Subjects are forced to place a predetermined number of closely related items into distinct piles and may make mechani-

TABLE 5-1. *Continued*

Method	Essential characteristics	Aspects to consider before using and/or constructing
	3. For example, a Q sort might be developed to determine what subjects believe to be the most important to the least important characteristics of a nurse practitioner. Fifty statements, each describing one characteristic of a nurse practitioner are typed on cards and presented to the subject(s). The subject is then asked to sort the 50 items into 10 piles containing 5 items each, ranging from most to least important.	cal rather than conceptual choices simply to complete the procedure. The reliability and validity of Q sort data are improved when directions are clearly specified and when the subject understands and accepts the importance of the study.
Questionnaires	1. Subjects are provided with a brief, clear explanation of why they are being asked to respond to the questionnaire. 2. Subjects are provided with an explanation of what value the questionnaire results will have for them personally. 3. The purpose for each question is explicitly identified. 4. An objective format is preferred, i.e., possible categories of responses are anticipated and offered as alternatives. 5. Provisions are made for followup (a high return rate is desirable).	1. How will respondents be convinced of the importance of completing the questionnaire? 2. What is the purpose to be served by the questionnaire, and how will the information it produces be used in the study? 3. What means will be used to encourage subjects who do not respond initially to complete the questionnaire?
Rating scales 1. Summated	1. A summated rating scale contains a set of scales all of which are considered approximately equal in attitude or value loading. 2. The subject responds to the scale with varying degrees of intensity, such as: a. Agree/disagree. b. Like/dislike. c. Accept/reject.	1. All the statements in the item pool should concern a particular attitudinal object. 2. Since it is usually easy to obtain a homogeneous scale for the measurement of attitudes, seldom are more than 40 items required in the item pool. 3. Since the purpose for each item on a summated scale is

TABLE 5-1. *Continued*

Method	Essential characteristics	Aspects to consider before using and/or constructing
	3. Scores for all scales are summated to yield an individual's score. 4. Frequently employed in combination with the observation method.	to obtain reliable variance with respect to the attitude, most of the items should be either moderately positive or moderately negative, i.e., there is no place for neutral statements in summated scales. Statements that are very extreme in either direction tend to create less variance than statements that are less extreme. 4. The pool of items should be evenly divided between positive and negative statements. 5. In the development of summated scales, it is very important that reliability and validity information be obtained under circumstances very similar to those in which the final scale will be employed (i.e., similar subjects, same administration procedures, same instructions, etc.).[10]
2. Semantic differential	1. A semantic differential scale employs direct rating of concepts anchored on the extremes by bipolar adjectives. 2. It provides a flexible approach to obtaining measures of attitudes and other sentiments. 3. Numerous factor analytic studies of semantic differential scales have suggested there are three major factors of meaning involved. The most frequently found factor is evaluation, which is defined by pairs of adjectives, such as: a. Good-bad. b. Fair-unfair.	1. The meaning of the scale does not depend on the concept being rated. Interaction of scales with concepts, when it occurs, places a limit on the extent to which individual scales can be interpreted the same when applied to different concepts, and it also limits the extent to which factors in semantic differential scales can be employed as general yardsticks (e.g., to measure evaluation) regardless of the concepts in a particular study. Less scale concept interaction is likely to occur when all the concepts in a study are selected

TABLE 5-1. *Continued*

Method	Essential characteristics	Aspects to consider before using and/or constructing
	c. Positive-negative. d. Honest-dishonest. e. Successful-unsuccessful. f. Valuable-worthless.	from the same domain of interest. 2. The concepts to be rated should be relevant to the research problem and sensitive to differences or similarities among the participants. 3. When the scores are summed over a number of scales, the logic of constructing semantic differential measures is the same as for the construction of summated scales, i.e., a homogeneous group of scales that meets the requirements of reliability is sought, and is not usually difficult to attain. 4. It is usually good to employ numbers to designate steps on semantic differential scales. The meanings of numbers should be carefully defined and illustrated in the instructions to the inventory. For example, subjects can be told that on the scale good-bad, 5 means "slightly good" rather than "bad," 4 means "slightly bad" rather than good, etc. 5. Although in many studies it has been the practice to reverse the polarity of scales to prevent subjects from being influenced from scale to scale by ratings made on previous scales, the weight of the argument is for keeping scales pertaining to any factor all pointing in the same direction. (e.g., making the "good" pole of all evaluation scales either on the left or the right.) 6. In addition to summing scores over groups of scales,

TABLE 5-1. Continued

Method	Essential characteristics	Aspects to consider before using and/or constructing
		in many studies it is also instructive to compare concepts on individual scales.[10]
Simulation	1. The situation imitates (does not duplicate) some aspect of reality. 2. Simulation requires the active participation of the respondent. 3. The respondent's participation can trigger appropriate feedback that may or may not modify the situation but can, in any case, be utilized for subsequent decisions about pending action. 4. This action of the respondent may modify the problem.[7-9]	1. Currently available formats include: a. Paper and pencil measures. b. Computer simulations. c. Human interaction. d. Models.

some of the pitfalls encountered when methods and devices are not adequately evaluated at the time of their selection. In considering the information in Table 5-1, the reader is encouraged to keep in mind the basic concepts and principles of measurement discussed in Chapter 4. That is, methods and devices cannot be considered in isolation. Constant attention must be directed to the measurement framework to be employed in a specific study and to how a particular method's reliability and validity will be assessed within the context of a specific study.

EVALUATING THE INSTRUMENT

Whether developing a device or employing an existing one, the researcher should pause to systematically evaluate the instrument prior to using it for data collection. The content of this and the preceding chapter has addressed the many considerations to be taken into account by the researcher in designing the measurement component of the study. For convenience, the major considerations are summarized in question form below:

1. What is the cost of utilizing this instrument in terms of dollars as well as time and energy expenditure on the part of both researcher and subjects? Will the information obtained justify the cost?
2. What are the qualifications of the author of the device in the content area addressed by the device?

3. Has the author developed the device utilizing the appropriate measurement theory and concepts for this type of instrument?
4. Does the author explicitly state the purpose for which the device was designed? In what ways if any does the author's purpose differ from the current study purpose? Are modifications necessary and, if so, feasible?
5. Does the author clearly describe the type of subjects for which the device is applicable? How are subjects in the current study the same or different from those for which the device was designed?
6. Has the author identified the objective and/or rationale for each item included on the device?
7. What method (rating scale, multiple choice, and so forth) is employed? Is the method employed correctly?
8. Is the scoring procedure described in sufficient detail?
9. Is the administration procedure clearly described?
10. What is the level of measurement of the resulting scores?
11. Is there any special training required to use the device?
12. Was the instrument pretested? How? Does the author's report of results include information regarding time to complete, type of subjects, justification and rationale for modifications made on the basis of findings?

TABLE 5-2. Form for Evaluating an Instrument

Title: _____

Author: _____

I. *General Information*
   A. Cost _____
   B. Author's qualifications:
      1. content area _____
         _____
      2. measurement _____
         _____
   C. Purpose for which developed, note ways in which current study purpose differs_____
      _____
      _____
   D. Type of subjects to which applicable, relate to subjects for current study____
      _____
      _____
      _____
      _____

II. *Design Information*
   A. Author's rationale for items included _____
      _____
   B. Method employed (i.e., rating scale, multiple choice, etc.) _____
      _____
   C. Considerations in Table 5-1 reflected in design?
      _____
      _____
      _____
   D. Scoring procedure _____
      _____
      _____
   E. Level of measurement of resulting scores_____
   F. Note special training required to score _____
      _____
   G. Administration procedure _____
      _____
      _____
   H. Procedures for taking and administering adequate? _____
      _____

III. *Practical Concerns*
   A. Pretest procedure_____
      _____
   B. Pretest results including time to complete, modifications made ___
      _____
   C. Reliability determination _____
      type(s) _____
      author procedure_____
      # of cases_____
      results _____
   D. Validity determination
      _____
      type(s) _____
      outline procedure_____
      _____
      # & type subjects _____
      _____
      results _____
      _____

13. Does the author report estimates of the instrument's reliability and validity? What procedures were employed?
14. What reliability and validity determinations are indicated in the current study?

If the answers to the majority of these questions are positive and the design of the device closely parallels the researcher's current needs and interests, the researcher can feel some confidence in employing the method in the current research. If, on the other hand, responses to the majority of the questions are negative or unknown or if the author's design does not parallel the researcher's needs and interests, the researcher may find it possible to modify the method or, more likely, may find it more feasible to search for another form of instrumentation.

Table 5-2 presents a form for recording the answers to the questions posed. If such a form is completed each time an instrument or method is considered by the researcher, over time the researcher will accumulate a convenient and handy measurement file for future use.

REFERENCES

1. Bloom, B. S. (ed.): *Taxonomy of Educational Objectives: Handbook I: Cognitive Domain.* David McKay, New York, 1956.
2. Cummins, R. E.: *Some applications of Q methodology to teaching and educational research.* Journal of Educational Research 57:96, 1963.
3. Fivars, G. and Gosnell, D.: *Nursing Evaluation: The Problem and the Process.* Macmillan, New York, 1966.
4. Gronlund, N. E.: *Measurement and Evaluation in Teaching.* Macmillan, New York, 1965.
5. Lindeman, C. A.: *Delphi Survey of Clinical Nursing Research Priorities.* Western Interstate Commission for Higher Education, Western Council on Higher Education for Nursing Regional Program for Nursing Research Development, Colorado, 1974.
6. Linstone, H. A. and Turoff, M.: *The Delphi Method, Techniques and Applications.* Addison-Wesley, Menlo Park, Calif., 1975.
7. McGuire, C.: *Simulation in the Assessment of Clinical Judgment and Problem Solving.* (mimeo.) University of Illinois, Chicago, 1976.
8. McGuire, C.: *Simulation in the Assessment of Technical and Interpersonal Skills.* (mimeo.) University of Illinois, Chicago, 1976.
9. McGuire, C.: *Simulation in the Assessment of Observation and Interpretation.* (mimeo.) University of Illinois, Chicago, 1976.
10. Nunnally, J.: *Psychometric Theory.* McGraw-Hill, New York, 1967.
11. Phaneuf, M. C.: *The Nursing Audit: Profile for Excellence.* Appleton-Century-Crofts, New York, 1972.
12. Schweer, J. E.: *Creative Teaching in Clinical Nursing,* ed. 2. C. V. Mosby, St. Louis, 1972.
13. Staropoli, C. and Waltz, C.: *Developing and Evaluating Educational Programs for Health Care Providers.* F. A. Davis, Philadelphia, 1978.
14. Weed, L. L.: *Medical Records, Medical Education, and Patient Care.* Case Western Reserve University, Cleveland, 1969.
15. Wesman, A. G.: *Writing the test item.* In Thorndike, R. (ed.): *Educational Measurement,* ed. 2. American Council on Education, Washington, D.C., 1971.

CHAPTER **6**

DATA ANALYSIS

Data analysis is planned in advance of a study and is a function of the research question and methods of instrumentation employed. When data collection and analysis are not planned concurrently and are not viewed in light of the research question, the researcher runs the risk of discovering at the data analysis stage that some of the information needed to perform the kind of analysis desired has not been collected. To avoid this problem, at the time the researcher decides on the data collection method, the researcher must plan the method of data analysis as well, taking into account (1) the type of data that needs to be collected, (2) how it can be collected, (3) whether or not data will be analyzed via the computer, (4) the type of statistical procedure(s) that will allow the researcher to answer the research question(s) or demonstrate whether the hypothesis was accepted or rejected, and (5) the design of tables, graphs, and the like that will facilitate a clear and concise presentation of the data analysis findings.

TYPES OF STATISTICAL PROCEDURES

Like the field of measurement, that of statistics is also abundant with esoteric terms utilized to differentiate among the types of statistical methods. The most frequently encountered schemes for classifying statistical procedures are by: (1) their purpose (summary, inferential, Bayesian), (2) the nature of the assumptions underlying their utilization (nonparametric, parametric), (3) the number of variables simultaneously analyzed (univariate, bivariate, multivariate), and (4) the interpretation of probability underlying their development (classical, nonclassical). These categories are not mutually exclusive and, thus, a given statistical method may be classified in one or more ways depending on the framework being used.

101

Purpose

When methods are classified on the basis of their purpose, they are labeled as summary, inferential, or Bayesian. *Summary statistics* attempt to organize, summarize, describe, and communicate a picture of the data. Procedures employed generally involve counting, describing, tabulating, or ordering. Examples of summary statistics are measures of central tendency (mean, median, mode), measures of dispersion (variance, standard deviation, range), and indicators of the shape of a distribution of scores (frequency distributions, kurtosis, skewness).

Inferential statistics allow the researcher to make statements about an entire population using information collected from a small subset or sample of the population. Probability theory, sampling, and hypothesis testing form the basis for inferential procedures. Examples of inferential statistics are the t-test, analysis of variance, and covariate analysis.

Bayesian statistics employ Bayes' theorem to allow the researcher to combine all available information about a problem in order to make decisions, that is, to choose from among a number of alternative actions. The basis for Bayesian statistics is statistical decision-making theory.

Assumptions

When alternative statistical procedures are available for a given research design, it is necessary to employ some rationale for choosing among them. The considerations that are used to select a statistical test are: (1) power, that is, the probability that the test will reject the null hypothesis when in fact the null hypothesis is false, (2) the manner in which the sample of scores was drawn, (3) the nature of the population from which the sample was drawn, and (4) the level of measurement employed in obtaining scores. Every statistical test has a model and a measurement requirement. The statistical model for a test is established by the nature of the population and the nature of the sampling used to select subjects. The model and measurement requirement specify the conditions under which the test results are valid. Since it is not always possible to directly test whether the conditions of a particular statistical model are met, one has to assume that they are met. Hence, the conditions of the statistical model for a test are called the "assumptions" of the test.[1]

Parametric statistical procedures have a variety of assumptions underlying their use. When these assumptions are valid, parametric statistical tests are the most powerful of all statistical tests. The assumptions that usually are components of the parametric statistical model are:

1. The observations must be independent. That is, the selection of any one case from the population for inclusion in the sample must not bias the chances of any other case being included, and the scores assigned to any one case must not bias the scores assigned to any other case.
2. The observations must be drawn from normally distributed populations.

3. These populations must have the same variance, that is, must be homogeneous.
4. Variables are measured at least at the interval level.[1]

Examples of parametric statistical tests are the t-test, F-test, and the product moment correlation coefficient (r_{xy}).

Nonparametric statistical procedures are tests whose models do not specify conditions about the population from which the sample was drawn. Fewer assumptions are associated with nonparametric tests than with parametric tests, and nonparametric tests can be used with very small numbers of subjects while most parametric tests cannot. The assumptions usually associated with nonparametric tests are:

1. The observations are independent.
2. The variables are measured at the nominal or ordinal level.[1]

Examples of nonparametric statistical tests are chi-square, the contingency coefficient, and the point biserial correlation coefficient.

Number of Variables

Statistical procedures that are concerned with the analysis of one variable are *univariate* statistical procedures, *bivariate* statistical procedures involve the simultaneous analysis of two variables, and *multivariate* techniques involve the analysis of three or more variables simultaneously. For example, a nurse investigator undertook a study to ascertain the effect of age and socioeconomic status on attendance at a Pediatric Diabetic Clinic. The nurse investigator collected data from 50 subjects who were registered at a particular clinic using a random sampling technique to obtain the data. During the first stage of data analysis, a univariate statistical procedure was employed when subjects were tabulated by age as shown in Table 6-1.

This univariate analysis was then expanded to a bivariate analysis when the nurse investigator simultaneously considered the frequency and percent of missed appointments by age of subject as shown in Table 6-2.

The nurse investigator then performed another bivariate analysis when a regression procedure was used to assess the effect of age on the number of

TABLE 6-1. Frequency and Percent of Subjects by Age (n = 50)

Age of subject	Number of subjects	Percent of total
Under 10 years	10	20
10 to 13 years	12	24
14 to 17 years	15	30
Over 17 years	13	26
Total	50	100

TABLE 6-2. Frequency and Percent of Missed Appointments by Age (n = 50)

Number of missed appointments	Age				Total
	Under 10	10 – 13	14 – 17	over 17	
None	5				5
1 to 4	5	5	6	3	19
5 or more	—	7	9	10	26
Total	10	12	15	13	50

missed appointments. During the next stage of the analysis, a multivariate regression procedure was used to consider the effect of age and socioeconomic status on the number of missed appointments, that is, three variables were considered simultaneously.

Probability Interpretation

Classical and nonclassical statistical methods are developed using different interpretations of probability. *Classical approaches* employ a *relative frequency* interpretation of probability and *nonclassical approaches* are based on *subjective* probability.

The *classical* approach to statistics is exemplified by the null hypothesis testing decision model discussed in Chapter 2. By testing the null hypothesis and establishing the level of significance, the researcher is setting odds on the number of times a correct decision will be made in the long run. In other words, when a hypothesis is tested at the 0.05 level of significance, one assumes that if the same experiment were repeated an infinite number of times under identical conditions, one would make a correct decision 95 times out of every 100 repetitions. This relative frequency interpretation of probability is based on a theorem referred to as the Law of Large Numbers. The *Law of Large Numbers*[4] states that if an experiment is repeated many times under identical conditions, the relative frequency of occurrence of any event (for example, rejecting the null hypothesis) is likely to be closer to the probability of that event (for example, the null hypothesis is false). Furthermore, the law states that the relative frequency and the probability are more likely to be close as the number of repetitions of the experiment increases. The Law of Large Numbers formally expresses in mathematical terms what might be thought of as statistical regularity. A problem with the relative frequency interpretation is that technically it requires a long series of experiments under identical conditions to determine probabilities with reasonable accuracy. In nursing, the researcher is interested, frequently, in the probability of an event, but is unable to observe repeated experiments under *identical* conditions. In this sense, the nonclassical statisticians argue, the relative frequency interpretation is a conceptual interpretation, but not an operational one.

Nonclassical statistical methods grew from the belief that the relative frequency interpretation of probability is but one interpretation, an interpretation of an abstract model, and as such there is no universally agreed upon interpretation.[2] Nonclassical methods are devised on the premise that there are many events that can be thought of in a probabilistic sense, but that cannot have a probability in terms of the relative frequency interpretation. Such events are unique in that the situation in which they occur cannot be duplicated. Although some information may be available regarding past occurrences in similar situations, no information in the form of observed frequencies is available regarding repeated trials under identical conditions. *Bayesian analysis* exemplifies nonclassical statistical approaches. The subjective interpretation of probability[2] employed in Bayesian statistics provides for the description of the researcher's own degree of belief about a situation that will occur once and only once. In this approach, a probability is interpreted as a measure of degree of belief or as the quantified judgment of a particular individual. As a result, one can think of a probability as representing what will happen in a single trial or experiment of interest, rather than a statement about what will happen in the long run. It is not necessary, however, for an experiment to be nonrepetitive for the subjective interpretation of probability to be applicable. Bayesians argue that subjective probabilities are operationally more useful than relative frequency because they allow a person to consider individual situations rather than long run outcomes or statistical regularity. Thus, they contend, subjective probabilities are both conceptual and operational.

The justification for frequency interpretations of probability is based on certain assumptions that are necessary for the proof of the Law of Large Numbers. Although some techniques are available for assessing these assumptions, the decision as to whether or not the assumptions are reasonable for a given experiment is ultimately a subjective decision made by the researcher. Thus, Bayesians contend that there is an element of subjectivity in the relative frequency interpretation of probability. Some Bayesians go a step further and espouse that subjective probability can be thought of as an extension of frequency probability. That is, if a researcher feels that the assumptions of relative frequency probability are reasonable, it is perfectly acceptable to make the researcher's own subjective probability for a given experiment equal to the probability determined by the frequency approach. If the researcher does not believe relative frequency assumptions are reasonable or if the researcher has additional information (other than frequencies) about the experiment in question, the researcher's subjective probability may differ from the frequency probability.

CONDUCT OF THE DATA ANALYSIS

In data analysis, the initial steps undertaken by the researcher regardless of the specific study design are (1) the tabulation of data and (2) the selection and employment of appropriate summary statistics. Since these two activities are germane to descriptive studies, they are discussed in detail in Chapter 8. In addition, the researcher who is interested in making statements about an entire population using information collected from the sample will employ a third step, that is, the researcher will select and employ an appropriate inferential statistical procedure. Inferential statistical procedures are discussed in depth in Chapters 9 and 10 dealing with experimental and correlational studies, respectively. Bayesian analysis is introduced in Chapter 11.

USING THE COMPUTER FOR DATA ANALYSIS

Not too long ago analysis of research data was the most tedious, time consuming, and difficult constituent of the research process. Researchers were forced to tabulate their data by hand, or at the most use the old omnipresent Frieden mechanical calculators to perform intricate operations upon long columns of numbers using even longer algebraic formulas for the various statistical tests.

The introduction of high speed electronic calculators with memory capability aided the process greatly, but their use still required considerable mathematical and computational skill on the part of the researcher. Even then, certain statistical procedures required hours of laborious computations during which it was quite easy for the most competent statistician to err. Also, due to the enormous amounts of time involved, many multivariate statistical procedures were completely impractical. Small wonder, therefore, that during this era few individuals without rigorous statistical training dared venture into extensive empirical research projects.

Even though high speed digital computers were becoming more and more available to researchers during this time, their advent did little to change the situation. The reason for this was that it often required even more mathematical and statistical sophistication to analyze data via computer than by "hand," simply because the researcher often had to communicate to the computer each step it was to perform on the data and these steps had to be communicated in esoteric languages developed especially for the purpose. This process is referred to as *programming* the computer; it requires very specialized training and can be more difficult than the analysis of the data itself.

Fortunately the situation has changed radically. Today computer programs have been written for every conceivable research purpose and they have been written in such a way that all the researcher normally need do is tell the computer which program to utilize and to then feed the data directly into the machine.

There is a carefully orchestrated myth that has grown up around computers, however, and this myth often causes great trepidation in the novice who has never seen or used a digital computer. The simple truth of the matter is that anyone who can use a hand held calculator can use the most formidable computer in existence. The only difference is that the latter is *easier* to use and *much, much* faster.

The Myth of the Computing Center

To the uninitiated the utilization of computers and their attendant machines conjures up images of manikin-like technicians dressed in white coats solemn-

ly and quietly moving from multilighted display to flashing panel authorita-
tively pressing appropriate buttons. Riding on the outcome of these flashing
lights lies the fate of the civilized world, the future of countless unborn children, or at the very least, the key to a major scientific breakthrough. How could
a novice researcher, who may never have seen an electronic computer, be so
presumptious as to intrude upon this august scene with data collected to ascertain, say, nursing attitudes toward working the night shift? Probably all that is
necessary is for this same person to set aside these images accruing from a doz-
en movies and television shows and to actually walk through a typical university computing center and look around for a few minutes.

In the first place, the computer probably won't even be in sight; if it is, it will
be in a glass encased, hermetically sealed room attended not by the envisioned
serious manikin-like technicians but by bored undergraduates working part-
time for spending money and casually dressed high school or technical school
graduates, also bored, and also underpaid. Neither group seemingly cares a
great deal about the earth shaking outcomes harbingered by the flashing lights
on the control panel, mainly because computer operators are often simply electronic babysitters who have no knowledge or interest in what the computer is
analyzing. Their job is to simply make sure that the machine functions properly, and, as evidenced by "authorized personnel only" signs, to save computer
users the inconvenience of ever having to operate or come in contact with the
machines themselves (which is one advantage the computer has over the calculator).

The computer operators, in fact, seldom even see the results of their charge's
labors. These results, called *output*, are normally printed in a separate room to
which researchers and other users do have access. This output comes from an
incredibly quick printer on special paper with which everyone is now familiar,
and is normally available to the user fairly soon after data have been fed into
the computer. This latter step is accomplished by placing a deck of computer
cards (to be described below) in a special machine called a *card reader* and
pushing a button. The cards quickly disappear one by one into the reader
(where their contents are fed to the computer itself) and reappear in an adjacent
hopper in the same machine.

What about the hubbub of activity in the other rooms, however? Surely some
higher level, more technical operations are going on there! Continuing the tour,
the first room that the researcher is likely to enter will contain rows of odd
looking machines resembling typewriters more than anything else. Closer examination does reveal them to be quite similar, in fact. The main difference lies
in the fact that the typists (or operators) are typing on cards rather than on paper, and that the machines are not only printing on these cards but they are also
punching holes in them as well. Watching the operators "punch cards" on
these *keypunch machines*, as they are called, indicates that the process is really
no more difficult than typing. In some ways it is easier since, when an operator
is through punching a card, a simple touch of a button replaces the finished
card with a fresh one, automatically stacking the punched cards in order.

Other rooms contain other mundane machines. Machines that duplicate
cards, machines that automatically count cards, or that sort them into different

stacks according to the particular holes punched in any given column. Simply reading the instructions posted over each machine or asking someone using one, usually enables a novice to use any of them on the first try.

By the time the researcher reaches the rows of teletype machines (typing back voluminous messages to their users) and terminals with green television-like screens (lit up with displays of weird geometric shapes) the researcher has probably become jaded and suspects that there is really nothing magical or sacred here either. Careful observation of their users will surely confirm this suspicion, especially when the researcher finds that some of the weird geometric shapes represent computerized games and that the majority of the remaining users are undergraduates simply trying to complete the next day's assignment in Computer Science 101.

The point of this little fantastical visit to a hypothetical computing center is that the mythology built up around electronic computers is just that: myth. Although exceedingly complex technologically, their use and operation has been made very simple so that they could be made available to as large a variety of uses and users as possible. In fact, secretaries, clerks, undergraduates, and high school students probably account for the bulk of their use, employing the machines as rote counters and enumerators (such as keeping track of enrollments and bills), as learning aids, and as recreation.

Data Coding Procedures

To take advantage of the computer's enormous time saving computational capacity, two things must be communicated to it. The researcher must present data to the computer in an organized, systematic format and must tell it what to do with that data. Both steps are extremely easy and neither requires knowledge of any special computing language.

DATA CODING SHEETS

Although the first step is the most simple, it is also far and away the most time consuming. To understand the process of preparing data to present to the computer it is first necessary to understand the function of the data card and data coding sheet presented in Figure 6-1.

There are several ways to communicate with the computer. The most basic and commonly used method is via small holes punched in a 4 × 8 inch card as depicted in Figure 6-1. Other methods are by typing data and instructions directly into the computer with a teletype machine, or using combinations of the two methods to direct attention to information (data or instructions) already stored in the computer itself in the form of electrical impulses or stored on magnetic tapes that can be attached to and read by the computer. The mode of communication with the computer is heavily dependent upon the researcher's particular set of circumstances. Communication via teletype is often the most convenient format, simply because teletype machines are often located in the

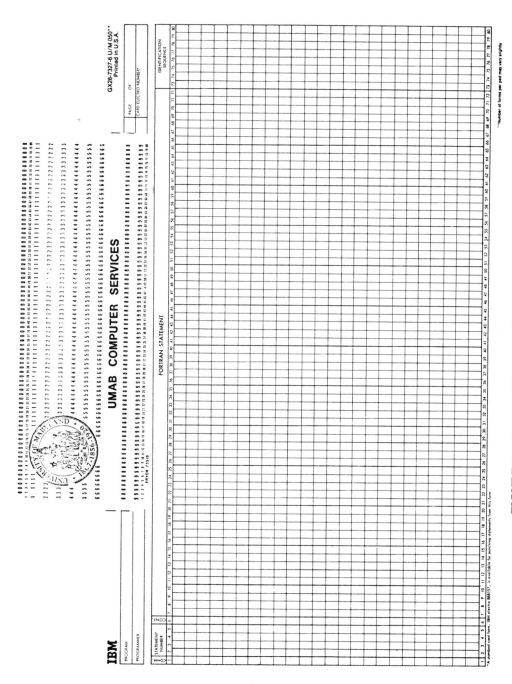

FIGURE 6-1. Data card (*top*) and data coding sheet (*bottom*).

researcher's institution which negates the necessity of physically going to the computing center. Many investigators, in fact, have access to portable terminals that can be used anywhere a phone can be used (since they connect directly to the computer via ordinary phone lines), including the home. By the same token, storing data in the computer itself for relatively short periods of time (called storing it on file or on *disk*) or on magnetic tape (especially helpful for permanent storage of very large amounts of data) can be extremely convenient and time saving regardless of the mode of communication.

When cards are used as the medium of communication, the first step is to transcribe collected data to data cards that can be read by the computer. (In fact even when data are stored on disk or tape they are often read into both via cards in the first place.) The most commonly used way to accomplish this is through the use of data coding sheets such as illustrated in Figure 6-1. An examination of that figure should indicate one basic similarity between the coding sheet and the data card: both have 80 columns, thereby implying that columns on the coding sheet correspond to columns on the card. By the same token, each row on the coding sheet (there are 24 on the one pictured in Fig. 6-1) corresponds to *one* data card, hence one coding sheet can be used to represent the information contained on 24 cards.

For example, suppose the first card in a set of data represented Mary Smith's age and attitude toward working the night shift. Suppose further that there were fewer than 100 Ss in the study (with each S being given a consecutive number starting with 01 as an identifier) and that the attitudinal score in question was always represented by a number less than 100. The data coding sheet for this study and the first data card representing Mary Smith (that is, S #01) might look as shown in Figure 6-2, with the S's number punched in the first two columns (actually this is optional, since these numbers will never be analyzed by the computer and are only for the researcher's convenience), her age in columns 4 and 5 (skipping column 3 for ease of proofreading the cards), and her attitude score in columns 7 and 8 (again skipping a column; a strategy which is completely optional, incidentally).

Examination of Figure 6-2 indicates that all numbers on the data coding sheet have holes punched in the row corresponding to the particular number belonging in each particular column. The important point to remember about this figure is that although different cards may be used to represent different people, the same columns on each card *must* contain information relevant to the same variables. For example, since S #01's age was placed in columns 4 and 5, S #02's (and all other respondents') age must be placed in columns 4 and 5, because when the time comes for the computer to analyze the data it must be told not only which columns are allocated to which variables, but also which columns represents the ones digit, which the tens digit, and so forth.

In Figure 6-2, for example, some of the Ss' attitudinal scores are two digits, some only one (that is, less than 10). S #02, the second respondent, recorded an attitude score of 9; hence the 9 was placed in column 8 and nothing was put in column 7. This procedure is called *right justifying*, and is invariably practiced in data coding for a very simple reason. If S #02's 9 had inadvertently been placed in column 7, the computer would read the value as 90 (blanks in a col-

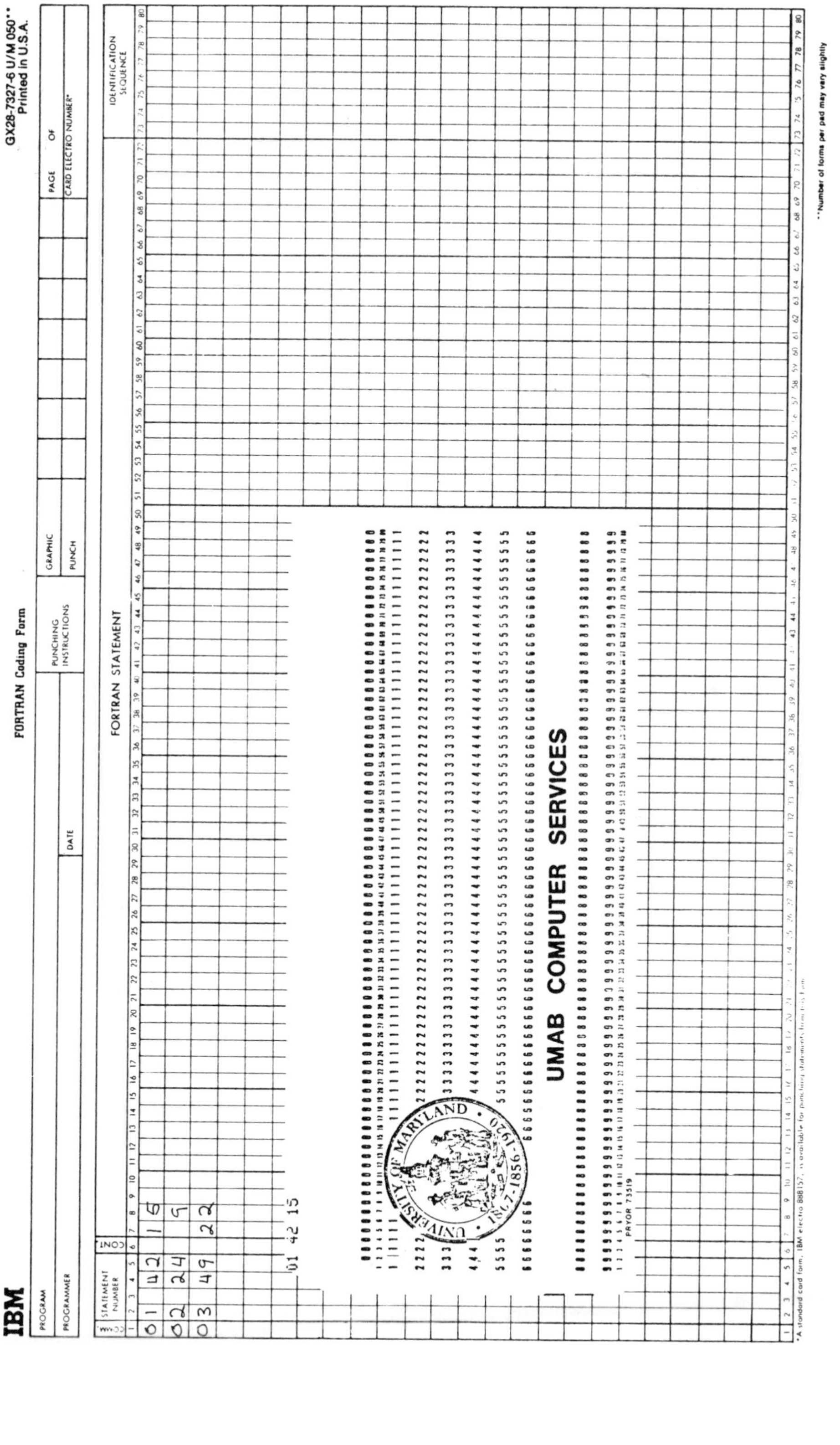

FIGURE 6-2. Data coding sheet and data card for Subject #01 (see text).

umn are read as zeros) because column 7 is reserved for the tens digit of *each* S's attitude score. By the same token, if one of the Ss had recorded an attitudinal score of more than 99, it would have been necessary to reserve three columns for all Ss' attitude scores even though the leftmost column would be used only once. Finally, at the risk of being repetitious, none of the columns 1 to 3 or 6 will be read by the computer; they are included only to enable the researcher to check and proofread data—a process which should be undertaken with great care since one number in the wrong column is capable of invalidating an entire analysis.

Coding and punching data can be quite time consuming if there is a great deal of data, but it is conceptually a very simple process analogous to neatly writing down all the information collected in numerical form and then typing it. Actually, researchers normally do not even have to keypunch their data in most computing centers. If they have sufficient funds in their computer accounts they can simply code their data on coding sheets (or have someone else do it if clerical help is available) and turn them over to the appropriate person at their computing center. In a few days, the sheets will be returned along with correspondingly punched cards with the fee billed to the researcher's computer account. Since this account is usually supplied compliments of the institution for which the researcher works, the only real disadvantage to the procedure lies in the time it takes to get the cards punched. If only a few cards are involved, most individuals prefer to punch them themselves; students are almost always required to punch their own cards when conducting exercises and assignments, partly for the experience, mostly to save money for actual data analysis.

SCAN SHEETS

Although the use of data coding sheets is the most commonly used method to transcribe data to punched cards, there is an easier way. In those cases in which the data accrues from a study consisting of Ss' responses to multiple choice or true/false test items, or to Likert scales as with attitudinal or personality questionnaires, Ss can be asked to respond directly on a specially constructed sheet of paper called a *scan form* (or computerized answer sheet). Everyone is familiar with these forms, which provide spaces in which the respondent shades in the answer with a No. 2 pencil. The chief function of scan forms is to permit machine scoring of tests, but most computing centers also contain equipment that permits their contents to be punched directly on cards, thus negating the necessity of human keypunching. Although circumstances exist in which machine punching from scan forms is not feasible, researchers would be well advised to consider this labor saving device where applicable.

Communicating with the Computer

Once data cards have been prepared, a few additional cards must be punched to tell the computer (1) what the user's account number and password are to

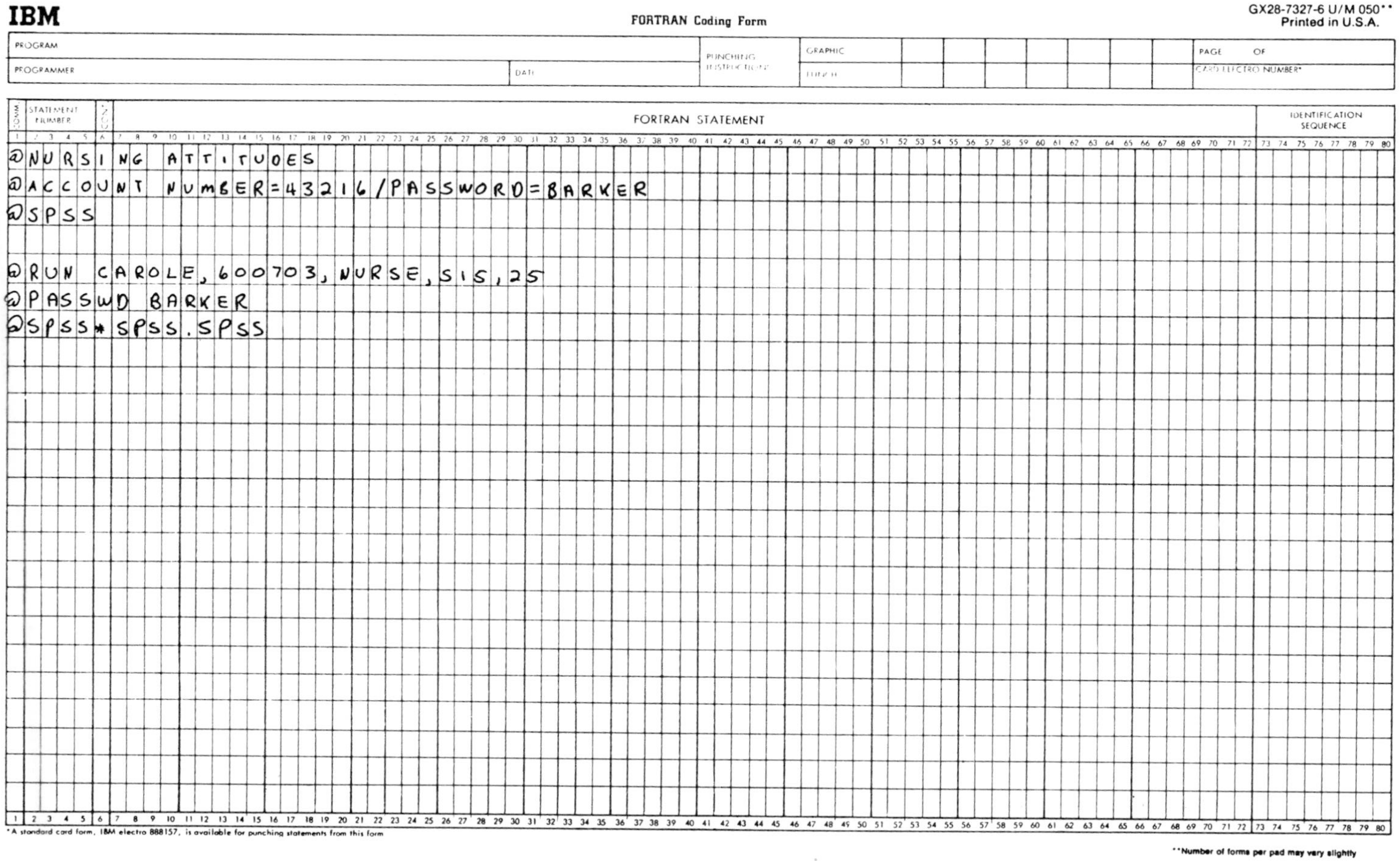

IBM — FORTRAN Coding Form — GX28-7327-6 U/M 050** Printed in U.S.A.

PROGRAM | PUNCHING INSTRUCTIONS | GRAPHIC | PUNCH | PAGE OF
PROGRAMMER | DATE | CARD ELECTRO NUMBER*

STATEMENT NUMBER | CONT. | FORTRAN STATEMENT | IDENTIFICATION SEQUENCE

```
@NURSING ATTITUDES
@ACCOUNT NUMBER=43216/PASSWORD=BARKER
@SPSS

@RUN CAROLE,600703,NURSE,SIS,25
@PASSWD BARKER
@SPSS*SPSS.SPSS
```

*A standard card form, IBM electro 888157, is available for punching statements from this form

**Number of forms per pad may vary slightly

FIGURE 6-3. Data card showing account number, user's identification, password, and program to be used in analyzing data.

assure it that it will be paid for its labors and (2) what general statistical program should be used in the analysis. This information is communicated via system cards (the reader will remember that anything that can be punched on a card can also be entered directly into the computer by teletype), which simply means that their function is to convey information to the particular computer (system) being used. The specific format of these cards varies from center to center, but it is always readily available, usually on a bulletin board near the keypunch machines. If not, a consultant can be asked. One is usually on duty specifically to answer questions such as this.

Figure 6-3 gives some examples of what these cards will generally look like, but very few computing centers use exactly the same format. The first example consists of three cards. Card #1 simply allows the user to give the data a name; Card #2 tells the computer the account number to which the run (analysis) should be charged and its password (designed to keep unauthorized people from using funds from said account); Card #3 tells the computer which program (already on file in the computer) to use to analyze the data. The second example uses a slightly different format to convey almost identical information. (There is provision for identifying the user, in this case "Carole;" it is assumed that each user has a separate account number and password.) There are occasions when additional communication is necessary (such as for analyses that require a great deal of time or computing memory to complete), but information concerning these special instances is also readily available.

Statistical Programs

As stated earlier, not very long ago it was essential for any serious computer user to know at least one computer language and be able to program in it. Digital computers are not flexible enough to communicate directly in human languages; they operate on a binary system with exactly two values, 0 and 1, hence necessitating languages that can be easily translated into these terms. This constraint, plus the fact that complicated statistical procedures require an inordinate number of minute step-by-step directions, combined to make routine statistical analysis unavailable to the vast majority of medical and health related researchers not having direct access to a programmer.

Again, over the past two decades this situation has altered radically. Today preprogrammed packages (also called canned or library programs) exist for almost every conceivable statistical analysis and some are almost universally available. This book will deal chiefly with the most comprehensive and flexible of these, the *Statistical Package for the Social Sciences* (SPSS). Only when a particular procedure is not available in SPSS will sample output from other, less universally available, programs be used.

After the discussion of each of the more commonly used statistical procedures presented in subsequent chapters, examples of computer output from one of these packages will be given to facilitate the reader's own use and interpretation of output. Readers are strongly urged to become familiar with the program library at their facilities, since each computing center has many excellent and easy to use statistical programs which have been created to augment the large commercial packages.

All programs in common use possess manuals containing detailed instructions on the preparation of cards to communicate to the package itself what is to be done with the data. In other words, the system cards call up the package and once called, a few additional cards are used to specify which particular program in the package is desired, which variables (or data card columns) are to be used, the number of data cards to be analyzed, and so forth. These cards normally follow the system cards in a clearly specified order and precede the data itself, and, along with an "end" card telling the computer that all cards have been read, constitute a *deck*, which is fed into a card reader as described above.

SPSS

SPSS is rapidly becoming the most widely used statistical package in the country for very good reasons. The manual, *Statistical Package for the Social Sciences*[3] is clearly written and contains not only detailed instructions for the preparation of necessary control cards and excellent statistical overviews for the available programs, but also options that allow the researcher to manipulate data by creating new variables via the combination of existing ones, by collapsing cells in contingency tables, automatically throwing out missing data, and a host of other transformations. SPSS further allows multiple analyses using divergent statistical techniques with different variables in the same run (that is, requiring the researcher to submit data to a card reader only once) and has features that facilitate its use via teletype and tape. In the opinion of the authors, no other statistical package gives clearer or more cosmetically attractive output, or allows its user more control over the appearance of output (as with labelling options). More importantly, however, no other statistical package contains as wide a range of useful statistical procedures with as clear, explicit instructions for their use.

Minicomputers

As convenient as electronic computers can be, many researchers prefer an even more convenient (and sometimes quicker) tool: the mini- or tabletop computer. These fascinating little machines are becoming more readily available all the time and, partly because of almost continual technologic improvements, are one of the few commodities whose price has been consistently and drastically reduced over time.

There are many, many brands and models of minicomputers available that can be conveniently used for statistical analysis. The genre of machine that is currently most useful to the widest range of researchers, however, is that which is both programmable (that is, for which specific step-by-step instructions can be written) and comes equipped with statistical routines already available on magnetic cards or permanently wired into the machine.

Those computers that can be directly programmed by inserting small magnetic cards directly into the machine are probably the most flexible and have the widest range of statistical procedures available. Once the machine is programmed, the operator only has to punch the data directly into the machine as with a calculator, one entry at a time. Upon command, statistical results are printed out almost instantaneously, saving the researcher hours of laborious computations with a calculator (or a trip to the local computing center if a teletype is not available).

Depending upon the model available, these machines perform a truly impressive number of statistical procedures. If the researcher has a relatively small amount of data, and if the analyses planned are relatively simple, then minicomputers can actually produce quicker results than the large computer. They do have disadvantages, however, which are primarily all size-related.

The advantages of using a large digital computer emanate from its enormous memory capacity. Minicomputers are severely limited with respect to the number of steps they can be programmed to perform and the amount of data upon which they can operate. A researcher with over 100 subjects in a study and several separate analyses to run on them, for example, will find entering data for each separate analysis very tedious, especially when the researcher realizes that a large computer using a program such as SPSS could perform them all in one run.

Deciding whether to use a system such as SPSS or a minicomputer involves deciding exactly how the data from a study should be analyzed and considering the complexity of said analyses. Certainly if several statistical procedures are to be run on several variables, then using the digital computer is the only sensible choice. Furthermore, once data have been punched on cards, the researcher has the option of performing auxiliary and exploratory analyses, or of re-analyzing the data at another time with relatively little effort. Another consideration is the fact that many of the more complex statistical routines are not available on the small machines because of their limited memory capacity. Nevertheless, minicomputers are a valuable adjunct used by many researchers in pilot or exploratory work and their use can often supplement analysis via the larger computer.

REFERENCES

1. Siegel, S.: *Nonparametric Statistics for the Behavioral Sciences*. McGraw-Hill, New York, 1956.
2. Winkler, R. L.: *Introduction to Bᵣyesian Inferences and Decision*. Holt, Rinehart and Winston, New York, 1972.
3. Nie, N. H., et al.: *Statistical Package for the Social Sciences*. McGraw-Hill, New York, 1975.
4. Glass, G. V. and Stanley, J. C.: *Statistical methods in education and psychology*. Prentice-Hall, Englewood Cliffs, New Jersey, 1970, pp. 201–202.

CHAPTER **7**

THE RESEARCH REPORT

Once completed, research must be communicated. This is customarily accomplished via a research report whose audience may be (1) other researchers, (2) scholars, and (3) interested professionals. The function of the research report is to delineate to its readers the study's purpose (that is, the problems being investigated, hypotheses, and so forth), the rationale for this purpose (that is, practical, theoretical, or empirical), the way in which this purpose was accomplished, the results, and the interpretation of those results. The researcher should write the report with the realization that the audience may wish not only to be apprised of all these points, but also to evaluate the study and possibly even *replicate* it for themselves. These last two points make it incumbent upon the researcher to communicate the procedures used in the study in considerable detail.

COMPONENTS OF A RESEARCH REPORT

Regardless of the medium through which the report is published, all research reports have four basic components in addition to an abstract (whose purpose is, in a few hundred words or less, to simply give the reader an overview of the research question, the results, and a sentence or two regarding implications). The first element is an *introduction* to the research problem and a statement of that problem. When the report appears in a scholarly journal the introduction usually takes the form of a few sentences discussing the general area of concern, followed by a relatively brief review of prior research that has bearing on this area. Results of past studies should then blend smoothly into a statement of the specific problem to be investigated, often rather overtly such as "The purpose of the present study, therefore, is to investigate. . . ."

Once the background of the problem and the problem itself have been presented, the report normally proceeds directly into a discussion of the *procedures* (methodology) used to effect the study's purpose. The researcher should attempt to present these procedures in sufficient detail to permit a colleague to replicate the study *exactly* as well as to evaluate the efficacy of the procedures employed. Unfortunately, many writers forget to include this level of detail.

Following the procedures section comes the report of the *results* of the study. This section contains not only a description of the statistical procedures employed, but an explanation of why those procedures were chosen and a *statistical* interpretation of their results. The scientific interpretation of the results occurs in the final section.

The *discussion* and/or *conclusions* section of the report ties the entire study together, relating the results to the problem and to the prior studies reviewed. This part also typically states whether or not the hypotheses were rejected and presents the researcher's own evaluation of the study through a discussion of limitations inherent in the research just reported.

Before pursuing these constituent parts of a report in greater detail, some general comments on writing style and the medium in which a report is to appear will be discussed.

STYLE

The first rule that must be learned in preparing research results for scholarly publication, regardless of the medium in which the final report is to appear, is that the *purpose of a research report is to communicate factual information in as concise and clear a method as possible.* Its purpose is not to entertain and not to provide an esthetic experience for the reader.

This does not imply that a research report need be dull. It should be concise, to the point, and should communicate as much information as possible in as few words as possible. A reader who is interested in the topic will find the procedures designed to answer the research question and the results themselves interesting if they are clearly presented. A reader who is not interested in the problem will probably find the report dull because the embellishments used by esthetic writers (metaphors, poetic prose, amusing anecdotes, and so forth) have absolutely no place in a research report whose audience is *not* the general public, but rather, as stated above, scholars, other researchers, and interested professionals.

The stylistic goal of the writer of a research report should be primarily clarity of communication. Once that is achieved, a secondary goal should be the communication of as much information in as few words as possible. This not only saves the reader time and effort, but also saves space which is always at a premium in scholarly publications. An exception to this might seem to be the thesis or dissertation that is published as a separate entity. The truth of the matter is, however, that the shorter the report the more likely it is to be read, hence the researcher should always be as parsimonious as possible.

Anyone planning to write a research report for the first time should avail themselves of three references in addition to a dictionary. (A thesaurus is not routinely recommended because of the temptation for the beginning writer to use it to try to sound erudite, often with disastrous results.) The first and most general of these is Strunk and White's *The Elements of Style*.[4] This "little book" should be owned by anyone planning to write for publication, research or otherwise; it gives excellent advice on every aspect of the writing process but is especially helpful concerning clumsy constructions, common misusages, and strategies for achieving brevity of communication.

A *Manual of Style*[1] published by the University of Chicago Press is probably the most popular reference of its sort in use. Although relevant to research reports, its scope is much more ambitious and it is used by many professional writers. (The same press also publishes *A Manual for Writers of Term Papers, Theses, and Dissertations*[5] which can be of incomparable value to graduate students, although anyone planning to write a dissertation or thesis should first check with their graduate school to make sure that institution-specific guidelines are not available in their schools.)

A third reference whose scope is more specifically focused upon the research report is the American Psychological Association's *Publication Manual of the American Psychological Association*.[2] Although this publication is geared specifically to APA journals, many other scholarly journals follow its guidelines. Its suggestions for the construction of tables and graphs are especially helpful.

As useful as these references and guidelines can be, however, nothing can substitute for concentrated effort on the part of the writer to make the report as succinct and readable as possible. This effort normally takes two forms. One is constant revision. Even the most experienced writer never considers submitting the first draft for publication; most completely rewrite their first drafts and then make extensive revisions on their second attempt. It is usually a good idea to allow a few days to elapse between drafts—objectivity comes with time.

Once something approximating a final draft has been completed, the next step is to submit the report to a knowledgable, critical colleague with the request to point out (in writing) anything that is not clear or that could be presented better. Sometimes this strategy is hard on the ego, but it can be very helpful. A disinterested party can spot weaknesses in both the study and its reporting that the author can never bring himself to see. The author is, of course, not obligated to take the reviewer's advice; the author is obligated, however, to take any criticisms graciously since their submission was done as a favor.

MEDIUM

There are many appropriate places to publish a research report. If the research was undertaken as a thesis or dissertation requirement, then it will be duplicated, bound, and registered in its author's university library. In addition, doctoral dissertations are abstracted and microfilmed (*Dissertation Abstracts* in Ann Arbor, for example, as well as various professional abstracting services). Because the stylistic requirements for the writing of dissertations and theses are so rigidly prescribed by the student's institutions and thesis chairman, the present chapter will not dwell on this medium.

Many institutions provide an internal publishing service for staff members in the form of technical reports and ongoing paper series which allow results of research studies to be permantly archived. Although such reports usually have a very limited circulation, they can be referenced in other media and abstracting services and made available to outside researchers upon request. There is usually considerable flexibility in preparing such reports, although some institutions have very specific guidelines for their technical reports. As with dissertations and theses, more space is usually available for greater detail although, as suggested above, brevity of exposition should remain an objective.

A third medium in which the researcher can communicate research findings is provided by professional conferences. Many opportunities are provided by these professional meetings both on national and regional levels for the presentation of research findings. Typically, the researcher is given from 15 minutes to an hour to discuss the findings and answer questions from the audience. This particular medium has the advantage over all others of allowing the consumer the opportunity to directly ask the researcher for clarification of points not covered or not clear in the presentation. Most conferences further require a written report to accompany the talk, and even when not required, the researcher should have a written document available for interested members of the audience as well as interested professionals who were not able to attend the session. In fact, a written report of some sort is essential for anyone with a serious interest in the study, because research is basically a written rather than an oral medium. The truth of this generalization should be apparent to anyone attempting to follow the oral presentation of a complicated study at a professional conference.

As important as the foregoing media are for the communication of research, the scholarly journal is by far the most important and widely used medium. Journals typically have very large circulations, and more importantly, they tend to reach professionals who are most interested in, and who can most fully utilize, the reported research. Research reports in scholarly journals are also indexed in numerous sources according to the subject matter, hence making the study indirectly available to a much larger audience than the publication's subscribers.

There are many types of scholarly journals in nursing, only a few of which regularly devote a substantial amount of space to formal research reports. Nurse researchers, however, should not confine their publishing outlets to nursing journals. Many interdisciplinary research journals exist whose audiences are equally interested in topics relevant to nursing.

The professional journal contains one other very definite advantage over the other media discussed. If the journal is refereed, the researcher has access to critiques of different aspects of the study by colleagues knowledgeable in the particular area of endeavor. These critiques can be especially valuable for subsequent revisions of the report.

Although other media exist for reporting research (for example, in edited books, annuals, and so forth), the scholarly journal remains the avenue of choice for most researchers. If the medium has a disadvantage, it probably lies in the premium many editors must place upon space (hence requiring researchers to be even more concise than they *should*), since the best journals are forced to reject many times the number of articles they accept. This limitation is usually most severely felt by readers who wish either to replicate a study or to very thoroughly evaluate it. However, this particular shortcoming can usually be overcome by direct communication with the author, who is usually flattered by the fact that someone is taking so active an interest in the study.

PREPARING THE REPORT

The first step in writing a research report is to decide upon the medium in which it will be published. This requires a certain amount of objective and realistic evaluation on the part of the researcher. Researchers who are unsure of their ability in this respect should seek a colleague's opinion.

Generally, the medium of choice for most academic researchers is the refereed journal. Since this is the first choice, however, it follows that there is a good deal of competition for the limited space available. If the study in question is seriously flawed in some way, then the researcher is probably being unrealistic in expecting it to be published in a prestigious journal. However, there are so many journals available (many of which are not refereed), that persistence will usually be rewarded if the researcher does a good job in both writing the report and selecting an appropriate journal.

Once a journal is selected, it is mandatory for the researcher to (1) study the format of published articles in that journal and (2) obtain the publication's style sheet. Although most journals use one of the references listed above as a general style guide, almost all have some individual idiosyncracies that the writer would be wise to heed. Specific instructions are usually available to the author somewhere in the publication. If not, then a letter to the editor will result in such specifications being sent to the prospective author. Once the format of the chosen journal is ascertained, the researcher should tailor the report to that specific publication. In other words, the researcher should write the article for that journal and that journal alone. The following suggestions for preparing the four constituent parts of the research report are, therefore, only general guidelines that must be interpolated to the specific ones of the medium actually chosen for the final report.

Introduction

PURPOSE

The most important element of the introductory part of any research report is a clear, concise statement of the purpose of the study. This statement should not be couched in vague, general terms but should specify the variables under consideration, the hypothesized relationship between them, and the conditions under which this relationship is to be studied. The purpose should probably be preceded by a general discussion of its significance to the overall area under study.

LITERATURE REVIEW

The literature review, which is also contained in this introductory section, should be designed to provide a theoretical and empirical rationale for the study's purpose. Although many published literature reviews contain general, nonempirical remarks by authorities in the area touting the importance of a topic, these references should be kept to a minimum. (An exception is a reference to the *relationship* hypothesized in the study under consideration.)

References should usually be limited to specific studies bearing upon the variables, relationships, and conditions stated in the purpose of the study. Previous research involving the variables under consideration that has no bearing on the study should not be mentioned in the literature review. Any study cited should be tied directly to the purpose at hand; if such a tie cannot be explicitly made, then that reference should not be cited. (Media other than journal articles, while admitting more flexibility in this regard, operate under basically the same rules.)

Nursing research is replete with strings of references, sometimes 10 to 15 on a single page, that bear no apparent relationship to the study in which they are cited. Many writers feel that they should cite every study they have reviewed in the area to convince the reader of their knowledgeability. This is not the purpose of a literature review, however. It should be assumed that researchers are experts in the literature relevant to their areas (theses and dissertations being an exception). Actually, a good test of this assumption is not the number of studies cited, but their overall relevance to the problem at hand. The function of the literature review is threefold: to bring knowledge to bear on the overall purpose of the study, to enhance the meaningfulness of this purpose, and to help generate predictions for the likely outcomes of the study.

HYPOTHESES

Although not required by many very good journals, it is often helpful to explicitly state the major hypotheses to be tested, either in null or alternate forms. This usually occurs at the end of the introductory section.

Methodology

This may well be the most important part of the research report. The more detail the author is able to supply, the better the study can be evaluated. The main function of this section is to permit an intelligent evaluation of how the purposes of the research were accomplished.

SAMPLE

The first part of the methodology section should describe who the participants in the study were, relevant characteristics of this sample, the population from which they were drawn, how they were selected from this population, and any mortality that may have occurred over the course of the study.

INSTRUMENTATION

Any tests, scales, or other data collection devices should be described in as much detail as possible. The number of items and their formats should be given. Sample items should be presented and detailed psychometric information offered (for example, indication of the reliability of the measures used and how that reliability was obtained).

PROCEDURES

This section should detail exactly what transpired in the study. Timetables for testing, detailed instructions to participants including procedures for insuring informed consent, conditions (where the study was conducted, environmental factors, and so forth), and precise operational definitions of treatments should be delineated. The design should be graphically described even if the researcher feels that it should be obvious from the above descriptions. This entire section should be written as though the researcher's chief purpose were to help the reader replicate the study under identical conditions. Finally, and most painfully, any aberrations or mistakes that occurred in the conduct of the study must be mentioned herein. No study is perfectly run, and the reader must be able to evaluate the discrepancy between intent and reality.

Results

The first part of this section should describe which analytic procedures were chosen to test which hypotheses. Many times, the results section contains not only statistics that have bearing upon the specific hypotheses listed in the introduction but subsidiary findings as well. This is as it should be, but the researcher should make a special effort to tie statistical tests to specific hypotheses for the reader's benefit (again even though it may seem obvious) and to explain why auxiliary analyses were undertaken.

The reader should not only be apprised of the results of the hypotheses testing, but also should be given the means to "see" these results. To this end, summary statistics should always be included, either within the text or presented in tabular or graphic form.

Most studies will require the use of tables and/or figures (although journals do not afford as much opportunity for the latter as other media) to facilitate the explication of the study's results. These aids should be kept to a minimum, however, and used only when the text cannot adequately present all the available data. The *Publication Manual of the American Psychological Association* and the University of Chicago's *A Manual of Style* cited earlier contain excellent suggestions for using these devices.

The results section should be kept as concise as possible. Just as the researcher will review many more studies than will be cited in the literature review, so will the researcher conduct many more analyses (especially if a computer is used) than will be reported in the results section. The same criterion must be used to select the ones reported: they must bear directly upon the stated purposes of the study and this relevance should be clearly delineated for the reader.

Discussion

Although often the shortest section in the report, the discussion is also often the most difficult to write. It must show how the purposes of the study were met, review and amplify the results that have a bearing upon these purposes, and explain how these results fit into the previous body of knowledge on the subject cited in the literature review. Limitations of the study must be discussed and *evaluated* with respect to their relationship to the fulfillment of the purposes of the study and to the *implications of the study to theory and/or practice.*

SUMMARY

This chapter has presented a very brief overview of the characteristics of a good research report as well as suggestions for writing one. Hopefully, the reader will find this discussion and the selected references helpful. In the final analysis, however, the only way to learn to write a competent research report is to actually write one, modeling it upon positive examples gleaned from the literature. As with most behaviors, performance is a function of practice. For those who wish to read further about preparing a research report, Kerlinger[3] may be helpful.

REFERENCES

1. *A Manual of Style*, ed. 12. University of Chicago Press, Chicago, 1969.
2. *Publication Manual of the American Psychological Association*, ed. 2. American Psychological Association, Washington, D.C., 1974.
3. Kerlinger, F. N.: *Foundations of Behavioral Research.* Holt, Rinehart and Winston, New York, 1973.
4. Strunk, W. and White, E.: *The Elements of Style*, ed. 3. Macmillan, New York, 1978.
5. Turabian, K. A.: *A Manual for Writers of Term Papers, Theses, and Dissertations*, ed. 4. University of Chicago Press, Chicago, 1973.

CHAPTER **8**
DESCRIPTIVE STUDIES

The researcher conducts a descriptive study in order to construct a picture or account of events as they naturally occur. Most descriptive studies employ survey or case study methods to accomplish this purpose. Data are usually collected by questionnaires, interviews, observational techniques, literature reviews, or the critical incident technique. Results are then analyzed using summary statistics. Computer programs useful in descriptive studies are characterized by the SPSS programs CONDESCRIPTIVE and FREQUENCIES.

DESIGNS FOR DESCRIPTIVE STUDIES

Descriptive studies may be guided by research questions and/or research objectives rather than a research hypothesis per se. That is, the statement of a research hypothesis is optional in conducting a descriptive study. Similarly, because the researcher makes no attempt to introduce something new or to in any manner modify or control the situation being studied, independent and dependent variables are not specified. The definition of variables in a descriptive study requires the researcher to delineate the variables or events the researcher seeks to describe in such a manner that the researcher and others may recognize them when they occur. Thus, variables and events are best described as behavioral acts.

The specific type of descriptive design employed by the researcher will depend upon the type of research question and/or the research objectives. Usually, descriptive studies are designed as surveys or case studies. A *survey* is intended to provide an accurate description of a small number of variables across a large number of subjects. Surveys can be obtained by sampling all or part of a population. Specific types of surveys are simple descriptive, comparative, correlational, and developmental. *Case studies,* on the other hand, are intensive systematic investigations of a small number of subjects across a large number of variables and/or conditions. Table 8-1 illustrates research questions and objectives and the types of descriptive designs generally employed to investi-

TABLE 8-1. Research Questions and Objectives Leading to Specific Types of Descriptive Designs

Research question	Research objective	Type of descriptive design
How do students who participate in a human sexuality course use the content in subsequent clinical work?	To describe how students who participated in a course use its content in their clinical work.	Simple descriptive survey.
What are the attitudes of adolescent diabetics who fail to comply with their diet regimen?	To describe the attitudes of an intact group of patients who fail to comply with their diet regimen.	Simple descriptive survey.
How does the clinical performance of students who participate in a human sexuality course compare with the performance of students who do not?	To compare the clinical performance of a group of students who participate in a particular course with a group of students who do not participate.	Comparative descriptive survey.
How do the attitudes of adolescent diabetics who fail to comply with their diet regimen compare with the attitudes of those who do comply?	To compare the attitudes of a group of adolescents who comply with their diet regimen with the attitudes of a group of adolescents who do not.	Comparative descriptive survey.
What factors in a human sexuality course explain students' attitudes toward sexuality at the completion of the course?	To identify and describe the relationship between various factors included in a human sexuality course and students' attitudes at the completion of the course.	Correlational descriptive survey.
What factors explain adolescent diabetics' compliance/noncompliance with their diabetic regimen.	To identify and describe the relationship between various factors common to adolescent diabetics and their compliance/noncompliance with their diet regimen.	Correlational descriptive survey.

TABLE 8-1. *Continued*

Research question	*Research objective*	*Type of descriptive design*
What are the trends and patterns of utilization of primary health care services by rural clients during the initial year of program development?	To describe trends and patterns of utilization in a rural primary care program over the first year of its development.	Developmental descriptive survey.
How are nursing students in baccalaureate nursing programs socialized into professional nursing?	To describe the professional socialization of baccalaureate nursing students.	Developmental descriptive survey.
What are the personal, physical, and cognitive needs of a paraplegic patient during the first six months postdiagnosis?	To describe in depth the needs of two newly diagnosed paraplegics during the first six months after they are made aware of their prognosis.	Descriptive case study.
What facilitates or hinders students graduating from doctoral programs in nursing from becoming active nurse researchers?	To describe in detail the characteristics, attitudes, and environmental influences operating to facilitate or hinder a small number of nurse graduates of a doctoral program from becoming active nurse researchers.	Descriptive case study.

gate them. When the designs in Table 8-1 are discussed in greater detail in subsequent sections of this chapter, it will become apparent that they are by no means mutually exclusive. For example, all types will include aspects of the simple descriptive design and correlational designs may also involve comparisons between two or more groups of subjects or vice versa. Similarly, the steps carried out in relation to all types of descriptive designs will closely parallel each other.

The *primary objective* for conducting the study should be the deciding factor in the selection of one type of design over another. By linking the research question or objective to a specific design and then proceeding according to the steps outlined for that design, the researcher will increase the probability that at the completion of the study the results will in fact provide the information necessary to answer the research question and/or attain the research objective. By not systematically following the steps for a specific design, the researcher runs the risk of completing the study only to find that a great deal of information has been acquired, but not necessarily information that (1) allows the researcher to answer the research question or meet the research objective, (2) is appropriate for analyzing the data using desirable statistical procedures, or (3) is cost effective and efficient in terms of its utility in providing meaningful results.

Surveys

The first step in conducting any survey is to define the purpose and objective for the study in readily observable behavioral terms. A knowledge and skill in writing behavioral objectives is thus essential for the researcher who employs such studies. The reader who requires a review of behavioral objectives will find the work by Staropoli and Waltz[12] a helpful reference. Depending upon the specific objective for the survey, it can then be characterized as simple descriptive, comparative, correlational, or developmental.

SIMPLE DESCRIPTIVE SURVEYS

Simple descriptive surveys are employed when the aim is to describe an intact situation or area of interest factually and accurately. Van Dalen and Meyer[13] point out that the information obtained by a simple descriptive survey may: (1) provide detailed factual information that describes existing phenomena, (2) lead to the identification of problems with current conditions and practices, (3) provide justification for current conditions and practices, (4) form a basis for making judgments and/or (5) determine what others are doing with similar problems or situations and allow the researcher to benefit from their experiences in making future plans or decisions. Thus, simple descriptive studies are particularly suitable for conducting the early stages of a comprehensive program evaluation.

The specific steps involved in designing a simple descriptive study are:

1. State objectives for the survey in observable behavioral terms.
2. Review literature related to the objectives.
3. Identify the facts and characteristics being sought by the study.
4. Select a method for obtaining a representative sample of subjects or events.
5. Select a data collection method.
6. Select an appropriate descriptive statistical procedure and a computer program for analyzing results.
7. Identify the audiences for study results and plan how results can best be presented to them.

A published example of a simple descriptive survey is presented in Example 8-1.

EXAMPLE 8-1. Published Example of a Simple Descriptive Survey

Title: *Training in induced abortion by obstetrics and gynecology residency programs.*

Source: Lindherm and Cotterill, Family Planning Perspectives, vol. 10, no. 1, January–February, 1978, pp. 24–28.

Purpose: To determine the extent to which instruction in induced abortion is incorporated into the clinical training provided to future obstetricians and gynecologists (p. 24).

Design:
1. Research questions were formulated and operationalized in questionnaire form.
2. Literature was reviewed in the areas of U.S. abortion statistics and institutional guidelines for evaluating ob-gyn specialists.
3. Specific information regarding training offered to residents in four areas was sought: techniques of abortion complications, observation of abortion, performance of first trimester abortions, and performance of second trimester abortions.
4. Directors of all 438 hospital-based residency programs in obstetrics and gynecology were identified in the AMA Directory of Approved Residencies 1974–1975.
5. Directors were surveyed by mail utilizing the questionnaire developed to obtain the information cited in #3 above.
6. Responses to the questionnaire were summarized by number and percent in order to answer the research questions.
7. Results were presented in a journal whose aim is to disseminate information to professionals with concern for research, policy analysis, and public education regarding family planning.

COMPARATIVE SURVEYS

A survey is comparative if the same information is obtained from a representative sample of two or more groups of subjects and the results are compared. An important consideration in this design is the selection of groups in such a manner as to allow the researcher to focus on the study variables without confusion caused by extraneous variables not addressed by the study. In other words, it is desirable to select groups that are alike as much as possible in areas not addressed by the study, yet different in regard to the study variables. Sampling representativeness is also important in a comparative study. That is, those subjects selected for study should as nearly as possible represent the population from which they are selected. For this reason, random sampling and stratified random sampling are usually preferred.

The researcher carries out the following steps when designing a comparative survey:

1. State the objectives for the survey in observable behavioral terms.
2. Review the literature related to the objectives.

3. Identify two or more groups of subjects and/or situations to be described and compared.
4. Select a method for obtaining a representative sample from each of the groups.
5. Select a data collection method that will be used for all groups.
6. Select an appropriate statistical procedure and computer program for analyzing results.
7. Specify the audiences for results and plan how results can best be disseminated to them.

A published example of a comparative descriptive survey is presented in Example 8-2.

EXAMPLE 8-2. Published Example of a Comparative Descriptive Survey

Title: *Factors associated with rapid, subsequent pregnancies among school-age mothers.*

Source: Jekel, Klerman, and Bancroft, American Journal of Public Health, vol. 63, no. 9, September, 1973, pp. 769–773.

Purpose: To answer the research question: Can family planning services be offered to school-age mothers in the same way as to other, older patients or must new approaches be tried to overcome the special problems of this group? (p. 769)

Design: 1. Subjects were 180 girls entered through a young mothers clinic and 160 through a special school operated by an Interagency Services Program located in the same state.
2. Criteria for selection of subjects were that each participant had to be in the program, and at registration be under 18 years of age, unwed, and a resident of the local area served by the respective program.
3. Interviews with subjects were scheduled at 2, 13, and 24 months postpartum to obtain information regarding the reproductive performance of the participants in both programs and relate this performance to characteristics of the programs, certain pre-existing characteristics of the participants, the degree of their participation in the programs and other findings at postpartum.
4. Responses of subjects in both groups were tabulated and then compared using numbers and percents.
5. Results were reported in a journal whose aim is to disseminate information to professionals from a variety of public health fields and settings.

CORRELATIONAL SURVEYS

In a correlational survey the researcher investigates the extent to which changes in one factor correspond with changes in one or more other factors. A correlational survey design is especially appropriate in situations in which variables are complex and/or do not lend themselves to the use of more precise experimental methods. Specifically, because the correlational survey permits the assessment of several variables and their interrelationships simultaneously in a realistic setting, it is particularly valuable in conducting clinical studies.

Steps involved in designing a correlational survey are:

1. State the objectives for the survey in observable behavioral terms.
2. Review the literature pertaining to the objectives.
3. Specify the variables or factors to be investigated.
4. Select appropriate subjects.
5. Select or develop measuring devices.
6. Select the correlational procedure that is appropriate for assessing the objectives.
7. Plan for the collection of data.
8. Select a computer program appropriate for analyzing the results.
9. Plan for reporting the results.

A published example of a correlational descriptive survey is presented in Example 8-3.

EXAMPLE 8-3. Published Example of a Correlational Descriptive Survey

Title: *Preexisting correlates of hospital stress.*

Source: Volicer and Burns, Nursing Research, vol. 26, no. 6, November–December, 1977, pp. 408–415.

Purpose: To identify predictors of the level of hospital stress that patients experience in an acute hospital setting.

Design: 1. Research questions were formulated, e.g., one such question to be answered was "whether high life stress patients have high hospital stress scores regardless of the severity of the diagnosis."
2. Literature surveyed related to the theoretical basis for the relationship between stress and illness, measurement of stress, and prior research on psychosocial stress and illness.
3. Several variables, demographic characteristics, prior hospitalization experiences, life stress preceding hospitalization, and seriousness of current illness, which might affect the level of hospital stress were considered.
4. Included in the study were all patients on the medical and surgical wards of a community hospital who were able to complete the interview (according to the nurse in charge) and who were willing to participate.
5. An instrument was developed by the researchers as a method for quantifying psychosocial stress that results from the experience of hospitalization. For a detailed description of the instrument's development and testing for reliability and validity see p. 409 of the article.
6. To consider factors which might be correlates of hospital stress, study variables were classified into four groups: demographic data, prior hospital experiences, life stress preceding hospitalization, and present

EXAMPLE 8-3. *Continued*

illness. A stepwise multiple regression procedure was then employed to consider the relative importance of the variable in each of these groups in explaining or predicting hospital stress.

7. Data were collected by interviews. Medical patients were interviewed on the third day of hospitalization, surgical patients on the second or third day postsurgery. In addition, each patient was contacted by phone two weeks following discharge and information was obtained from patient charts.

8. Results were presented in a nursing journal whose aim is to inform members of the nursing profession and other professionals of the results of scientific studies in nursing and to stimulate research in nursing.

DEVELOPMENTAL SURVEYS

A developmental survey is undertaken when the aim is to describe the patterns of growth or change as a function of time. A developmental survey may be cross-sectional or longitudinal.

In a *longitudinal* survey the researcher studies the same subjects over an extended period of time. For example, a researcher who studied the professional socialization of nursing students by following the same 200 baccalaureate nursing students from time of entry into their nursing program until five years post-baccalaureate, that is, studied the same 200 subjects over a nine year period, would be conducting a longitudinal survey. Babbie[2] identified three variations of longitudinal designs for survey research: (1) trend studies in which the general population is studied at different points over a long period (data may be collected by the researcher or the researcher may utilize data collected by other investigators), (2) cohort studies in which the focus is on the same specific population each time data are collected, but samples may be composed of different subjects, and (3) panel studies in which the same subjects are used at each progressive time period that the data are collected. The length of time for conducting a longitudinal study will depend upon the specific phenomena being investigated and may range from a number of weeks to a number of years.

Cross-sectional surveys differ from longitudinal surveys by a time factor. In a longitudinal study, a group of subjects is followed for a period of time, whereas in a cross-sectional survey several groups of subjects in various stages of development are studied simultaneously. For example, if a researcher studied the professional socialization of nursing students by sampling groups of nursing students at nine different educational points (for example, freshmen, sophomore, junior, senior years, and one, two, three, four, and five years postbaccalaureate), the study would be a cross-sectional one.

Whether it is desirable to utilize a cross-sectional or longitudinal approach is determined on the basis of several considerations made by the researcher during the planning stages of the descriptive study. More specifically, a *cross-sectional survey* is preferable when the following conditions exist:

1. Resources for conducting the study are limited (that is, time, money, subjects, personnel).
2. It is necessary or desirable to complete the study in a relatively short period of time, that is, the researcher cannot wait years to obtain results.
3. The number of subjects available at the beginning of the study is limited and a loss of subjects over time may preclude completion of the study or in some manner diminish the importance of the results.
4. Financial restrictions and/or demands on subjects make it necessary or desirable to limit the number of data collections to a minimum, for example, one time.
5. The characteristics of subjects, for example, their geographic mobility, lead the researcher to anticipate problems in locating or contacting subjects for subsequent data collections.
6. The researcher is willing to accept the risks that:
   a. Subjects' recall may be biased.
   b. Accuracy of the composite picture of subjects' feelings and emotions may be diminished by the greater probability of error due to individual differences at measurement time.
   c. Observed changes may be the result of personality traits or a series of circumstances beyond the control of the subjects rather than the variables being investigated.
   d. Changing trends or patterns over time noted in the study may be biased because the method can only consider the present and past and not the future as well.

On the other hand, a *longitudinal survey* approach is desirable when:

1. Resources (money, time, personnel, subjects) are ample and there is little or no concern that they may be depleted before completion of the study.
2. The researcher finds it desirable and/or possible to:
   a. Follow subjects over time in order to note and interpret any variations near the time of their occurrence.
   b. Obtain more objective observations than are provided by subjects' recall.
   c. Have the flexibility within the design to study in depth a specific concern or trend that emerges during data collection at subsequent data collection points.
3. The researcher is willing to accept the fact that:
   a. Results of the study may not be available for a number of years.
   b. Repeated collection of data may influence the performance of the subjects and thus bias study results.

The researcher employing a *developmental survey* design undertakes the following steps:

1. State the objectives for the survey in observable, behavioral terms.
2. Review the literature to establish a baseline of existing information and to

compare research methodologies, instruments, and data collection techniques.

3. Design the approach, that is, cross-sectional or longitudinal.
4. Select appropriate subjects, data collection methodologies, times for data collection, and instruments.
5. Select the appropriate techniques for analyzing the data and the computer program(s) available.
6. Consider the audiences for results, their need for information, and plan for reporting results accordingly.

Published examples of longitudinal and cross-sectional descriptive surveys are presented in Examples 8-4 and 8-5.

EXAMPLE 8-4. Published Example of a Longitudinal Descriptive Survey

Title: *Patterns of reproductive health care among the poor of San Antonio, Texas.*

Source: Gibbs, Marin, and Gutierrez, American Journal of Public Health, vol. 64, no. 1, January, 1974, pp. 37–40.

Purpose: To obtain information on the amount and kind of family planning care obtained by patients whose babies were born at the only hospital in San Antonio providing obstetrical services for indigent women (p. 37).

Design: 1. Four research questions were identified seeking information regarding social and demographic characteristics, patterns of antepartum and family planning care, major deterrents to utilization of care, and the existing relationship between perinatal morbidity and mortality.
          2. Literature was reviewed regarding maternal and perinatal morbidity and mortality, utilization of health care by the poor, medical folklore, and existing patterns of prenatal care.
          3. Information was obtained from patients and medical records over a period of approximately 15 months.
          4. Every patient registered in the delivery book for a one-year period of time was selected for interview (n = 1500). In addition, subsequent interviews were conducted dealing specifically with family planning behavior during the next three-month period (n = 381). Basic information concerning the obstetrical and perinatal outcomes for each patient was obtained from medical records upon discharge.
          5. Responses to the research questions were tabulated by number and percent. The relationship between perinatal morbidity and mortality was examined by considering the joint frequency distribution of pregnancy outcome by antepartum care.
          6. Results were reported in a journal whose audience includes professionals from a variety of public health fields and settings.

EXAMPLE 8-5. Published Example of a Cross-Sectional Descriptive Survey

Title: *Faculty consensus as a socializing agent in professional education.*

Source: Gliebe, Nursing Research, vol. 26, no. 6, November–December, 1977, pp. 428–431.

EXAMPLE 8-5. *Continued*

Purpose: To assess the effectiveness of the professional socialization process in a school of nursing by describing emerging attitudes of students and comparing them to faculty attitudes, and by describing students' perceived limits of their role, nursing autonomy, and rights of patients (p. 428).

Design:
1. Four hypotheses were stated (p. 428).
2. Literature related to socialization in postsecondary educational settings and student socialization in nursing were reviewed.
3. A cross-sectional sample of 129 respondents was obtained in a diploma school of nursing. Included in the sample were 20 faculty, 43 first-year students, 41 and 25 second- and third-year students, respectively.
4. A three-dimensional attitude scale developed by Pankratz and Pankratz[11] was employed to collect data from all subjects at one point in time.
5. Scores for each subject group on each of the three dimensions were computed and the results compared utilizing frequency distributions, modal score categories, and a nonparametric measure of association, i.e., gamma.
6. Results were communicated in a journal whose audience is predominately nurses and whose aim is to inform members of the nursing profession and other professionals of the results of scientific studies in nursing and to stimulate research in nursing.

Case Studies

Case studies are intensive, systematic investigations of the background, current status, environmental characteristics, and interactions of an individual, group, or community. Case studies, because they examine a small number of subjects across a large number of variables, are particularly useful for: (1) providing background information for planning major subsequent research studies, (2) gaining insight into problems that deserve more extensive attention, and (3) providing examples to illustrate more generalized statistical findings. Case studies, because of their narrow focus, lack representativeness and thus do not allow the researcher to make generalizations to the population from which the subjects were drawn. The case study does, however, afford the investigator the flexibility to begin or stop the case study at any time, determine as the study proceeds the amount of data and degree of specificity to be obtained, as well as the sources from which it is to be obtained. It should be cautioned that for these same reasons, case studies are also particularly vulnerable to subjective biases to the extent that the researcher makes selective judgments ruling in or out certain data, placing them in one context or another, and seeking one source of data or another. The results of case studies should therefore be scrutinized carefully for biases and should be followed by research focusing on specific hypotheses generated by the case study and using a more precise research design.

The specific steps involved in designing a *case study* are:

1. State the objectives for the case study in observable behavioral terms.
2. Identify the unit of study, individual, group, or community.

3. List the characteristics, relationships, processes, and so forth that will direct the investigation, at least initially.
4. Review the literature.
5. Determine how subjects will be selected and identify potential data sources.
6. Specify the available data collection methods and plan as much as possible how data will be collected.
7. Develop a tentative scheme for organizing the findings into a coherent, well integrated description of the unit.
8. Plan for reporting results.
9. Anticipate hypotheses for further study that may result from the case study.

A published example of a descriptive case study is presented in Example 8-6.

EXAMPLE 8-6. Published Example of a Descriptive Case Study

Title: *Development of an abortion service in a large municipal hospital.*

Source: Walton et al., American Journal of Public Health, vol. 64, no. 1, January, 1974, pp. 77–81.

Purpose: To illustrate the problems encountered in creating a service to meet the objective of providing safe, ambulatory, and easily accessible service to patients and to ascertain whether or not the objectives were achieved (p. 77).

Design: 1. Objectives and measures of success were determined.
          2. Historical development of abortion service in New York and the hospital to be studied was described.
          3. Demography of the hospital center under investigation was described, including information regarding number and percent of requests for service over a two-year period, and characteristics of the population served.
          4. Delivery of service, routine screening procedures, financial screening, abortion scheduling, abortion procedures, and family planning techniques were described.
          5. Trends in the areas cited in #3 and #4 were examined by number and percent over a one-year period of time.
          6. Measures of success were applied to the information obtained in order to advance statements regarding attainment of the objectives and to identify continuing problems.
          7. Results were reported in a journal whose audience is comprised of professionals from a variety of public health fields and settings.

STATISTICAL PROCEDURES EMPLOYED IN DESCRIPTIVE STUDIES

Summary statistics allow the researcher to organize the mass of collected data in order to: (1) get some indication of trends and patterns and (2) answer a number of questions frequently raised by others regarding the research results. To accomplish these purposes it is necessary to: (1) tabulate data and (2) select and apply measures of central tendency, dispersion and shape. Although summary statistics are germane to descriptive studies, they are also employed by the researcher prerequisite to additional statistical procedures in other designs.

Tabulation of Data

A *raw score* is usually the number of points earned by a respondent on a particular measure. When items are each worth one point, the raw score is simply the number of correct responses made.[17]

A *distribution* of raw scores may be displayed as a table, graph, or polygon in which each score is paired with its frequency of occurrence in the set of scores. For example, if the same 10-item pretest were administered to 20 subjects and one received a score of 3, three received scores of 5, 10 received scores of 6, and six received scores of 9, the distribution of their scores could be represented by a *table* as shown in Table 8-2.

This table is called an *ungrouped frequency distribution* and is useful because it clearly illustrates how many subjects obtained each score. Sometimes it is desirable to carry the tabulation of raw score data one step further by using a *grouped frequency distribution*. That is, when there is a wide range of scores in a distribution and/or a number of scores are not received by respondents, it is economical to group scores according to size. For example, if the information in Table 8-2 were grouped, it would look like that in Table 8-3. Note that in practice more data points would normally be represented in tables such as these.

Each group in Table 8-3 is called a *score class*, and the complete grouping arrangement is called a *grouped frequency distribution*. The width of each score class interval in this case is 4.

TABLE 8-2. Ungrouped Frequency Distribution of Subjects' Scores on the Pretest (n = 20)

Score	Number of subjects
10	0
9	6
8	0
7	0
6	10
5	3
4	0
3	1
2	0
1	0

**TABLE 8-3. Grouped Frequency
Distribution of Subjects' Scores
on the Pretest (n = 20)**

Score	Number of subjects
11−8	6
7−4	13
3−0	1

Although there are no fixed rules for when a grouped frequency distribution is preferred to an ungrouped one, Glass and Stanley[5] suggest that the grouped frequency distribution be used when there is a large number of scores, 100 or more, and that it is usually best to construct not fewer than 12 nor more than 15 score classes. They state that with fewer than 12 classes the researcher runs the risk of distorting the results, whereas with more than 15 classes the table produced is inconvenient to handle.

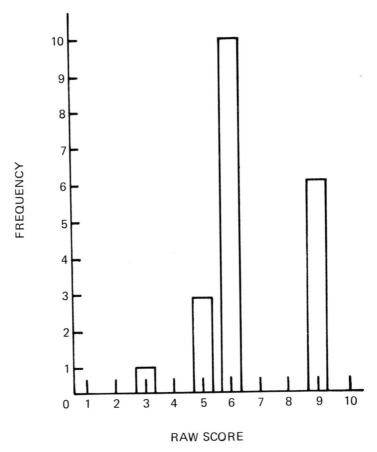

FIGURE 8-1. Graphic representation of subjects' scores on the pretest (n = 20).

In lieu of a frequency distribution, the researcher might opt to present scores using a *graph* such as that presented in Figure 8-1.

The graph in Figure 8-1 is a *histogram.* It not only displays all the information in the frequency distribution, but has the advantage of making information regarding the shape of the distribution more accessible to the reader.[17]

The histogram is a series of columns, each having as its base one score or class and as its height the frequency or number of subjects in that class. A column is centered around the mid-point of the score/class interval.

A *frequency polygon* is yet another way that the researcher may choose to represent the data. A polygon is very similar to a histogram.

In the histogram, the top of each column is represented by a horizontal line, the length of one score or class placed at the proper height to represent the number of subjects in that class. In the polygon, a point is located above the midpoint of each score or class and at the height that represents the frequency at that score. These points are then joined by straight lines. Figure 8-2 illustrates a polygon for the data represented by the histogram in Figure 8-1.

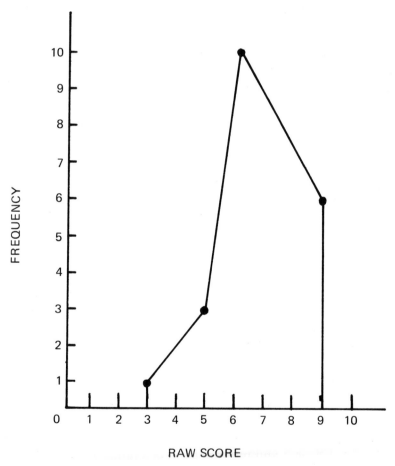

FIGURE 8-2. Frequency polygon of subjects' scores on the pretest (n = 20).

The main advantage of the polygon over the histogram is that it allows the researcher to superimpose up to three distributions on each other with a minimum of crossing of lines.[5] Thus, the polygon facilitates making comparisons among distributions.

Standards for constructing tables, graphs, and polygons were first published in 1915,[3] and have changed little through the years. That report still covers most of the points required for the proper representation of data, thus the following rules are cited from it:

1. The general arrangement of a diagram should proceed from left to right.
2. The horizontal scale should usually read from left to right and the vertical scale from bottom to top.
3. Whenever practical, the vertical scale should be selected so that the zero line appears on the diagram.
4. In diagrams representing a series of observations, whenever possible the separate observations should be clearly indicated on the diagrams.
5. All lettering and figures on a diagram should be placed so they easily read from the base as the bottom, or from the right-hand edge of the diagram as the bottom.
6. The title of a diagram should be as clear and complete as possible.

Additional information regarding the tabulating of data can be found in Kelley,[8] Walker and Durost,[15] or Arkin and Colton.[1]

Summary Statistics

When the researcher has tabulated the data, summary statistics are then employed to communicate information about the characteristics of the distribution of scores. Three types of summary statistics are of interest, measures of: (1) central tendency, (2) dispersion, and (3) the shape of the score distribution.

CENTRAL TENDENCY

Three indices of central tendency or averageness are the mean, median, and mode. Each has unique advantages and disadvantages in a particular situation and thus the relative merits of each should be considered whenever an index of central tendency is selected.

The *mode* is simply the score in a distribution associated with the largest number of subjects. The mode of scores on the 10-item pretest in Figure 8-1 is 6. Note that the mode refers to a score value and not the number of subjects receiving the score. The mode is the easiest to calculate of the three measures of central tendency, and in very large groups it is a fairly stable measure of the center of the distribution. The mode serves as the measure of central tendency basic to the development and interpretation of a number of the nonparametric statistics discussed in a later chapter.

The *median* of a distribution is the raw score value that separates the upper

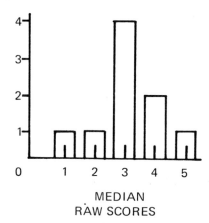

MEDIAN
RAW SCORES

FIGURE 8-3. When there is an unequal number of scores (1, 2, 3, 4, 5), the median is simply the middle score (3).

50 percent of the scores in the distribution from the lower 50 percent of the scores. When the researcher has an unequal number of scores, (for example, 1, 2, 3, 4, 5) as in Figure 8-3, the median is simply the middle score.

If, on the other hand, there is an equal number of scores, the median is determined in the following manner.

1. If there is an even number of untied scores, for example, 2, 3, 7, 8, the median is the point halfway between the two central values when the scores are ranked.

$$Md = (3 + 7)/2$$
$$= 5$$

2. If tied scores occur in the data, (as in Table 8-4), particularly at or near the median, a *frequency tabulation* of the scores will be necessary.

The median score will be the n/2 = 12th score from the bottom. The 12th score however lies in the interval from 5 to 6. Since 6 scores have been accumulated up to the lower limit of this interval, move through

TABLE 8-4. Frequency Tabulation of Subjects' Pretest Scores (n = 20)

Score	Frequency	Cumulative frequency
10	0	20
9	6	20
8	0	14
7	0	14
6	10	14
5	3	4
4	0	1
3	1	1
2	0	0
1	0	0
	n = 20	

10 − 6 = 4 frequencies in the interval. Since there is a total of 10 frequencies in the interval (that is, 16 − 6 = 10), the median will be taken to be the point (4/10 = 0.4). The interval extends from 5 to 6, a width of one unit, 4/10 of this distance is 0.4 unit. Hence, the median is the value 5 + 0.4 = 5.4.

Unlike the mode, the median may be a value which is *not* a member of the set of scores in the distribution. That is, in Table 8-4 no one actually obtained a score of 5.4. The value of the median is not influenced by extreme scores. For example, given the three scores 1, 2, 3, the median is 2. Given the three scores 1, 2, 100, the median is 2. This is not true, however of the arithmetic mean. For purely descriptive purposes, researchers working with small samples will find the median serves them well as a measure of central tendency.

The *arithmetic mean* is the sum of the scores in the distribution divided by the number of scores entering the sum.

(Formula 8-1)
$$\overline{X} = \frac{\Sigma X}{n}$$

where:
$\overline{X}$ = the arithmetic mean of the distribution of scores
Σ = the sum of
X = raw score
n = number of scores entering the sum

Example:

$$\begin{array}{c} \underline{X} \\ 1 \\ 2 \\ \underline{3} \end{array}$$

$\Sigma X = 6$ $\dfrac{\Sigma X}{n} = \dfrac{6}{3}$

$n = 3$ $\overline{X} = 2$

By locating these values on a number line, it can be seen that the mean is the fulcrum or balancing point of the distribution. That is, if the line in Figure 8-4 were thought of as a ruler and objects of equal weight were placed at points X_1, X_2, and X_3, the balancing point (∧) would be at the point associated with the score value 2. On the other hand, if X_1, X_2, and X_3 were of unequal weight and positioned as in Figure 8-5, the value of the mean would be affected by the extreme score or outlier (X_3) and the balancing point (∧) or mean would move toward the extreme score. The mean has two interesting properties.

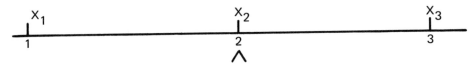

FIGURE 8-4. If the values for X_1, X_2, and X_3 are equal, the mean would be at the point associated with the score value 2.

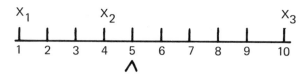

FIGURE 8-5. If the values for X_1, X_2, and X_3 are not equal, the value of the mean would move toward the extreme score.

1. If some number (a constant) is added to every score in a set of scores the resulting scores have a mean equal to the mean plus the constant.

   Example: The mean of the scores 1, 2 and 3, is 2.

X	C	X + C
1	5	6
2	5	7
3	5	8

   The mean of the new set of scores is 7 or 2 + 5.

2. If every score in a set of scores is multiplied by some number (a constant) the resulting scores have a mean equal to the mean times the constant.

   Example: The mean of the scores 1, 2 and 3 is 2.

X	C	XC
1	5	5
2	5	10
3	5	15

   The mean of the new set of scores is 10 or 2 × 5.

DISPERSION

When the arithmetic mean is used as the measure of central tendency, there are three indices that may be used to measure dispersion: (1) range, (2) variance, and (3) standard deviation.

The *range* is the simpliest of the three measures. It is calculated by finding the difference between the largest and smallest scores in the distribution.

Both the *variance* and the *standard deviation* are based on *deviation* or *difference scores.* A deviation score represents the distance between a subject's performance and the arithmetic mean of the distribution. For example, on a 20-item test, John received a score of 5, Sue 10, and Barker 18. The mean of this distribution of scores is 11. John's deviation score is 5 − 11 or −6, Sue's deviation score is 10 − 11 or −1, and Barker's is 18 − 11 or +7.

The *sign* of a deviation score indicates whether the performance it represents is below (−) or above (+) average, that is, the mean. The size of the number or numerical portion of the deviation score indicates the distance between "average" performance and that represented by the raw score under consideration.

The *variance* of a distribution of raw scores can be computed in one of two ways: (1) directly, using difference or deviation scores or (2) indirectly, using a computational or raw score formula. The results are the same for a given set of data regardless of which of the two methods is employed.

(Formula 8-2) The variance of a distribution using deviation scores:

$$\sigma^2_x = \frac{SS_x}{n}$$

where:

σ^2_x = variance of the distribution of X scores
SS_x = the sum of the squared deviation scores
n = the number of scores going into the sum

Example: Given the scores 5, 10, and 18 with $\overline{X} = 11$

$$
\begin{aligned}
SS_x &= (5 - 11)^2 + (10 - 11)^2 + (18 - 11)^2 \\
&= (-6)^2 + (-1)^2 + (7)^2 \\
&= 36 + 1 + 49 \\
&= 86 \text{ square points} \\
\sigma^2_x &= \frac{86}{3} \\
&= 28.66 \text{ square points}
\end{aligned}
$$

It should be noted that the variance is actually an average, that is, it is the average of the sum of the squared deviation scores.

(Formula 8-3) The variance of a distribution using the computational formula or raw score formula:

$$\sigma^2_x = \frac{\Sigma X^2 - \dfrac{(\Sigma X)^2}{n}}{n}$$

where:

σ^2_x = the variance of the distribution of raw scores
ΣX^2 = the sum of the squared raw scores
$(\Sigma X)^2$ = the square of the sum of the raw scores
n = the number of scores used in the computation

Example:

X	X²
5	25
10	100
18	324
$\Sigma X = 33$	$\Sigma X^2 = 449$

$(\Sigma X)^2 = 33 \times 33$
$ = 1089$

$$
\begin{aligned}
\sigma^2_x &= \frac{449 - \dfrac{1089}{3}}{3} \\
&= \frac{449 - 363}{3} \\
&= \frac{86}{3} \\
&= 28.66 \text{ square points}
\end{aligned}
$$

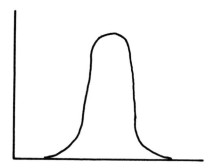

FIGURE 8-6. Polygon of a distribution of raw scores that displays little variance.

The polygon of a distribution of raw scores that displays very little variance looks bunched as in Figure 8-6 while a set that displays considerable variation is spread out as in Figure 8-7.

The variance has the following properties:

1. Adding a constant to each score in a group will not change the variance of the scores.

   Example: The variance of the scores 5, 10 and 18 is 28.66 square points.

$$
\begin{array}{ccc}
\underline{X} & \underline{C} & \underline{X+C} \\
5 & 5 & 10 \\
10 & 5 & 15 \\
\underline{18} & \underline{5} & \underline{23} \\
 & & \overline{X}_{x+c} = 16
\end{array}
$$

$$
\begin{aligned}
SS_{(x+c)} &= (10 - 16)^2 + (15 - 16)^2 + (23 - 16)^2 \\
&= (-6)^2 + (-1)^2 + (7)^2 \\
&= 36 + 1 + 49 \\
&= 86 \text{ square points}
\end{aligned}
$$

$$
\begin{aligned}
\sigma^2_{(x+c)} &= \frac{SS_{(x+c)}}{n} \\
&= \frac{86}{3} \\
&= 28.66 \text{ square points}
\end{aligned}
$$

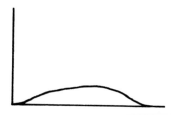

FIGURE 8-7. Polygon of a distribution of raw scores that displays considerable variation.

2. Multiplying each score by a constant makes the variance of the resulting scores equal to the constant squared times the variance.

Example: The variance of the scores 5, 10 and 18 is 28.66 square points.

X	C	XC
5	5	25
10	5	50
18	5	90

$$\overline{X}_{xc} = 55$$

$$
\begin{aligned}
SS_{xc} &= (25 - 55)^2 + (50 - 55)^2 + (90 - 55)^2 \\
&= (30)^2 + (-5)^5 + (35)^2 \\
&= 900 + 25 + 1225 \\
&= 2150 \text{ square points}
\end{aligned}
$$

$$
\begin{aligned}
\sigma^2_{xc} &= \frac{SS_{xc}}{n} \\
&= \frac{2150}{3} \\
&= 717 \text{ square points (rounded)}
\end{aligned}
$$

The variance of XC is equal to 717 square points or σ^2_x (28.66) times the constant squared $(5)^2$.

The *standard deviation* of a distribution of raw scores is simply the square root of the variance.

(*Formula 8-4*) $$\sigma_x = \sqrt{\sigma^2_x}$$

where:
σ_x = standard deviation
σ^2_x = variance

Example: The variance of the scores 5, 10 and 18 is 28.66 square points.

$$
\begin{aligned}
\sigma_x &= \sqrt{28.66 \text{ square points}} \\
&= 5.11 \text{ points}
\end{aligned}
$$

Like the variance, adding a constant to each score in a group will not change the standard deviation of the scores. The standard deviation is often useful because in many distributions it is known approximately what percent of the scores lie within one, two, or more standard deviations of the mean. For example, the researcher might know that 70 percent of the scores lie between $\overline{X} + \sigma_x$ and $\overline{X} - \sigma_x$.

It is frequently desirable to describe the position of a score in a set of scores by measuring its deviation from the mean of all scores in standard deviation units. This can be accomplished by converting the raw scores of each subject to a *standard score*. Any set of n scores with mean $\overline{X}$ and standard deviation σ_x can be transformed into a different set of scores with mean zero and standard deviation 1 so that the transformed score immediately tells one the deviation of the original score from the mean measured in standard deviation units. This is accomplished by subtracting the mean ($\overline{X}$) from the score (X) and dividing the differences by σ_x. The resulting set of scores are called Z scores.

(Formula 8-5)
$$Z = \frac{X - \overline{X}}{\sigma_x}$$

where:

Z = a standard score

X = the subject's raw score

$\overline{X}$ = the mean of the raw score distribution

σ_x = the standard deviation of the raw score distribution

Example: The mean and standard deviation of the scores 5, 10 and 18 are 11 and 5.11, respectively.

$$Z_5 = \frac{5 - 11}{5.11}$$
$$= \frac{-6}{5.11}$$
$$= -1.17$$
$$Z_{10} = \frac{10 - 11}{5.11}$$
$$= \frac{-1}{5.11}$$
$$= -0.19$$
$$Z_{18} = \frac{18 - 11}{5.11}$$
$$= \frac{7}{5.11}$$
$$= 1.36$$

The resulting Z scores are −1.17, −0.19, and +1.36.

Aside from being a convenient means for communicating the position of a subject's score, Z scores are a step toward transforming a set of raw scores to an arbitrary scale with a convenient mean and standard deviation. There are many scales of measurement (arbitrary means and standard deviations). For example, intelligence test scores are often transformed to a scale with mean 100 and standard deviation 15 or 16. Similarly, t scores with mean 50 and standard deviation 10 are used widely.

(Formula 8-6) To transform a Z score to any scale of measure:

$$\text{Transformed score} = (\sigma_{sm} Z_x) + \overline{X}_{sm}$$

where:

σ_{sm} = the desired standard deviation

Z_x = the Z score that results from $\dfrac{X - \overline{X}}{\sigma_x}$

$\overline{X}_{sm}$ = the desired mean

Example: To transform the Z score 1.36 to a t score with mean 50 and standard deviation 10:

$$t = (10)(1.36) + 50$$
$$= 13.60 + 50$$
$$= 63.60$$

The Z score is sometimes referred to as a derived score. Two additional derived scores obtained from a raw score distribution using specific arithmetic operations are *percentage scores* and *percentile ranks*. A *percentage score* is the percentage of the total number of points available that have been earned by the subject.

(Formula 8-7) To convert a raw score to a percentage score:

$$\text{Percentage score} = \frac{\text{subject's raw score on a measure}}{\text{the maximum possible raw score on the measure}} \times 100$$

That is, the percentage score is the subject's raw score on a measure divided by the maximum possible raw score on the measure times 100.

Example: A raw score of 10 on a 20-item tool is equivalent to a percentage score of:

$$\text{Percentage score} = \frac{10}{20} \times 100$$
$$= 0.50 \times 100$$
$$= 50$$

The percentage score indicates where the individual's performance is in relation to the minimum and maximum possible values on the raw score scale. The percentage score is a measure of absolute performance. That is, the percentage score obtained by one subject is completely independent of the percentage scores of all other subjects in the group. Therefore, it is a useful measure of performance in a criterion-referenced context.

The *percentile rank* of a particular raw score is the percentage of area in the histogram located to the left of the raw score in question. To determine the percentile rank:

1. Determine how many subjects obtained scores exactly equal to the subject's raw score value.
2. Divide the number obtained in Step 1 by half.
3. Count the number of subjects who obtained scores less than the subject's raw score value.
4. Add the results obtained in Steps 2 and 3.
5. Divide the result of Step 4 by the total number of scores in the distribution.
6. Multiply the resulting value by 100.

Example: Find the percentile rank of the raw score 2 in the following distribution:

<table>
<tr><td colspan="2" align="center">Distribution</td></tr>
<tr><td>*Raw Score*</td><td>*Frequency*</td></tr>
<tr><td align="center">5</td><td align="center">0</td></tr>
<tr><td align="center">4</td><td align="center">3</td></tr>
<tr><td align="center">3</td><td align="center">2</td></tr>
<tr><td align="center">2</td><td align="center">4</td></tr>
<tr><td align="center">1</td><td align="center">1</td></tr>
</table>

1. Four subjects obtained scores exactly equal to 2.
2. One half of 4 is 2.
3. Exactly one subject had a raw score less than 2.
4. Adding the results from Steps 2 and 3, 2 + 1 = 3.
5. Since there are 10 scores in the distribution, $\dfrac{3}{10} = 0.30$.
6. Multiplying 0.30 × 100 = 30, indicating 30 percent of the area of the distribution is located to the left of the raw score 2.

The percentile rank is an indicator of relative performance. The percentile rank of a subject is totally dependent upon the quality of the subject's performance as compared with the performances of the other subjects in the group. Thus, it is an excellent measure in a norm-referenced context and totally inappropriate for use with criterion-referenced measures. (A *percentile* is simply a point on the raw score continuum.)

The Xth percentile is the point or value on the raw score scale that separates the left-most X percent of the histogram area from the remainder of the graph. If a subject scored at the Xth percentile, the subject's performance was better than or equal to exactly X percent of the performances in the group.

Selected percentiles are sometimes referred to as *quartiles.* That is, the 25th percentile may be called the first quartile, the 50th percentile the second quartile, the 75th percentile the third quartile. The first, second, and third quartiles are symbolically designated as Q_1, Q_2, Q_3, respectively. Q_2 is the median of the distribution. Quartiles are useful for summarizing data because simply reporting that P_{50} is 10 and P_{25} is 15 tells the reader immediately that 50 percent of the observations are less than 10 and that 25 percent of them lie between 10 and 15. For large groups of data, knowing the quartile values may enable the reader to readily envision the entire collection of observations.

SHAPE

The more common distribution shapes are illustrated in Figure 8-8. The *normal distribution* (Fig. 8-8E) is a symmetric distribution. *Symmetric* means the left half of the distribution is a perfect mirror image of the right half. The normal curve will always be symmetric around its mean, it is *bell shaped,* begins and

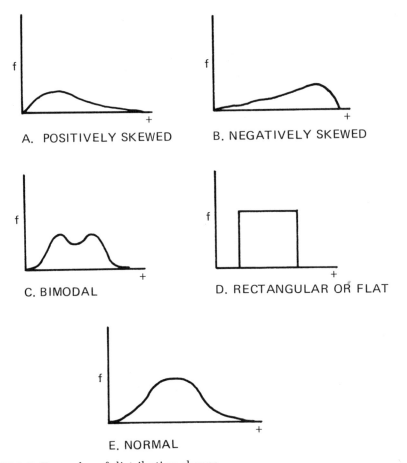

FIGURE 8-8. Examples of distribution shapes.

ends near the baseline, but never quite touches it and therefore is unbounded, meaning there is no beginning and no end. The normal curve is a mathematical construct first used as a mathematical exercise. In practice, it is used as a model for distributions that closely approximate its characteristics or would if a very large sample were used. There are many normal curves. The one most often encountered is the unit normal curve illustrated in Figure 8-9. It is a distribution of Z scores and is called the *unit normal curve* because the area under the curve is 1. Its mean and standard deviation are 0 and 1, respectively, and any other normal curve can be moved along the number scale and stretched or compressed by using a simple transformation.

It is often desirable to find the height of the curve above the Z axis for any value of Z on the unit normal curve or the area under the curve, between any two values of Z. Statistical Table 1 in the Appendix gives the area under the unit normal curve to the left of any point on the Z axis from −3.00 to +3.00. Appendix Table 1 also provides the height of the unit normal curve for values of Z from −3.00 to +3.00. Appendix Table 1 is used in the following manner.

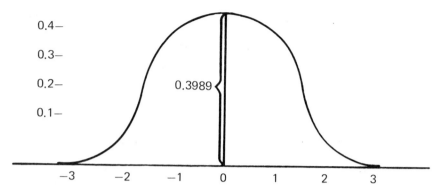

FIGURE 8-9. The unit normal curve (mean = 0, standard deviation = 1).

Example:

1. To find the area under the unit normal curve to the left of Z = −2.67. The value −2.67 is found in the first column of Appendix Table 1. To the right of this entry in the second column, title "Area," the number 0.0038 is found. Thus, 38 ten-thousandths of the area under the unit normal curve is contained to the left of Z = −2.67. The height of the unit normal curve at the point Z = −2.67 is found in the "Ordinate" column to the right of the "Area" column. For Z = −2.67, X = 0.0113.
2. Since the total area under the curve is 1, the areas (but not the ordinates) can be interpreted as proportions or percents of the total. Ninety-seven and five tenths percent of the area under the unit normal curve lies to the left of Z = 1.96.
3. To find the area under the unit normal curve between any two values of Z, (for example, between the values Z = −2.67 and Z = 2.50) first determine the area to the left of both Zs as in Step 1. The area to the left of Z = −2.67 is 0.0038 and the area to the left of Z = 2.50 is 0.0062. Therefore, the area between −2.67 and 2.50 is 0.0062 − 0.0038 = 0.0024. That is, $^2/_{10}$ percent of the area lies between these two points.

There is an infinite number of normal curves, a different one for each different pair of values for the mean and standard deviation. The most important property they have in common is the amount of the area under the curve between any two points expressed in standard deviation units. In any normal distribution approximately:

1. 68 percent of the area under the curve lies within one standard deviation of the mean either way (that is, $\overline{Z} \pm 1\sigma$).
2. 95 percent of the area under the curve lies within two σs of the mean.
3. 99.7 percent of the area under the curve lies within three σs of the mean.

It is useful if all references to normal distributions are in terms of deviations from the mean in standard deviation units. That is, when the normal curve is employed, one wants to know how many standard deviations a score lies above or below the mean. The deviation of a score from its mean is $X - \overline{X}$, the number of standard deviations X lies from its mean is $\dfrac{X - \overline{X}}{\sigma_x}$ and is called the unit normal deviate. The shape of the normal curve does not change when one subtracts the mean and divides by the standard deviation.

Example: What proportion of the area lies to the left of a score of 30 in a normal distribution with mean 35 and standard deviation of 10?

It is the proportion of the area that lies to the left of $\dfrac{(30 - 35)}{10} = -0.5$

in the unit normal distribution or from Table 1, 0.3085.

The normal distribution is important in both descriptive and inferential statistics. Discussion of the utility of the normal distribution in inferential statistics will be deferred until later. In descriptive statistics, the normal curve is an excellent approximation to the frequency distribution of a large number of observations taken on a variety of variables. For example, frequency polygons of heights of adult males and females both look quite similar to a normal curve, and psychometric tests of general and special mental abilities (e.g., IQ tests) are approximate normal distributions.

Skewness is the degree to which the frequency distribution of a group of scores is asymmetrical. In Figure 8-8, distributions A and B are skewed distributions. Note that the direction of the skewness is determined by the direction in which the tail points. Various summary statistics that measure the type and degree of asymmetry of a group of scores have been devised. The best measure of skewness, derived by Karl Pearson, is simply the average of the Z scores which have been raised to the third power.[5]

(Formula 8-8)   Skewness $= \dfrac{\Sigma Z^3}{n}$

$$= \overline{Z^3}$$

where:
  $Z^3 = Z \times Z \times Z$ for every Z score
  n = number of scores entering the sum

Distribution A in Figure 8-8 is positively skewed because its measure of skewness is positive. A positively skewed distribution has scores that extend further above the mean than the small scores extend below it. Distribution B in Figure 8-8 is negatively skewed. The value of the skewness statistic for this distribution is negative.

In a symmetric distribution, the value of the skewness statistic is zero. This is true because exact symmetry implies that one half of the distribution is a perfect mirror image of the other half. The values of the skewness statistic will range generally between -3 and $+3$. A negative value indicates that scores are clustered more to the right of the mean with most of the extreme scores to the left. A positive value indicates clustering to the left. The statistic is used to compare the relative skewness of different distributions.

Distribution C in Figure 8-8 is a bimodal distribution. Large sets of scores are often referred to as bimodal when they present a frequency polygon that looks like a Bactrian 2-humped camel's back—even though the frequencies at the two points are not equal. A distinction can be made between major and minor modes. In a group of scores, the major mode is the single score that satisfies the definition of the mode. Several minor modes may exist at points throughout the group of scores.

Figure 8-10 illustrates the relationship between the shape of a distribution of scores and the values of its measures of central tendency. In the normal distribution (A) the value of the distribution's mean, median, and mode are identical. In a positively skewed distribution (B), the mean is the largest value, then

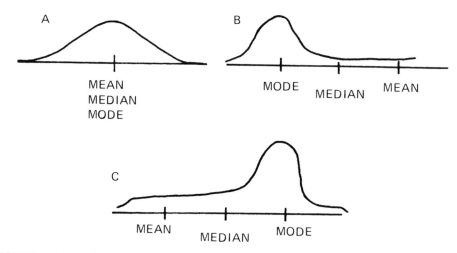

FIGURE 8-10. Relationships between the shape of a distribution of scores and the values of its measures of central tendency.

the median, and the mode is the smallest, while in a negatively skewed distribution the order is reversed (that is, mean is smallest, then median, and mode is largest).

Kurtosis refers to the peakedness of a curve. In Figure 8-11, three curves differing in peakedness are presented. Curve C is a normal curve and is used as the standard against which the kurtosis of other curves is compared. It is called *meso*kurtic, meaning intermediate. Curve A is very peaked and is called *lepto*kurtic, meaning slender. Curve B is *platy*kurtic, meaning flat or broad. Kurtosis applies only to unimodal distributions and concerns the peakedness of the curve in the vicinity of the single mode. If a distribution is bimodal, it is appropriate to talk about the kurtosis of the curve in the area of each mode. Kurtosis is measured by finding the average of the Z scores taken to the fourth power.[5]

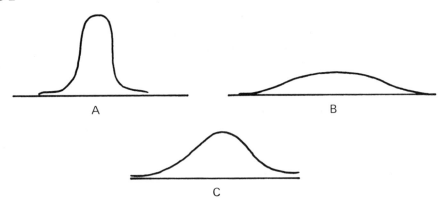

FIGURE 8-11. Examples of various degrees of kurtosis.

(Formula 8-9) $\text{Kurtosis} = \dfrac{\Sigma Z^4}{n}$

$= \overline{Z^4}$

where:
   $Z^4 = Z \times Z \times Z \times Z$ for every Z score
   n = number of scores entering the sum

The value of the kurtosis statistic for the normal curve is zero. Leptokurtic curves have positive signs and their numerical values can become quite large. Platykurtic curves have a kurtosis statistic with a negative value.

There is an inverse relationship between the variance of a distribution and its kurtosis. That is, as the variance of a distribution increases its kurtosis decreases, whereas as the variance decreases, kurtosis increases.

Summary

The initial data analysis steps undertaken by the researcher, regardless of the study design, are (1) the tabulation of data and (2) the selection and employment of appropriate summary statistics. Summary statistics allow the investigator to (1) get some indication of trends and patterns and (2) communicate information regarding the central tendency, dispersion, and shape of the score distribution. Measures of central tendency include the mean, median, and mode. In large samples the mode is a fairly stable indicator of "averageness." The median is useful for descriptive purposes with small samples. The mean is the most frequently employed because it serves as the basis for measures of dispersion and the bulk of the available inferential statistical procedures. When the mean is used as the measure of "averageness," three indices may be used to measure dispersion, (1) range, (2) variance and (3) standard deviation. The shape of a score distribution is characterized by the skewness and kurtosis statistics.

USING THE COMPUTER TO ANALYZE DATA FROM DESCRIPTIVE STUDIES

SPSS has two programs, CONDESCRIPTIVE and FREQUENCIES, each containing numerous options for obtaining basic summary statistics, that exemplify available library computer programs. CONDESCRIPTIVE provides the user with the capability of obtaining means, standard errors, standard deviations, variances, skewness, kurtosis, range, minimum, and maximum statistics for any set of variables that are continuous and approach interval level data. It also has a number of useful options, one of which permits the user to transform raw scores to standardized Z scores for any set of variables for which statistics have been requested.

TABLE 8-5. Sample Output for Summary Statistics

CONDESCRIPTIVE

Variable — Highest Education Attained

Mean	2.605	Std. Error	.086[a]		Std. Dev.	.801	
Variance	.642	Kurtosis	−.164		Skewness	−.686	
Range	3.000	Mimimum	1.000		Maximum	4.000	

Valid Observations — 86[b]   Missing Observations — 0[c]

FREQUENCIES

Variable — Highest Education Attained

Code[d]
1. *******[e] (11)[f]
   Assoc
2. ********* (18)
   Diploma
3. ************************ (51)
   Bacc
4. **** (6)
   Masters

Mean	2.605	Std. Error	.086	Median	2.775
Mode	3.000	Std. Dev.	.801	Variance	.642
Kurtosis	−.164	Skewness	−.686	Range	3.000
Minimum	1.000	Maximum	4.000		

[a]Standard error of the mean. This statistic is an estimate of the probable distance of the sample mean from the population mean. A standard error of 0.086 indicates that the researcher can assume that the population mean is 2.605 ± 0.086 with approximately 68% accuracy.
[b]Number of Ss completing this item.
[c]Number of Ss not completing the item.
[d]The way in which the data were coded: 1 = associate degree, 2 = diploma, etc.
[e]The asterisks are simply the computer's way of drawing a histogram.
[f]Number of Ss who received an associate degree.

FREQUENCIES provides one-way frequency distribution tables and summary statistics for discrete variables. A frequency distribution table or a histogram can also be obtained as an option. Summary statistics available as output from FREQUENCIES include means, standard errors, medians, modes, standard deviations, variances, kurtosis, skewness, range, minimum, and maximum. It should be noted that the summary statistics obtained with the FREQUENCIES program are the same as those obtained with CONDESCRIPTIVE with the addition of the median and the mode.

It is usually a good idea to run either CONDESCRIPTIVE or FREQUENCIES prerequisite to data analysis in any study, not just descriptive ones. The reason for this is twofold: (1) errors in transcribing or recording data may be identified by scrutinizing the output and (2) factors that may affect the findings when inferential procedures are employed may be anticipated. For example, a primary aim of most research and hence most statistical procedures is to "explain" variance. In other words, most research attempts to locate variables that may account for or explain variance in other variables, or equivalently, explain why a case is not exactly equal to the mean. In order to do this, in most instances, it is essential that variables be measured in such a way that their variance is relatively large. If the variance in the variables being examined is limited, this may preclude the ability to detect statistically significant results. Thus, the variance is an example of a summary statistic that warrants attention prior to more sophisticated data analysis.

The reader who desires specific instructions regarding the utilization of the CONDESCRIPTIVE and FREQUENCIES programs will find them in the SPSS manual.[10] Examples of SPSS output from each are presented in Table 8-5.

REFERENCES

1. Arkin, H. and Colton, R. R.: *Graphs: How To Make and Use Them.* Harper, New York, 1936.
2. Babbie, E. R.: *Survey Research Methods.* Wadsworth, Belmont, California, 1973.
3. Brinton, W. C.: *Preliminary Report by the Joint Committee on Standards of Graphic Representation.* Quarterly Publications of the American Statistical Association, 14, 1915, pp. 790–797.
4. Gibbs, C., Marin, H., and Gutierrex, M.: *Patterns of reproductive health care among the poor of San Antonio, Texas.* Am. J. Public Health 64(1):37, 1974.
5. Glass, G. V. and Stanley, J. C.: *Statistical Methods in Education and Psychology.* Prentice-Hall, Englewood Cliffs, New Jersey, 1970, pp. 28–29, 89, 91.
6. Gliebe, W.: *Faculty consensus as a socializing agent in professional education.* Nurs. Res. 26(6):428, November–December, 1977.
7. Jekel, J., Klerman, L., and Bancroft, D.: *Factors associated with rapid, subsequent pregnancies among school-age mothers.* Am. J. Public Health 63(9):769, 1973.
8. Kelley, T. L.: *Fundamentals of Statistics.* Harvard University Press, Cambridge, Mass., 1947.
9. Lindherm, B. and Cotterill, M.: *Training in induced abortion by obstetrics and gynecology residency programs.* Fam. Plann. Perspect. 10(1):24, 1978.
10. Nie, N. H., et al.: *SPSS—Statistical Packages for the Social Sciences,* ed. 2. McGraw-Hill, New York, 1975, pp. 181–202.

11. Pankratz, L. and Pankratz, D.: *Nursing autonomy and patients' rights: Development of a nursing attitude scale.* J. Health Soc. Behav. 15:211, 1974.
12. Staropoli, C. and Waltz, C.: *Developing and Evaluating Educational Programs for Health Care Providers.* F. A. Davis, Philadelphia, 1978.
13. Van Dalen, D. B. and Meyer, W. J.: *Understanding Educational Research.* McGraw-Hill, New York, 1966.
14. Volicer, B. and Burns, M.: *Preexisting Correlates of Hospital Stress.* Nurs. Res. 26(6): 408, November–December, 1977.
15. Walker, H. and Durost, W.: *Statistical Tables: Their Structure and Use.* Teachers College, Columbia University, New York, 1936.
16. Walton, L., et al.: *Development of an abortion service in a large municipal hospital.* Am. J. Public Health 64(1):77, 1974.

CHAPTER 9
EXPERIMENTAL STUDIES

An experimental research study possesses three characteristics, the combination of which differentiates it from all other types of research discussed in this book. Experimental research involves (1) a manipulation of some sort which (2) some Ss receive and some do not *and* (3) it contains a mechanism, called random assignment, for maximizing initial equality between those Ss receiving the manipulation and those not so receiving. (Actually there can be any number of different manipulations within the same study, but for ease of exposition only two will be assumed unless otherwise noted.)

The manipulation itself is called the experimental treatment or the independent variable when considered in conjunction with whatever it is being compared with (that is, no manipulation, which is called a control group, or a completely different treatment of some sort). An experimental manipulation can involve anything that the researcher can directly control. It can be a surgical procedure, a type of analgesic, or an instructional method. Its effect is studied upon something that the researcher would like to be able to directly manipulate but cannot, such as recovery rate, surcease of pain, or student learning; all of which as a class are called dependent variables.

The purpose, then, of an experimental study is for the researcher to attempt to indirectly manipulate a dependent variable by directly manipulating an independent variable. This is accomplished by dividing Ss into two groups, performing the experimental manipulation on one of the two, and measuring everyone with respect to the dependent variable. If the manipulated group differs from the other with respect to its constituents' possession of whatever attribute was represented by the dependent variable, then it may be assumed that the manipulation was effective (or detrimental, depending upon the direction of the difference) if this difference was not attributable to (1) something else intervening within the experimental environment, (2) an initial disparity

159

between the two groups on some relevant attribute, or (3) a simple chance fluctuation of scores.

None of these possibilities can ever be completely ruled out, but the probability that any particular one is true can be minimized. The first two, that some extraneous variable or initial discrepancy between groups resulted in the observed differences, may be minimized by the *design* that the researcher chooses, much as an architect or engineer designs a structure to withstand certain environmental pressures and still serve its appointed function. The likelihood of the third contingency, that the observed difference is a function of nothing more than chance, may be assessed via the inferential procedures discussed later in the chapter.

The purpose of an experimental design is to allow the researcher to answer the crucial question: "What was the effect of the experimental manipulation?" or more precisely "What effect did the manipulation of the independent variable have upon the dependent variable?" The degree to which this question can be accurately answered is known as the *internal validity* of a study, to which there are so many threats that it is never possible to completely vitiate them all. Fortunately, all are not equally threatening in all situations, hence the researcher may estimate which factors are most likely to operate in the study's particular set of circumstances and correspondingly choose a design to withstand these threats. Before considering the relative strengths and weaknesses of the more commonly used experimental designs with respect to each threat however, the most powerful tool available to the researcher in the quest for internal validity must be discussed.

RANDOM ASSIGNMENT

In order to ascertain the effect of an experimental manipulation upon a dependent variable, a comparison of some sort is necessary. As tautological as this statement sounds, the principle underlining it is not yet in the realm of common sense. Intuitively, many well educated people are quite satisfied with simply observing the effect of some phenomenon upon a single group of Ss, not realizing that a multitude of other factors could have operated concomitantly with or against the phenomenon of interest.

As an extreme example, suppose a researcher, interested in the effect of a protein supplement added to infants' diets (the independent variable) upon their subsequent weight gain (dependent variable), administered said supplement for a four-week period measuring weight gain over the interval. If the researcher documented a substantial weight increase in the Ss, the question becomes: "Can the gains be ascribed to the new dietary regimen?" Obviously not, since infants have a well known tendency to gain weight over time on any adequate diet. In order to ascertain the effect of this manipulation, as indeed with all experimental manipulations, a comparison group is needed. In this particular case, babies fed traditional diets during the same period in similar environments would probably suffice quite well *if* the babies in the comparison group could be assumed to have the same propensity to gain weight over time as the experimental infants. If this assumption were tenable, the researcher could conduct the experiment and ascertain which group of babies gained *more* weight during the four-week period. A troublesome question is, however, how can anyone be sure that two groups of infants had "the same propensity to gain weight" irrespective of the applied experimental treatment?

The answer, unfortunately, is that no one can ever be completely sure. The *best* way to increase the probability of initial comparability, however, is to allow each participant in the study an *equal* chance of being either in the experimental or the control group. This process is known as *random assignment*; its function is to protect the interpretability of an experiment (that is, increase its internal validity) by insuring comparability between groups prior to the experimental manipulation. It is accomplished in one of two ways: by simply assigning Ss to groups in such a way that no systematic bias is possible (such as by flipping a coin or rolling a die) or by using a third variable (that is, over and above the independent and dependent variables) to further insure the complete absence of bias. The former strategy is termed *simple random assignment* and the latter is termed *stratified random assignment*.

Simple Random Assignment

Simple random assignment is by far the most commonly used method of deciding which Ss will participate in which treatment in experimental research. If two groups are involved, the experimenter simply lists the available Ss prior to the study and flips a coin (allowing one side to represent one group, the reverse to represent the second group) until *half* of the Ss have been assigned to one of the two groups (which means of course that the other half will be assigned to the second group). If Ss cannot be prelisted, then the order in which they become available can be randomly assigned (for example, if Ss are to consist of the first 30 patients admitted to a hospital, then a coin can be flipped to decide to which group the first patient admitted will be assigned, which group the second will be in, and so forth until one group has 15 patients assigned to it, at which point the remaining patients are assigned to the other group). This strategy fulfills the definition (*each S had an equal chance to be assigned to each group*), and the assignment was conducted in such a way that no systematically different or biased group of Ss should have accrued to one of the groups and not the other. For more sophisticated randomization procedures involving more than two groups and large numbers of Ss, the use of tables of random numbers or computer generated random numbers can be used.

As suggested above, random assignment does not guarantee equality between groups. It is conceivable that all the brightest, healthiest, biggest, or most cooperative Ss could still be assigned to one group by chance alone. The probability of this happening is miniscule, however, especially for relatively large numbers of Ss (that is, 30 or more) and can be reduced further by a strategy known as stratified random assignment or, more simply, blocking.

Stratified Random Assignment

Stratified random assignment is almost always preferable to simple random assignment if two conditions can be met: (1) Ss must be capable of being pre-listed before the start of the experiment and (2) an additional score must be available for each on some measure that is *related* to the dependent variable. If these conditions can be met, Ss are rank ordered on the blocking variable (that is, the measure related to the dependent variable) and then randomly assigned in pairs to one of the two groups. In the original example involving infant weight gains, Ss might be rank ordered, for example, according to their chronologic ages (if it could be assumed that age in days would be related to weight gain over and above the experimental manipulation — in other words related to weight gain in both the experimental and control groups) from youngest to oldest. The two youngest babies would then be identified and a coin flipped to assign one member of the pair (or block) to the experimental treatment, the other going into the control by default. The process would then be repeated for the next two youngest Ss and so forth through the entire sample to the two oldest babies. This strategy possesses an overriding advantage to simple random assignment in that each S has an equal chance of being assigned to each group *and* the resulting two groups are *practically identical* with respect to a measure related to the dependent variable, hence tangentially almost identical on the dependent variable itself. The procedure results in matched pairs of Ss being present in both groups, and it enables the researcher to later use more precise and powerful statistical analyses. It is only effective, however, if a blocking variable can be found that is *related* to the dependent variable. If no such relationship exists, then stratified random assignment is not superior to simple random assignment and will actually be detrimental if the more powerful statistics alluded to above are employed.

Sometimes the blocking variable is not continuous, as was assumed in the infant weight example, but is dichotomous (such as sex), trichotomous, or takes on some other number of discrete values. The above procedure cannot be used in such circumstances per se, because Ss cannot be rank ordered according to scores on a variable taking on only a few discrete values. If the variable is suspected of being related to the dependent variable however, the researcher would still be wise to ensure equality between groups with respect to it, both to insure internal validity and to increase statistical power and precision (see the section on factorial ANOVA later in this chapter). Using sex as an example, this could be accomplished by identifying the males in a sample and randomly assigning them to the experimental and control groups and repeating the process for the females. This strategy would, in effect, result in four groups of Ss instead of two: (1) males assigned to the experimental group, (2) males assigned to the control group, (3) experimental females, and (4) control females. As with stratified random assignment using a continuous blocking variable, this procedure should always be applied when (1) there is *good* reason to believe that the blocking variable is related to the dependent variable and (2) there are enough Ss for each level of the blocking variable to make the process worthwhile (for example, if a sample consisted of 36 females and only four males, assigning two males to the experimental group and two to the control would accomplish very little). Also as with stratified random assignment using a continuous blocking variable, the procedure will be no better than simple random assignment if the chosen variable is not related to the dependent variable (and will also result in a statistical penalty). It has the advantage, however, of not requiring prelisting. Ss can be assigned to groups as they become available if the researcher has some idea of the relative frequencies of the attributes in the general population from which the sample is drawn.

Matching. These stratified random assignment procedures should in no way be confused with nonrandomly matching Ss, a strategy often used in educational and psychologic research several decades ago in which the researcher *started* with an intact group whose members had been designated to receive the experimental manipulation. A "comparable" group was then identified and a S as similar as possible to each experimental S was found to serve in the control condition. Although possessing intuitive appeal, matching possesses a fatal flaw even when it can be assumed that two groups have been equated on one variable. There exists such a multitude of parameters upon which individuals can differ that to choose only one and leave all the others completely uncontrolled is really relatively ludicrous. Intact groups, in fact, are almost never chosen randomly, they are usually selected *because* they can be more conveniently enlisted for the experimental treatment for some reason, and it is often this very reason that guarantees that they are different in some systematic way from other groups. Even when this is not true, there is no way to minimize the risk of nonequated groups comparable to random assignment simply because of the experimenter's ignorance concerning possibly confounding differences between Ss. Because of this ignorance, and because of the very real possibility of unconsciously systematically selecting different Ss into groups if done personally, random assignment of some form is a prerequisite to true experimental research. No compromises are accepted, mainly because no good ones are known, partly because none are necessary.

Many variations upon the random assignment theme exist, such as alphabetizing a list of names and allowing the first half of the list to be in one group, the second half in another, or selecting every other person admitted to a hospital to be members of one group. Strategies such as these, however, possess potential sources of bias and hence should not be used, especially given the fact that if the experimenter possesses the power to assign Ss on one of these bases, he also possesses the power to randomly assign Ss. In those rare cases (rare in research, unfortunately not so rare in evaluation) in which a researcher does not possess the power to randomly assign Ss, the researcher might be well advised to choose another topic to study. If the researcher decides not to take this course, then one of the quasi-experimental designs that affords the best possible chance to achieve some degree of internal validity should be chosen.

INTERNAL VALIDITY

Campbell and Stanley[2] in their classic *Experimental and Quasi-Experimental Designs for Research* list "eight different classes of extraneous variables . . .

(which) if not controlled in the experimental design, might produce effects confounded with the effect of the experimental stimulus." Most of them are controlled to some extent by what the authors refer to as "true experimental designs" (that is, designs that permit the random assignment of Ss to groups); some are controlled only in the sense that *false positive results* are precluded. *False negative results*, not really addressed by Campbell and Stanley, are quite troublesome and require special care on the part of the researcher over and above choosing an appropriate design. Strategies for their control will be discussed under the appropriate class of extraneous variable before the different experimental and quasi-experimental designs are presented. Seven of Campbell and Stanley's eight classes of extraneous variables are discussed below.

1. *History*, which is defined as events occurring during the course of the experiment over and above the experimental manipulation, owes its prevalence to the fact that the world does not come to a halt during an experiment. Relevant to the present definition are historical events that are capable of *influencing performance on the dependent variable* in lieu of, in conjunction with, or in opposition to, the independent variable. An example might be a television special dealing with alcoholism broadcast during a week-long experiment designed to ascertain whether or not an instructional unit could influence attitudes toward alcoholics. If no comparison group existed, and if the television special were quite effective, the experimenter might conclude that the observed positive shift in attitudes resulted from the experimental treatment when in reality it may have resulted from Ss watching the television special. A randomly assigned control group would negate this possible occurrence, since Ss receiving and not receiving the experimental manipulation would be equally likely to have viewed, hence profited, from the television special.

A randomly assigned control group would not, however, protect the experiment from a false negative result. It is possible, for example, that the television special might contain similar elements to the instructional unit, elements that were effective in changing attitudes. In other words, deterioration or contamination of the independent variable would occur; thus, if no difference existed between groups following the experimental manipulation, the failure might not be due to a deficiency in the experimental manipulation but directly due to the intervention of a historical variable without which a difference would have occurred.

2. *Maturation*, which Campbell and Stanley defined as "processes within the respondents operating as a function of the passage of time *per se*," (p. 5) is a very similar type of phenomenon to history (and could be subsumed thereunder). An obvious example is growing older, which was operative in the example involving infants' weight gains used above. Special cognizance of developmental changes in Ss must be taken in longitudinal studies, but equal attention should be paid to less obvious types of maturation in shorter term studies involving testing at different times during the day or under different conditions, where Ss may be relatively more fatigued, distracted, or bored.

Again, the use of a randomly assigned control group negates the possibility that one group of Ss may have registered different scores on the dependent variable because of greater developmental changes, fatigue, and so forth, but it does not negate the possibility that differences might have accrued if such factors had not existed. As with historical variables, the best insurance against false negative results lies in (1) being aware of the existence of possible extraneous variables, (2) mitigating their influence whenever possible, and and (3) completing the experiment in as short a time as possible, commensurate of course with the objectives of the experiment.

3. *Testing*, which is defined as "the effects of taking a test upon the scores of a second testing" (p. 5), operates only when Ss are measured more than once during the course of an experiment and then usually only for tests with items possessing right or wrong answers such as learning assessments, intelligence tests, and to a lesser extent certain personality measures (those which have responses possessing varying degrees of acceptability). What normally happens in these cases is that Ss learn from taking the test the first time. How this occurs is not precisely known, but it may accrue from recognizing and remembering errors made the first time, interacting with other test takers, and possibly even "looking up" answers. Ss can sometimes improve their scores as much as a half standard deviation by these methods, comprising a considerable gain which, in the absence of a control group, might be incorrectly attributed to the experimental treatment.

Testing as an extraneous variable is still not as potentially damaging to the internal validity of a study as are history and maturation because (1) the effect is usually quite small when it occurs, (2) does not normally occur with many tests used in nursing research (for example, physiologic and attitudinal measures), and (3) can be completely avoided by not employing multiple testing of the same Ss. When the latter option is not feasible, a good control group (which is, of course, tested the same number of times as the experimental group) does protect against false positive results, and, since the probable effect is so small, the possibility of false negative results is not a major concern.

4. *Instrumentation*, defined as changes in the ways numbers are assigned to a dependent variable (or as changes in the scorers themselves), is also a relatively easy extraneous variable to control. An appropriate control group again protects against false positive results *if* it is run concomitantly with the experimental group and *if* individuals administering or scoring the dependent variable are not aware which Ss are in which groups. This latter point is critical: scorers should never be aware of the group memberships of their tests or observations. When names are recognizable, they should be covered in some way and experimental and control Ss' tests or observations mixed together with identifying marks placed on the back. For other types of measures not so easily disguised (such as blood pressures), naive research assistants should be recruited. The same principles hold for the administration of the independent variable. Whenever possible, the experimenter should be ignorant of the experimental purposes, design, and group membership of Ss (such as in double blind procedures in medical research). When this is not possible, rigid standardized procedures and protocols should be instituted to guard against potential unconscious biases on the part of the experimenter(s).

Instrumentation effects can occur in many ways, most of which are avoidable. Scorers can, for example, become more expert (or less conscientious) with practice, hence possibly assigning different scores to similar performances across time. Whatever the causes, the phenomenon can be mitigated by (1) making the scoring of the dependent variable as standardized as possible thus relying as little as possible on scorer judgments, (2) giving scorers as much practice as possible before actually working with experimental data (which also permits the identification and replacement of low aptitude scorers), (3) scoring all measures at the same time when feasible (for example, after the completion of the study) and, when not feasible, by having some measures rescored at different intervals (even if it necessitates video- or audiotaping) to ascertain and measure shifts in instrumentation, (4) employing the same scorers throughout the course of an experiment, and (5) documenting similarities and differences among scorers by having some tests scored by the same people.

Instrumentation is usually not a serious concern simply because most dependent variables permit relatively objective scoring. There is practically no danger of instrumentation in a 50-item multiple choice test for example, nor is there much danger with most physiologic measures containing well defined protocols, such as the taking of blood pressure or body temperature. The use of such measures as interviews, behavioral observations, and open-ended questionnaires do carry a certain amount of risk in this regard however, and extreme caution must be exercised in their use.

5. *Statistical regression*, defined as the tendency for Ss scoring at the extremes of a distribution to exhibit less extreme scores upon retesting, is operative only when Ss are selected for an experiment *because* they have exhibited extremely high or extremely low scores. It is perhaps the least obvious of all extraneous threats to internal validity, and it is completely vitiated through the use of a randomly assigned control group.

Statistical regression as a threat to internal validity owes its genesis to the fact that all scores on all dependent variables have an error component that is usually normally distributed. This error can be made up of many constituents: imperfections in the test, errors in scoring, fatigue or illness among certain Ss, environmental contamination such as noise, and so forth. Over the long run, however, this error can be considered randomly distributed because as many Ss will receive scores higher than they deserved (positive error) as Ss who will receive scores lower than they should (negative error).

When Ss are selected according to the criteria of having scored extremely high or extremely low on a measure however, error for these particular Ss can no longer be assumed to be normally distributed. If a test is administered to 100 Ss and the 10 highest scorers are selected to be tested again, their scores will be slightly lower the second time because relatively more positive than negative error was associated with their first score. Since error is assumed to be random, there is no reason to believe that their second score will contain more positive than negative error; hence, their overall scores will have a tendency to go down. The opposite would be true if the 10 lowest scores were selected for retesting.

At first glance neither the relevancy nor the veracity of this discussion may be apparent. Why would a researcher choose the sample on the basis of extreme scores and, even if the researcher did, why should this sample really be expected to score systematically differently the second time they were tested? In the first place, medical and nursing research are replete with examples of researchers focusing attention upon high or low scoring Ss, basically because doctors and nurses deal with sick as opposed to healthy people—people with high blood pressures as opposed to normal blood pressures, with high or low blood sugar levels as opposed to normal ones, and so forth. As for the *why* of the regression phenomenon, consider a situation in which an experimenter wished to ascertain the effectiveness of a yoga exercise upon the lowering of blood pressure. To obtain a sample of Ss with slightly higher blood pressures than normal, 200 undergraduates were tested and the 20 with the highest blood pressures were selected to participate in the evaluation.

Many, perhaps most, of these twenty Ss may actually have possessed chronically high blood pressure. A few, however, normally may have had no such condition but simply possessed high blood pressure at the particular moment it was measured for a number of reasons: one may have been late for class and forced to run up three flights of steps, one may have been under considerable tension because of an impending exam, one's blood pressure may have simply been recorded incorrectly by a harried research assistant, and so forth. Now certainly, it is also possible that some of these Ss may normally have possessed higher blood pressures than actually recorded on that particular day but, everything else being equal, the former condition is far more likely for these 20 Ss. If the researcher had no control group, then upon noting that more of the 20 Ss exhibited lower blood pressures the second time they were tested than the first (for example, the late student would probably not have to run up stairs this time, the tense student may have already taken the exam, the incorrectly recorded student's proper blood pressure was recorded the second time) the researcher would incorrectly conclude that the exercise regimen was solely responsible. If, on the other hand, the experimenter had assigned 10 of the 20 Ss to a control group, then the regression phenomenon would have affected both groups equally and would have been no threat to internal validity. If Ss are not selected on the basis of extreme scores, no regression artifact exists: as many scores go up as go down the second testing. This is even true when the Ss selected tend to have higher average scores for independent reasons; the regression artifact operates only when Ss are selected *because* of their extreme scores and even then it can be largely avoided if all Ss are measured twice and only Ss scoring very high or very low on *both* administrations are selected.

6. *Selection*, defined as a tendency for certain types of Ss with attributes related to performance on the dependent variable to be more likely to be present in one experimental group than another, is operative only when available Ss are not randomly assigned to treatments, and is therefore the chief advantage of random assignment. An extreme example of differential selection into treatments would be permitting Ss to choose which group they would rather be in, a strategy that would obviously result in unequated groups with respect to motivation if nothing else. A more likely contingency would be a strategy such as selecting the first 20 Ss to show up (or be admitted) to represent one treatment, the last 20 the second. This would of course most likely result in a bias of some

sort with the first group being more motivated, more desperate, less busy, or differing on any number of extraneous variables. The entire discussion concerning the advantages of random assignment is germane here, and there is simply no truly acceptable alternative to it because of the possibility of this selection artifact. If the researcher and the research consumer cannot have confidence in the original equality of treatment groups, then certainly no confidence can be had in the effects of the experimental manipulation.

7. *Differential experimental mortality,* defined here as a differential loss of Ss from treatment groups during the course of an experiment, can be the most troublesome of the potential threats to internal validity so far discussed. It can occur in several ways. In the first place, if Ss are assigned, even randomly assigned, to treatments before they are actually available, extremely high mortality rates can accrue. For example, 20 presurgical patients could be randomly selected from a larger pool to participate in presurgical education sessions and 20 Ss randomly selected to receive no instruction, with the effectiveness of the experimental manipulation being assessed by postoperative recovery rates. If only 10 of the experimental Ss were actually able (or willing) to attend the instructional sessions however, these 10 more healthy (or more apprehensive) Ss could hardly be veridically compared with all 20 controls of whom nothing was required. Faced with such a situation, a conservative but safe approach might be to compare all 20 experimental Ss with the 20 control Ss, even though only half of the former actually received instruction.[2]

Situations exist in which, even though all Ss are available at the beginning of an experiment and begin receiving the experimental treatment, so much more is required of experimental than control Ss (or one treatment is so much more palatable than the other), that differential mortality still occurs and a final measure is not obtained. Very little can be done about this phenomenon from a design perspective. About the only option open to the researcher is to document the loss, list it among the study's weaknesses, and let the readers draw their own conclusions. If additional data are available on Ss, the dropouts can be compared with nondropouts to describe the former's characteristics and possibly estimate how they might have scored on the dependent variable if they had remained in the study but, again, once differential mortality occurs there is very little the researcher can do.

Although there are no sure ways to either control or avoid differential mortality, the best preventive measures are to: (1) make all treatments as palatable as possible, (2) make all treatments as comparable as possible with respect to demands placed upon Ss, (3) impress upon Ss the importance of completing the study once started, suggesting that they not participate if they are not sure they will be able to compete the protocol, and (4) take every ethical action possible to persuade Ss not to drop out if they give indications of planning to do so. The final two suggestions, while often effective, can unfortunately be counterproductive by reminding Ss that they are participating in an experiment and thus produce atypical behavior, which when confounded with the experimental treatment, can result in a completely different outcome than would have occurred if Ss were unaware of what was going on. Since the primary purpose of an experiment is to assess the effect of an independent variable upon a dependent variable, such an occurrence would obviously serve as a source of experimental invalidity.

Although by no means the only threats to internal validity that can occur in the conduct of experimental research, the preceding seven classes of extraneous variables are probably the most common. Internal validity, it will be remembered, was defined as the degree to which the effect of the manipulation of the independent variable upon the dependent variable could be accurately ascertained. Methodologists have defined an entirely different category of experimental validity with attendant threats thereto. This category, called the *external validity* of experiments, is defined as the extent to which the results of an experiment can be generalized to different Ss, populations, settings, treatments, experimenters, and even dependent variables.

EXTERNAL VALIDITY

External validity is thus exclusively concerned with generalizability and in some ways it is not as absolute as internal validity. Most researchers have a general idea of the "universe" to which they are interested in generalizing their results as well as settings to which they do not aspire to generalize. The end effect, however, of the experimenter not being able to generalize an effect to a universe because of some source of external invalidity is the same as that of not being able to attribute that effect solely to the manipulation of an independent variable because of some source of internal invalidity: the goals of the study have not been fulfilled; the time, effort, and resources expended have been wasted.

In many ways, then, the dichotomization of experimental validity into external and internal sources is largely artificial. They could just as easily be viewed as being on a continuum in which extraneous variables threatening internal validity are dealt with first, chiefly because they are more easily controlled via experimental design than are many of the factors limiting external validity. Similarly, if a study does not possess acceptable internal validity then a consideration of how far the experimental results can be generalized is irrelevant, simply because invalid results should not be generalized. For present purposes, however, the appearance of this dichotomy will be preserved and it will be assumed, in subsequent discussions of external validity of experiments, that their internal validity has been preserved. For a more detailed discussion of external validity issues, the reader is urged to consult Glass and Bracht's[7] classic article, upon which much of this section is based.

Population Validity

As Kempthorne[11] has noted, the experimenter must normally generalize twice. The results must be generalized from the actual sample employed in the study to the population that was available when the sample was drawn, and then the results must be generalized from the available population to the target population, a most hazardous leap.

The first generalization is basically no problem *if* the experimenter has the patience and the resources to randomly sample* Ss from all those available and if the sample is of appreciable size. Unfortunately, experimental researchers seldom bother to define their available populations, and when they do, seldom bother to extend it by giving as many people as possible an opportunity to participate. A much more common practice is to simply decide approximately how many Ss are needed and then ask as many people as necessary to fill that quota. By so doing, even the opportunity to be able to generalize to all Ss who would be willing and able to participate has been squandered. A far better practice is to define the original accessible population as broadly as possible and then randomly select as many Ss as needed. If working in more than one hospital, for example, is truly not feasible, the next best option would be to randomly select one available hospital and then randomly select as many available patients as needed within it. Even if limited to only one hospital (such as the one in which the researcher is employed), the researcher should still attempt to randomly select Ss within that one hospital. Simply "grabbing" Ss as they become available, although often completely unavoidable, will quite likely result in a biased sample that is dissimilar from both the target and the accessible populations on some important attribute.

If the results cannot be generalized from the sample to an accessible population, they obviously cannot be generalized from the latter to the population that is of primary interest to the researcher. Even if the researcher does have a sample representative of Ss willing to participate in the experiment in the care of *cooperative* physicians affiliated with *liberal* hospitals, for example, it is often impossible to insure that the reactions of such patients will be similar to those of uncooperative patients (who may be more ill than their counterparts), under the care of uncooperative physicians (who may be using a different treatment plan), affiliated with unfriendly hospitals (which may have greater staff problems). About the best a researcher can do is to carefully examine the characteristics and attributes of the Ss and attempt to at least be aware of outstanding differences between them and the typical Ss to whom the generalization is desired.

This discussion is not intended to make the reader unduly pessimistic. Generally speaking, generalization of experimental effects is not as problematic as generalization of descriptive data. In the latter case, the researcher must assume that, say, a mean of 4.3 on a Likert scale is numerically close to the mean that would have been obtained if the entire target population had been tested, an assumption which necessitates random sampling of some sort. In experimental research, the researcher must only assume that the effect that an experimental manipulation had upon a sample will also occur when the manipulation is performed upon other Ss. In other words, even if the sample significant-

---

*Note again that the random selection of Ss is independent from their random assignment to treatments following selection. Random selection is relevant only to generalizing to a population and has no relevance to internal validity; random assignment is relevant only to enabling the attribution of an effect to the independent variable and does not insure generalizability to a population in the absence of random sampling.

ly differs from the target population with respect to several important variables, the study will still have external validity *if* the experimental manipulation would have a similar effect upon both groups. Fortunately, external validity of experimental research is usually considered relatively robust; the experimental researcher is given the benefit of the doubt and effects are normally assumed generalizable unless some outstanding feature of a study directly questions the reasonableness of said assumption.

The same is true of the second aspect of population validity that must be considered. Ignoring questions regarding the comparability of the experimental sample and the target population, another question remains: did the experimental effect accrue similarly for all subsets of the studied sample? To clarify, suppose the experimental treatment was superior to the control overall. Further suppose that it was also superior for, say, females in the experimental group as compared with females in the control. One would expect the same relationship to hold for the males in the study; if it did not, then the results would not have external validity with respect to all subgroups in the sample and hence probably the population.* This would be especially critical if (1) the order of the effect were reversed, meaning that the experimental treatment was efficacious for certain types of Ss and *detrimental* for others, and (2) if the accessible population happened to systematically differ from the target population with respect to the variable defining the subgroup in question, meaning that the treatment might work for the accessible sample but *not* the target population if the two groups had different constituencies. Fortunately, actual occurrences of this class of phenomenon, called aptitude by treatment interactions, are *extremely* rare. Their potential importance, however, makes a little a posteriori sifting of data worthwhile, especially in research involving manipulations with potentially serious consequences.

Ecologic Validity

While the burden of proof may rest upon critics of an experiment's external population validity, the burden of maximizing the type of external validity dealing with the "environment" in which an experiment is conducted rests squarely with the experimental researcher. First and foremost of these responsibilities is the operational definition of both independent and dependent variables in clear and explicit terms. It is a rarity indeed when said variables, especially independent variables, are defined in sufficient detail for another researcher to replicate an experiment.

Over and above exact replication, however, lies the assumption on the part

---

*A special caution is in order here. Ss in a sample can be broken down in so many ways that it is often possible to identify certain subgroups for which an effect was present and certain for which it was absent. Normally, only subgroups for whom there is some a priori reason to suspect that an experimental effect would be reversed *and* which contain sufficiently large numbers of Ss to make for meaningful comparisons are considered.

of both the researcher and the consumer that the effects can be replicated not only by employing different samples but also by employing similar but not identical procedures. Finding that an instructional unit delivered in a particular area changed relevant attitudes, for example, might be heralded with great enthusiasm by experts in that area, enthusiasm which would be greatly dampened if it were found that said instruction had to be repeated word for word and could never be altered to fit different audiences and changing circumstances in order to be effective. Furthermore, if it were found that these attitudinal changes could be demonstrated only on one set of items, the results of the originally heralded breakthrough would be considered completely trivial and ignored. Obviously, research is expected to generalize further than this; how far, however, can never be completely determined until an actual replication with the appropriate changes incorporated is attempted. *Replication is the final arbiter of all external validity questions.* Far more replications of important nursing research results should be attempted than presently are. In lieu thereof, the only course for guessing how far a given set of results will generalize is just that: *guessing,* aided perhaps by a thorough knowledge of, and experience in, the area in question.

Another aspect of the experimental environment often overlooked by beginning researchers accrues from the obtrusive nature of much experimental research. One example of the problems entailed with Ss knowing that they are participants in a study is a phenomenon known as the *Hawthorne effect.* It consists of a tendency for Ss to behave differently *because* they recognize themselves as participants in a study. There is a reported tendency, for example, for terminally ill patients to be especially cooperative with researchers, perhaps because of an altruistic hope that the results of the experiment will aid future patients, perhaps simply because of a value for personal, normalized interaction with someone other than family or treatment staff. Whatever the reason, it is possible that such Ss may "try" harder than their control counterparts (since it is often more difficult to wax enthusiastic over an unimaginative control treatment), hence resulting in an effect which would not have accrued if Ss had not been aware that an experiment was taking place. Remediation of this artifact is obvious: either disguise the fact that an experiment is being conducted (which is being made increasingly difficult by ethics legislation requiring informed consent on the part of all experimental participants) or use creative control treatments that are as appealing and *credible* to Ss as the experimental treatments.

In a similar vein, researchers themselves should be most careful to prevent communicating their enthusiasm for the experimental treatment. As suggested for avoiding instrumentation effects, the best tact is to employ naive research assistants when possible, rigid operationalized procedures when not. Hopefully, at this stage, the reader is beginning to note the convergence of external versus internal validation concepts. As mentioned above, they are not natural dichotomies but more descriptive of a continuum in which the center boundaries are more than a little blurred. A study in which an experimental effect was aided and abetted by a Hawthorne effect, for example, is certainly not generalizable to a setting in which Ss are more accustomed to novel disruptions; hence, the study is externally invalid. By the same token, the problem could be conceptualized from an internal validity framework, since an extraneous variable worked in concert with (or in lieu of) the experimental manipulation, thus denying the attribution of the accruing effect solely to the independent variable. The same conceptual blurring is also apparent in the last classification of external validity threat, pretest sensitization.

Pretest Sensitization

This phenomenon, like the Hawthorne effect, has seldom been empirically documented and then only with certain types of attitudinal measures. As its name implies, it accrues only when (1) Ss are pretested, and (2) the taking of this pretest sensitizes them to the experimental manipulation that follows. It is probably safe to say that pretest sensitization need be considered only in extreme cases in which the pretest itself is likely to "tip participants off" with respect to socially desirable answers. The present authors noted a trend toward such an effect in a study designed to measure the effectiveness of Swine Flu propaganda by the administration of an attitudinal instrument immediately following instruction. Half of the Ss had been pretested with the same instrument, half had been administered a different type of questionnaire containing only factual items. The randomly selected Ss receiving the attitudinal pretest manifested a definite tendency to respond more favorably after instruction than the Ss not receiving the pretest. Unfortunately, there was no control group in this experiment so it may well be that the observed tendency was simply a function of the testing artifact discussed in the internal validity section (that is, a tendency for Ss to register higher, or more socially acceptable, scores on a second testing). If this study had possessed a control group not receiving instruction in which half of the Ss had been pretested and half not, and if the pretested control Ss had not registered a trend toward superior attitudes to the nonpretested control Ss, then the results would have had to be explained as a function of the pretest differently affecting experimental Ss (since control Ss were not affected at all). Exactly why such a phenomenon would occur is difficult to explain, one possible explanation is that some Ss may have a tendency to miss the "point" of a presentation, hence not be affected by it. A pretest, on the other hand, could serve to underline or tip this type of purpose off to the presentation's underlying theme, hence giving Ss a chance to be affected by the independent variable.

When operative, studies in which pretest sensitization has occurred cannot be generalized to settings in which no pretest is present. For this reason, the phenomenon is listed under factors affecting external validity. It could just as easily be conceptualized as a situation in which an extraneous variable worked in concert with the experimental manipulation, denying the attribution of an effect solely to that manipulation. However viewed, pretest sensitization is not a prevalent phenomenon. To the authors' knowledge, it has not been documented in an important study in the last 10 years and it is definitely not a substantive threat with physiologic or cognitive (as opposed to affective) measures.

EXPERIMENTAL DESIGNS

Since there is no good way to estimate the likelihood of any particular threat to internal or external validity being operative, good researchers usually assume that if something can go wrong it will (Murphy's Law). Given this masochistic propensity, the only course open then is to design their studies as tightly as possible to vitiate as many rival hypotheses as possible. No matter how carefully a study is designed, however, rival hypotheses are always present. No matter how carefully a study is executed, human error always creeps in. A perfect crime is far more common than a perfect experiment, thus to categorize some designs as "true" and hence acceptable and others as "quasi-" and hence something less than acceptable makes very little sense in the real world. It is far more reasonable to visualize different types of designs as overlapping bands on a continuum in which results obtained from well planned, well executed quasi-experimental designs can possess far more credibility than those accruing from poorly designed and executed experimental designs.

True Experimental Designs

As stated earlier, experimental research involves four elements: (1) a manipulation that (2) some Ss receive and some do not, the identity of whom is (3) randomly decided, followed by some form of (4) measurement. In subsequent discussions concerning design, emphasis will be placed upon the random assignment of Ss to groups (item 3) for it is this mechanism or characteristic that differentiates variables that can serve as manipulations or treatments and variables that are primarily correlational in nature: any groups to which Ss *can* be randomly assigned *could* function as the independent variable in an experimental study; any groups to which Ss cannot be so assigned (for example, sex, age, race, religion, health status, and so forth) cannot serve as an experimental manipulation, only as a correlational variable. Random assignment to groups assumes further importance due to the fact that although it is most definitely fallible, especially for small numbers of Ss, it is by far the least fallible method available for insuring initial equality between groups.

An experimental study, therefore, involves the randomized assignment of Ss to groups that differ with respect to their treatment at the hands of a researcher. This treatment must be a priori operationally defined, and the various groups must differ *only* with respect to this treatment. If said groups differ in some superfluous respect in addition to the treatment, then changes in the dependent variable must be attributed to both the treatment *and* these superfluous differences. If no changes are observed between groups with respect to the dependent variable, then this lack of effect may be attributed to *either* (1) the impotence of the experimental manipulation *or* (2) the confounding effect of the superfluous variables. Obviously, therefore, random assignment and an experimental manipulation are not sufficient conditions for credible experimental research; they must be combined in a design that excludes the operation of superfluous or extraneous variables.

POST-TEST ONLY, PRETEST/POST-TEST, AND SOLOMON FOUR-GROUP DESIGNS

The *post-test only design*, presented schematically in Figure 9-1, combines the basic elements that must be present before a study can be labeled *experimental*. A published example of this type of design is presented in Example 9-1.

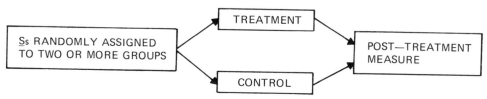

FIGURE 9-1. Post-test only design.

EXAMPLE 9-1. Published Example of a Post-Test Only Design

Title: *Effect of free time the day prior to mastery testing on nursing students' scores.*

Source: Dean, Nursing Research, vol. 28, no. 1, January–February, 1979, pp. 40–42.

Purpose: To determine if mastery test score averages of students who had a seven-hour hospital laboratory experience the day preceding the test (i.e., using a mastery criterion) were significantly different from scores of students who did not attend class on the day prior to testing.

Design: Students were randomly selected to serve in either the experimental group (n = 43) or the control group (n = 36). The only difference between the two conditions entailed the scheduling of a seven-hour laboratory experience the day prior to testing for the experimental Ss.

Results: t-Tests indicated no significant difference between groups with respect to mastery test scores.

Interpretation: The lack of significant difference in test means may support the nursing faculty's belief that mastery learning required sufficient comprehension and retention of information, so that timing of test administration did not appreciably affect student scores.

It should be kept in mind that this figure is only representative of the skeleton of a study, there is far more to the conduct of experimental research than these basic elements. As simple as this design is, it is the basis for all experimental research. All other designs are variants of it, such as the *pretest/post-test design*, in which Ss are measured prior to the experimental treatment on the same test (broadly defined) as they are following treatment. This design is shown in Figure 9-2 and a published example is presented in Example 9-2.

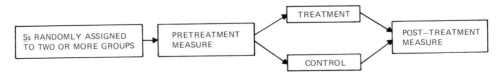

FIGURE 9-2. Pretest/post-test design.

EXAMPLE 9-2. Published Example of a Pretest/Post-Test Design

Title:	*Topical application of insulin in decubitus ulcers.*
Source:	Gerber and Van Ort, Nursing Research, vol. 28, no. 1, January–February, 1979, pp. 16–19.
Purpose:	To ascertain the effectiveness of insulin in the healing of decubitus ulcers.
Procedure:	Twenty-nine Ss were randomly assigned to experimental and control conditions. The experimental group received insulin therapy, the control group received any non-insulin therapy which was determined by physicians or nursing home standards. All Ss were suffering from decubitus ulcers, all ulcers were measured each day for the 15 days during which the study was conducted. The dependent variable consisted of changes in the size of the ulcers between the seventh and fifteenth days as well as of days to complete healing for those Ss whose ulcer surface areas went to zero. (In this study, therefore, the pre- and post-tests consisted of measures of the surface areas of decubitus ulcers).
Analysis:	One-way analysis of variance was computed for both the seventh and the fifteenth day ulcer sizes.
Results:	No significant differences were found in healing rate between those patients receiving insulin therapy and those receiving more conventional treatment.
Interpretation:	Although the experimental group registered numerically faster healing rates, no statistical significances were observed. The study indicated that insulin therapy could be safely administered, but "the observed clinical effectiveness of insulin therapy was not supported by this study."

In fact, an experimental design can even contain both Ss who did and did not receive pretreatment measurement, although this option necessitates the utilization of four groups (and is called the *Solomon four-group design* after its originator). This design is shown in Figure 9-3 and a published example is presented in Example 9-3.

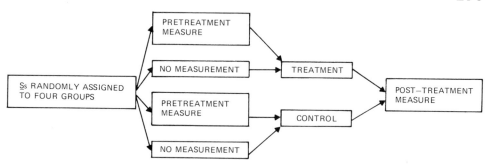

FIGURE 9-3. Solomon four-group design.

EXAMPLE 9-3. Published Example of a Solomon Four-Group Design

Title:	*Impact of a management-oriented course on knowledge and leadership skills exhibited by baccalaureate nursing students.*
Source:	Brock, Nursing Research, vol. 27, no. 4, July–August, 1978, pp. 217–221.
Purpose:	To evaluate the effectiveness of a management course taught to baccalaureate nursing students.
Procedure:	1. 80 Ss were randomly assigned to four groups. Groups I and II were officially enrolled in the management course, Groups III and IV were tested only and hence served as controls.
	2. Groups I and III were administered a knowledge pretest, Groups II and IV were not to control for pretest sensitization.
	3. All Ss were administered the knowledge post-test as well as a clinical evaluation some time after the course's completion.
Analysis:	1. A 2×2 ANOVA was conducted to test both the effect of pretesting and the effect of the course.
	2. A one-way ANOVA was used to ascertain whether or not the experimental treatment affected clinical evaluation ratings.
Results:	1. No effect was observed for taking the pretest alone (i.e., Groups I + III = II + IV.
	2. Students in the experimental group learned significantly more than students not taking the experimental course.
	3. Students taking the management course performed significantly better on the clinical evaluation tool than students not taking the course.
Interpretation:	A management-oriented course administered to undergraduate baccalaureate nursing students can result in increased knowledge and management/leadership behaviors.

The only difference between the post-test only design and the pretest/post-test design resides in the use of a pretreatment measure (referred to as a pretest) conceptualized as identical or equivalent (for example, an alternate form, see Chapter 4) to the post-treatment measure (that is, the dependent variable). There are both advantages and disadvantages to the use of a pretest. The disadvantages are: (1) its administration can be time consuming and expensive, depending upon the nature of the test and the characteristics of the sample, and (2) its use can feed the pretest sensitization threat to external validity, especially in situations involving socially acceptable attitudinal responses, hence restricting external generalizability to pretested populations, a rare phenomenon. Given the rarity with which pretest sensitization has been documented, however, the advantages of pretest use often outweigh its disadvantages. The advantages are: (1) the use of a pretest serves as a check upon the success of randomization with regard to the initial equalization of groups, and (2) the presence of a pretest permits the use of far more powerful statistical procedures, which greatly maximizes the chances of an experiment achieving its primary objective, (that is, rejecting the null hypothesis). Fortunately, alternatives to the pretest exist that allow the researcher to reap these advantages and completely avoid both of the above-mentioned disadvantages since there are occasions when the use of a pretest is most obviously not feasible, as when: (1) it is difficult or impossible to administer (for example, in a study of emergency room patients, or one in which the nature of the dependent variable precludes a meaningful premeasure, such as recovery time or postoperative medications), (2) pretest sensitization is a plausible possibility, or (3) the use of a pretest maximizes the artificiality of the experimental environment, thus maximizing the chances of creating some sort of Hawthorne effect (as with studies of very short duration, those in which nothing is asked of the control group, or in which control Ss are asked to perform a task totally irrelevant to the focus of the dependent variable).

The alternative to using the same measure twice in an experiment consists of collecting additional information about Ss prior to the experiment, information that is likely to be related to their performance on the dependent variable. As an example, suppose it were desirable to study the relative effects of two anesthetics upon postoperative recovery rates. Obviously a preoperative recovery rate could not be obtained, hence the concept of a pre-experimental measure is irrelevant. (Of the three designs presented so far, the post-test only design would be the only real alternative.) Suppose, however, that the total sample of patients to which the experimenter had access was relatively restricted; hence, the experimenter feared that random assignment might result in slightly uneven groups with respect to initial differential recovery propensities. The use of the post-test only design precludes both the initial detection of such a discrepancy and its subsequent *statistical correction* via the covariance procedures discussed later in this chapter, as well as the taking advantage of the incremental statistical power accruing from the use of more powerful statistical procedures.

POST-TEST WITH COVARIATE DESIGN

The pretest/post-test and Solomon four-group designs are indeed quite often not feasible, but it is almost always possible to obtain a pre-experimental measure that is *related* to the dependent variable. When the identity of the entire sample cannot be ascertained ahead of time (as when Ss are randomly assigned to treatments as they become available), then a variation of the pretest/post-test design must be used. One such variation, the *post-test with covariate design*, is presented in Figure 9-4 and Example 9-4.

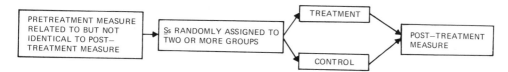

FIGURE 9-4. Post-test with covariate design.

EXAMPLE 9-4. Example of a Post-Test with Covariate Design

Title:	An experimental study of psychomotor skill learning of a nursing procedure using two methods of critique in instruction.
Source:	Harrison, O. A. Unpublished doctoral dissertation, University of Colorado, Boulder, Colorado, 1972.
Purpose:	To determine the relative effectivenesses of two forms of critique (self versus externally administered) with respect to the changing of sterile dressings.
Design:	Although both the effects of anxiety level and setting were also observed, the basic design consisted of randomly assigning Ss to two types of critiques while using scholastic aptitude as a covariate. The experimental critique procedure involved self-critique, observing a videotape, and practice in the use of a procedural checklist. The control critique procedure involved the verbal use of the checklist procedure by nursing graduate students.
Results:	All Ss were subsequently rated on their performance following the experimental manipulation. No significant differences were obtained.
Interpretation:	The nonsignificance between the methods could be attributed to a number of factors including the possibility that surgical asepsis is not a unitary domain, as it was treated in the study.

To the extent that the pretreatment measure is related to the dependent variable, this design can add a great deal of experimental precision and statistical power to a study.

When the entire sample can be prelisted and randomly assigned, however, additional initial information can be utilized even more effectively. The post-test with covariate design is amenable to statistical correction if indeed initial discrepancies result from the random assignment, but statistical correction does have certain drawbacks: it is obviously better to avoid the need for correction if at all possible. Fortunately, two methods do exist that *guarantee* equality between groups on a particular dimension when it is possible to obtain an appropriate pretreatment measure of some sort; these are discussed below.

RANDOMIZED BLOCK POST-TEST DESIGN

This simply entails rank ordering the entire sample with respect to the Ss' relative standings on some relevant information and randomly assigning matched Ss to the various treatments. If preoperative prognosis ratings had been obtained for the example used above, all 30 Ss could be ordered with respect to that variable. The two with the best prognoses could then be identified with one being randomly assigned (for example, via a coin flip) to the experimental group, one to the control. The process would then be repeated with the next two best prognoses and so forth until the entire sample of 30 had been randomly assigned as matched pairs. What would result, therefore, would be two groups practically *identical* with respect to rated prognosis. This genre of design is called *randomized block post-test design* and is presented in Figure 9-5 and Example 9-5.

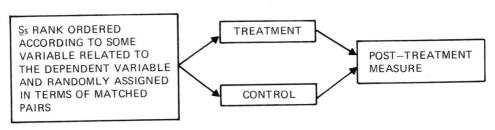

FIGURE 9-5. Randomized block post-test design.

EXAMPLE 9-5. Published Example of a Randomized Block Post-Test Design

Title:	*Psychological preparation of surgical patients.*
Source:	Schmitt and Woodridge, Nursing Research, vol. 22, no. 2, March–April, 1973, pp. 108–116.
Purpose:	To determine the effect of extra preparation for surgery upon patients' participation in treatment, their tension and anxiety level, and their postoperative recovery.
Design:	Fifty patients who were admitted to a VA Hospital for elective surgery were matched according to surgical procedure and "level of threat." From each matched pair of patients, one was randomly assigned to the experimental group, one to the control. The experimental group participated in carefully planned group discussions involving their surgery plus some individualized attention. The control Ss received only the usual hospital routine.

EXAMPLE 9-5. *Continued*

Results: Major differences were observed between the two groups: experimental Ss reported sleeping better, experiencing less anxiety as surgery approached (although no difference existed the night prior to surgery), and remembered surgical events as being less painful. Furthermore, experimental Ss registered shorter anesthesia duration, less urinary retention and difficulty voiding, and less elevation in blood pressure. Experimental Ss registered less medication intake on the second and third postsurgical days, returned to a regular diet sooner, and required less time to leave the hospital than Ss not receiving preoperative surgical preparation.

Interpretation: Giving the patient initial support and some skills to work with made him better able to cope effectively with the crisis of surgery. The results of this study indicate that the most effective nursing may be the most efficient as well, thus belying the belief that psychologic preparation for surgery is too time consuming for its potential benefits.

FACTORIAL POST-TEST DESIGN

A second strategy used with a discrete variable such as sex or socioeconomic class (high, upper-middle, lower-middle, low) is to randomly assign Ss within each discrete level of the variable to treatments. All males, for example, could be identified with half being randomly assigned to the experimental group, half to the control and the process being repeated for females. The strategy is very similar to the randomized block design discussed above in the sense that the groups' equality with respect to at least one variable (sex in the present case) is *assured*. This type of design is called a *factorial post-test design* and is presented in Figure 9-6 and Example 9-6.

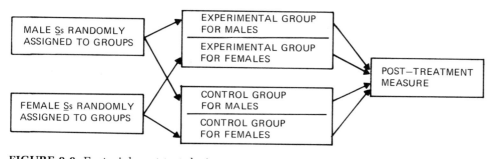

FIGURE 9-6. Factorial post-test design.

EXAMPLE 9-6. Published Example of a Factorial Post-Test Design

Title: *The effect of nursing interaction on patients in pain.*

Source: Diers et al., Nursing Research, vol. 21, no. 5, September–October, 1972, pp. 419–427.

EXAMPLE 9-6. *Continued*

Purpose:	To study the relative effectivenesses of three types of nursing interaction upon relief of pain.
Design:	Ss who complained of pain to a staff nurse were randomly assigned to one of three treatment groups. In Group A, patients were viewed as feeling, thinking, and doing persons, and the nurse tried to maintain approximately even distributions of her verbal behavior across all three dimensions. In Group B, the patient was considered a thinking and doing person with the nurse interacting accordingly. In Group C, interaction concentrated upon the doing dimension. *The study was conducted three times by three different nurses using different patients in each study.*
Analysis:	The main analysis consisted of a 3 (type of interaction) × 3 (study) analysis of variance conducted upon pulse and respiration changes for both an initial and a long-range relief period. Chi-squares were performed on nonverbal behavior and verbal statements.
Results:	Significant differences for nursing approach occurred for the initial period with respect to pulse changes, but not for the long-range period. The direction of the effect was not as predicted, however, with Group B registering higher pulse rates than either A or C. No effect was observed for type of interaction on respiration changes. Group A was generally superior to the other groups with respect to nonverbal behaviors and verbal statements.
Interpretation:	Both the use of replication (i.e., the three studies employing three different nurses) and the use of the three interaction categories seemed to offer methodologic rigor to the test of the effect of nursing. Taken individually or together, the three studies offer some support for the hypothesis (i.e., that the interaction employed in Group A would result in a significant decrease in pain as compared with Group B, which in turn would be superior to C). But there is enough variation among the studies in samples used, nursing approaches applied, and results to make interpretation and conclusions confusing.

Both the randomized block post-test and factorial post-test designs are variations of the pretest/post-test design. They are therefore subject to the same strengths and weaknesses with the considerable added advantage that they do insure greater internal validity to the extent that either the blocking variable (prerated prognosis) or the independent variable (sex) is related to the dependent variable. The randomized block post-test design, in fact, often results in the most powerful and precise tests of the null hypothesis available.

Before proceeding to other designs, two common sources of confusion should probably be discussed at this point. Researchers often question: (1) whether or not the factorial post-test design is truly experimental since one variable (sex in the present case) was not randomly assigned to treatments, and (2) whether or not a true experiment can exist without a control group. The answer to both of these questions is *yes*. The factorial post-test design described above is a true experimental design with respect to the type of anesthetic used and a correlational study with regard to sex. Secondly, as long as there are two or more randomly assigned groups of some sort that differ from one another in some way, then the conditions for experimental research have been met. A control group in the classic sense (that is, one receiving either nothing or a placebo) is often not feasible. Ss may need anesthetics of some sort, for example, or alternatively patients must receive treatment, negating the comparison of an innovative treatment to no treatment at all. Usually in these cases a novel drug or treatment is compared with a more standard one; hence, the researcher often visualizes the conventional treatment as the control group when in reality one treatment is being compared with another (or several others).

Pre-Experimental Designs

Since all the designs presented above are conceptually similar with the exception of their use of a premeasure, perhaps the most logical way of discussing exactly which threats to internal validity are and are not controlled via their use is to contrast the post-test only design with some less successful approximations containing either (1) no control, or (2) a nonrandomly assigned control, also called a nonequivalent control group, (Fig. 9-7 and Examples 9-7 and 9-8).

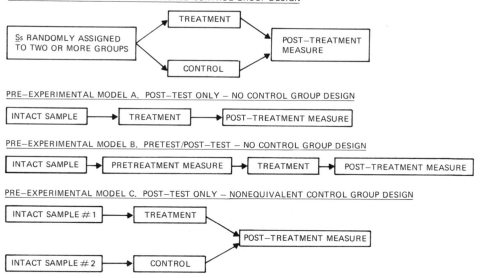

POST–TEST ONLY – RANDOMLY ASSIGNED CONTROL GROUP DESIGN

PRE–EXPERIMENTAL MODEL A. POST–TEST ONLY – NO CONTROL GROUP DESIGN

PRE–EXPERIMENTAL MODEL B. PRETEST/POST–TEST – NO CONTROL GROUP DESIGN

PRE–EXPERIMENTAL MODEL C. POST–TEST ONLY – NONEQUIVALENT CONTROL GROUP DESIGN

FIGURE 9-7. Post-test only – randomly assigned control group design and three pre-experimental models.

EXAMPLE 9-7. Published Example of a Pretest/Post-Test – No Control Group Design

Title: *Teaching strategies: A microteaching project for nurses in Virginia.*

Source: Crosby, Nursing Research, vol. 26, no. 2, March – April, 1977, pp. 144 – 147.

EXAMPLE 9-7. *Continued*

Purpose: To see whether or not ratings obtained by student-teachers for their
                lecture and group discussion performances in a microteaching proj-
                ect changed during the course of the project.

Design: Fifty-seven student-teachers were rated by five graduate students
                with respect to their performances in lecture and group discussion
                experiences three times during the course of a microteaching
                project.

Analysis: Two repeated measures analyses of variance were performed, one
                on lecture performance, one on group discussion performance at the
                beginning, middle, and end of the project.

Results: Large and significant behavioral changes were observed as a func-
                tion of time for both lecture and group discussion experiences.

Interpretation: The results indicate that microteaching, in conjunction with video-
                tape recording and immediate feedback and critique, provides a via-
                ble framework for facilitating positive change in teaching behavior.

EXAMPLE 9-8. Published Example of a Post-Test Only–Nonequivalent Control
Group Design

Title: *Increasing nurses' person-centeredness.*

Source: Wallston et al., Nursing Research, vol. 27, no. 3, May–June, 1978,
                pp. 156–159.

Purpose: 1. To assess the degree to which professional nurses respond effec-
                tively to patients.

                2. To determine whether a minimal intervention could increase
                nurses' effectiveness.

Design: Two samples of medical or surgical nurses drawn from different
                populations were asked to respond verbally to 24 patient statements
                in what they perceived as a helpful manner. The first group (n = 24)
                was simply so tested at two different times using 12 statements dur-
                ing the first testing, 12 others during the second. The second group
                (n = 20), in addition to the same testing schedule was administered
                a 450-word statement with suggestions and examples for increasing
                the helpfulness of their responses.

Analysis: Summary statistics were computed to address purpose 1 above; t-
                tests were computed both within samples and between samples to
                assess the effectiveness of the intervention.

Results: Significant changes were found between first and second testing for
                the group receiving the intervention but not the control group. Simi-
                larly, no difference was found between groups with respect to the
                first testing but the group receiving the intervention was more help-
                ful following the intervention than the control group.

EXAMPLE 9-8. *Continued*

Interpretation: Although not actually countertherapeutic, room was found for improvement after the first testing for both groups with respect to increasing nurses' person-centeredness. The brief intervention was judged effective for improving same.

POST-TEST ONLY – NO CONTROL GROUP DESIGN

The first pre-experimental alternative (the post-test only – no control group design) is not really a research design as such, but is very often (perhaps unconsciously) used as a basis for making causal inferences. Teachers, for example, even teachers of nursing research designs often use the results of an examination to infer how much or how little their students learned from a course. Such an inference is really based on data collected from Model A in Figure 9-7, in which instruction in the course is the treatment and the course exam is conceptualized as the post-treatment measure. Now although inferences based upon such a model are probably better founded than inferences made without the benefit of any data at all, there are serious logical and practical pitfalls that should be recognized.

Regardless of whether the hypothetical research students scored high or low on the exam, it is very difficult to ascertain to what these scores may be attributed without benefit of either a pretest or a comparison group. It may be, for example, that the students learned nothing at all from the course (even though they may have registered perfect exam scores) but came into the learning environment with the same amount of knowledge with which they left. Alternatively, it may be that their scores were as high as could be expected (although they may have missed most of the items) given their lack of preparation, previous experience, aptitude, and so forth. In research, a comparison of some sort is absolutely essential, but again this is not to say that Model A is worthless; usually a comparison group of some sort exists if the researcher is creative or persistent enough to ferret it out (for example, previous semesters' exam results after ascertaining similarities or differences between previous and present students prior to the course or with more standardized measures, or other students' scores registered under similar conditions). A study employing no comparison group whatever is the weakest possible type of research, but even here it is probably too strong to suggest that such a study would be better left unconducted. It can at least serve as a basis for refining the dependent variable or perhaps later serve as a comparison group in another study. It is the present authors' experience, however, that a comparison group of some sort is almost always obtainable, even if it is of the genre described in Model B of Figure 9-7.

PRETEST/POST-TEST – NO CONTROL GROUP DESIGN

Pre-experimental Model B (the pretest/post-test – no control group design) is probably the second weakest on the continuum of research designs, but it has several substantive advantages over the post-test only – no control group model in the sense that Ss' post-test scores can at least be compared with their pretest scores to measure gains occurring during the experimental interval. If gains do occur they may be attributable to any number of factors in addition to the treatment, such as:

1. History. The most obvious weakness inherent in this design is that something could have intervened between pre- and post-tests *in addition to* the treatment. In the case of the hypothetical research course, Ss could have learned certain concepts in other courses, on their own, or through exposure from other sources such as the media. A randomly assigned control group not receiving instruction would have been exposed to these same stimuli, hence preventing false positive results (the experimental group would have to gain *more* than the control group before anything could be inferred about instruction).

2. Maturation. If the pretest was given at a different time of day than the post-test, or at a less stressful time of the semester, then differences between pre- and post-test could be a function of these differences rather than the instruction. In this particular example, if extremely large gains were registered, then maturation as a rival hypothesis would lose some of its plausibility, at least as far as explaining *all* learning gains was concerned. There are situations in nursing research, however, in which maturation as a threat to the internal validity of the pre-experimental models must be taken very seriously. Suppose a medication's effect upon coughing needed to be ascertained with number of coughs in a 5-minute interval serving as the dependent variable and pretest. Following the initial observational period, further suppose that the medication (treatment) was administered for a 2-day period followed by a second 5-minute observational period. A dramatic reduction in frequency of coughs between the two "tests" might be indicative of medication effectiveness, but it might just as easily be a function of natural remission of common cold symptoms over time. A randomly assigned control could differentiate the effect if both groups were tested under the same conditions at the same time.

3. Testing. This particular design is especially sensitive to the testing artifact. Given that "practice effects" exist for many types of tests, a randomly assigned control is especially helpful in negating the effect of this common phenomenon: both groups can be expected to benefit equally from taking the pretest, hence experimental versus control differences may be attributed to the treatment alone. Again it should be emphasized that testing as a threat to internal validity is not relevant for all kinds of tests (for example, one would not expect a patient to cough more during the second observation solely as a function of being observed previously) and usually is a relatively small effect when it is operative (hence cannot be used to solely explain major differences between pre- and post-tests).

4. Instrumentation. This also remains uncontrolled in this design and may

be remedied by (a) the addition of an equivalent control group (at least insofar as data collectors are not aware of group identity and to the extent that experimental and control Ss are tested under identical conditions), and (b) by simply being very careful with respect to collecting data (for example, using rigidly defined operational procedures). Instrumentation effects can sometimes be especially pernicious because they often go undetected, hence giving the impression of an effect (either positive or negative) when none existed. In this regard, the use of a randomly assigned control group is especially helpful since said effects should predominate equally between groups, hence at least guarding against false positive results.

5. Regression. This is operative only if Ss within the one existing group are selected on the basis of their extreme scores on the dependent variable. When this occurs, the pretest/post-test – no control group model is far and away the most vulnerable design. If Ss are selected on the basis of extreme scores (as they are quite often in nursing research) a randomly assigned control group is almost essential in order to measure changes between pre- and post-tests attributable to treatment effects *over and above* those that will surely accrue as a function of regression toward the mean. Regression, too, can be a pernicious artifact in the sense that it is possible for a researcher who selects an intact available group to be unaware that these Ss may constitute an extreme group (with respect to the dependent variable) for some reason. This eventuality can be avoided when the researcher has the luxury of randomly selecting from a normally distributed population, an option that unfortunately is relatively rare. Fortunately, regression effects are usually small, and can be a priori estimated under certain conditions.

6. Selection. This is a very definite source of invalidity in this design simply because the researcher is likely to study Ss who are readily available: Ss who are more likely to register pre- to post-test changes due to enthusiasm, a desire to please, a Hawthorne effect, and so forth, than randomly sampled Ss from a general population unfamiliar with the experimenter. A randomly assigned control group at least insures that the same types of people with the same propensities will be measured across time with and without benefit of the treatment, although again care should be taken even here to minimize Ss' awareness of treatment-control differences.

7. Mortality. If mortality occurs, it is a serious threat to the validity of any study, but it is especially fatal in a one group model. It is extremely rare to end an experiment with the same number of Ss with which it was begun, and it is quite plausible to assume that Ss who dropped out along the way are different in some way from Ss who remained (for example, they might have been less motivated, more ill, and so forth). Some researchers attempt to "solve" this problem by demonstrating that dropouts were similar to those who persevered along certain dimensions, but by using this tact they mislead the research consumer. What must be demonstrated in order to totally discount the importance of substantial numbers of drop-

outs is that the Ss who left would not have *changed* more or less than those who remained and this, of course, is rather difficult to document without both a pre- and post-treatment measure on both groups of Ss. A randomly assigned control group can mitigate this problem *if* the mortality is not differential. If more Ss remain in the study in one group than the other, then the pretest/post-test design unfortunately does very little to address the problem. Actually, prevention is about the only cure for differential experimental mortality, and as discussed above, is best effected by requiring as much of control as experimental Ss.

Although many problems are entailed with Model B, it has certain advantages over designs employing nonequivalent control groups with no pretest. In the absence of both random assignment and a pretreatment measure, there is no truly adequate way to insure initial equivalence between groups, hence no way to know exactly to what post-treatment differences (or lack thereof) can be attributed. Pretreatment matching of groups on some measure other than the dependent variable in no way insures equivalence on the latter (in fact, pretreatment matching, when not accompanied by random assignment, on the dependent variable itself is not especially effective since Ss' performances on a post-test are normally only moderately correlated with their performances on a pretest), hence the design really gives less information in many ways than the single group pretest/post-test design. It is subject to most of the same threats to internal validity (with the exception of testing, and possibly instrumentation if care is exercised), but does not yield the gross pretest/post-test measure of gain inherent in the latter.

The reader should definitely not interpret this discussion of the relative weaknesses of these two pre-experimental models as indicative of total worthlessness. They are almost always better than no study at all, and often circumstances permit a reasonable degree of confidence in results accruing from their use (at least from an internal validity perspective). As an example, it is possible that although students may not have been randomly assigned to sections of the same nursing course, enough confidence could be had in their equivalency to give practically as much credence to their use in Model C of Figure 9-7 as in the true experimental design employing random assignment, especially if (1) other measures indicated no disparity between groups (for example, GPA, other standardized scores, and so forth), and (2) reasons for enrolling in one particular section as opposed to the other were ascertained to insure no known selection bias was present. By the same token, a one group pretest/post-test design might be quite adequate if (1) the experimenter had a good understanding of historical factors operating through the course of the study, (2) mortality was not a problem, and (3) the effect, if present, was too great to be explained solely in terms of artifacts such as regression or testing. The point, however, is that even though a certain amount of confidence is possible in results accruing from these rudimentary designs under certain circumstances, there are so many rival hypotheses possible that designs capable of controlling more extraneous factors are usually mandatory.

Quasi-Experimental Designs

There are of course situations in which true experimental designs are simply not feasible. Fortunately, alternative procedures exist that are superior to the three pre-experimental designs just discussed and can result in almost equal credence to the experimental designs themselves. These designs are often called *quasi-experimental designs*.

NONEQUIVALENT PRETEST/POST-TEST CONTROL GROUP DESIGN

The most rudimentary quasi-experimental design, the nonequivalent pretest/post-test control group design (Fig. 9-8 and Example 9-9) constitutes a major improvement over both the pre-experimental models presented above in the sense that initial equivalence or nonequivalence of the involved groups (with respect to the dependent variable) can be documented.

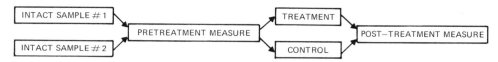

FIGURE 9-8. Quasi-experimental–nonequivalent pretest/post-test control group design.

EXAMPLE 9-9. Published Example of a Nonequivalent Pretest/Post-Test Control Group Design

Title	*Cognitive and affective consequences of formative evaluation in graduate nursing students.*
Source:	Huckabay, Nursing Research, vol. 27, no. 3, May–June, 1978, pp. 190–194.
Purpose:	Although the study had a dual purpose, the one relevant to the present design involved the implementation of a formative evaluation strategy to determine its effect upon affective behaviors of graduate nursing students.
Design:	Two samples of students were employed. One group of 25 graduate nursing students was enrolled in the first quarter and taught by means of formative evaluation using a mastery strategy. The second group of 32 students enrolled in the next quarter was taught by a conventional lecture-discussion technique.
Analysis:	The hypothesis that the group taught by formative evaluation methods would demonstrate affective behaviors significantly more than the group taught by lecture-discussion techniques was tested using a t statistic.
Results:	The hypothesis was supported with the innovative teaching technique apparently being associated with more positive affective behaviors.

EXAMPLE 9-9. *Continued*

Interpretation: Nursing students enrolled in a teaching strategy that implemented
                  formative evaluative techniques both learned significantly more and
                  exhibited more positive affective behaviors. The results are seen as
                  supportive of various educational theories.

There are, of course, exactly three possibilities with respect to how Groups 1
and 2 compare on the pretreatment measure. The experimental group may be
superior to the control group, in which case little credence can be placed in
either a positive effect or no effect as far as the post-treatment measure is concerned. The control group may be superior to the experimental, in which case
little credence can be placed in either a negative effect or no effect. Both groups
may truly be equivalent initially, in which case post-treatment differences can
be taken far more seriously. There are two basic problems with using a pretest
for establishing original equivalence or nonequivalence of intact groups: one
occurs when the pretest indicates an original discrepancy, the other occurs
even when none is indicated.

When two groups differ initially with respect to the premeasure, there is
very little that can be done about the problem other than to select two new
groups. Since this is usually not possible given the amount of preparation necessary to accomplish even the simplest experiments, researchers usually simply ignore the problem, compute gain scores by subtracting each S's pretest
score from that S's post-test score, and go on to compare gain scores between
the two groups. The fallacy in this procedure lies, of course, in the assumption
that Ss initially achieving different scores have an equal propensity to register
gains over time. They usually do not. From a measurement perspective, Ss
scoring near the low end of a distribution have a greater potential of improving
their scores than Ss scoring near the maximum possible on a test. The former
have "more room" to improve than the latter and hence, if nothing else is operative, are more likely to register positive gains. Sometimes the reverse is true,
however, with low scoring Ss having a *lower* probability of registering positive
gains than their high scoring counterparts (for example, low IQ children are
less likely to learn as much as a result of preoperative instruction than are children of higher intelligence). The point is that if two groups differ initially on an
attribute it *cannot* be assumed that they have equal propensities to register
gains on that attribute.

The second problem with using a premeasure to document initial equivalency or nonequivalence of intact groups ironically arises even when the two
groups do not differ initially. It must be remembered that initial equivalence on
a test score is not the issue, initial equivalence with respect to propensity for
gain is. Knowledge of a person's score on a pretest normally explains considerably less than 35 percent of the variance in that person's post-treatment score,
hence establishing equivalence on the former is only a small part of the task of
documenting overall equality.

The nonequivalent pretest/post-test control group design, though the weakest of the quasi-experimental designs that will be discussed in this chapter, can
nevertheless constitute an extremely useful strategy to the extent that selection

biases can be discredited (or at least discounted as the sole determinant of an effect). To the extent that this is possible, then, the nonequivalent pretest/post-test control group design is subject to the same strengths and limitations as its true experimental counterpart. As was true for that design, other information can be successfully substituted for the pretest per se, as long as these additional variables are equally good predictors of post-treatment performance.

TIME SERIES ANALYSIS

There are occasions when even a nonequivalent control group is not available. If it is possible to observe Ss over a period of time and record their behavior (or otherwise collect relevant data on them) periodically, then it is often possible to perform a relatively credible study involving one group of Ss. This genre of design is called *time series analysis,* and the chief criteria for its use are that (1) the testing (or observational) procedure not be excessively obtrusive, (2) a practice effect not exist for the measure (since if the testing artifact were present Ss might soon reach a ceiling effect on most tests), and (3) the treatment effect must be relatively transitory. There are many types of both independent and dependent variables that meet these criteria. Many illnesses, for example, are chronic and as such are never cured per se (for example, diabetes, high blood pressure, and so forth). Situations such as this are often quite appropriate for time series designs because by definition all treatments are relatively transitory and the physiologic measures used to assess symptoms are relatively nonreactive. Many other examples abound, however, such as the use of behavioral observations as dependent variables, and the manipulation of patient behavior itself (for example, compliance with treatment regimens), a most intractable and transitory variable.

Given a dependent and an independent variable meeting this criteria, however, the actual mechanics of a time series design are quite simple. There are as many variations as there are research settings, but the basic components of the design consist of a series of baselines of two or more observations on a single sample of Ss followed by the introduction of the experimental manipulation (Figure 9-9 and Example 9-10). The number of observations (measures), treatments, and intervals in between are determined by practical considerations.

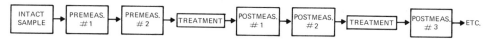

FIGURE 9-9. Time series design.

EXAMPLE 9-10. Published Example of a Time Series Design

Title: *The application and methodological implications of behavior modification in nursing research.*

Source: O'Neil, in Batey (ed.): *Communicating Nursing Research: The Many Sources of Nursing Knowledge.* Western Interstate Commission for Higher Education, Boulder, Colorado, 1972, pp. 179–191.

EXAMPLE 9-10. *Continued*

Purpose: To see if behavior modification techniques could be effectively used
                      with cerebral palsied children (especially those who display spas-
                      ticity) in the treatment of various motor problems.

Design: A single 5-year old female S with right spastic hemiparesis was
                      employed in a multiple-baseline design in order to measure the
                      effectiveness of three types of reinforcement: social, material, and
                      edible. Baseline data during 42 sessions were recorded with respect
                      to four behaviors: scooting, pulling up to a kneeling position, pull-
                      ing up to a standing position, and walking while holding to support.
                      In sessions 43 to 60 a spoonful of ice cream was given each time the S
                      successfully pulled up to a kneeling position; in sessions 61 to 75
                      when she pulled up to her feet; in 76 to 90 when taking supported
                      steps. In sessions 91 to 160 the ice cream was used as a reinforcer for
                      walking with crutch support; in sessions 161 to 180 for crutch walk-
                      ing; in 181 to 210 reinforcement was given for scooting *instead* of
                      crutch walking to see if a reversal would occur. From sessions 210 to
                      225 edible and social reinforcements were reinstated; in 226 to 240
                      edible reinforcement was replaced by social reinforcement.

Results: Edible reinforcement proved 100 percent effective for all behaviors
                      to which it was applied. When it was reversed to reinforce another
                      behavior, performance declined in the nonreinforced behavior and
                      increased in the newly reinforced one. When reinstated, behavior
                      level returned to 100 percent. Once established, the behavior (walk-
                      ing with crutch) could be maintained by social reinforcement alone.

Interpretation: Results support the efficacy of edible reinforcement and indicate
                      that some of the motor problems associated with cerebral palsy
                      which are of organic origin can come, at least in part, under the con-
                      trol of environmental events.

At first glance this particular design may resemble the single group pre-
test/post-test design to some degree, and it does share many attributes with that
model. The time series design, however, addresses many of the more serious
weaknesses of its predecessor, at least on an intuitive level. Let us examine the
differences between the two designs with respect to the way in which the various threats to internal validity are addressed.

1. History. This was largely uncontrolled in the pretest/post-test – no control
   group design in which the experimental manipulation followed a single
   administration of the premeasure (or a single observation or test of some
   kind). In a time series design, however, history is not a plausible threat *if*
   pre- to post-test gains are observed *each* time the treatment is administered and *if* similar gains are *not* observed between consecutive testings
   when the treatment is not present. Figure 9-10 indicates two of the many
   possible results that could occur from this model.

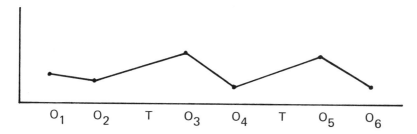

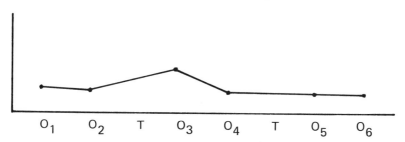

FIGURE 9-10. Examples of possible results of a time series design, where O indicates a measurement or test of some sort and T represents the treatment.

Beginning with the first graph, the task becomes the explanation of the jump in performance between Observations 2 and 3. Now certainly it might have occurred solely as a function of some extraneous historical variable that just happened to operate at the particular point in time at which the experimental manipulation was introduced. The fact that the same thing happened again at exactly the time the treatment was introduced the second time (that is, between O_4 and O_5) and not at O_2, O_4, and O_6, however, begins to strain the plausibility of history as a confounding variable. If, on the other hand, the results depicted by the second graph had occurred, then history as a rival hypothesis would have a good deal of credibility given the necessity of explaining why the treatment worked at one time and not another. It should be emphasized that just because the treatment "worked" twice in the study represented by the first graph in no way proves that it was the independent variable and not a historical one of some sort that was responsible for the effect (some extraneous occurrence *could have* happened twice at those particular instances), it is just that most people would find less difficulty in believing in the potence of the treatment instead. Certainly, a randomly assigned control group would still be preferable in order to completely rule out the possibility of an extraneous variable being responsible for the effects, but in lieu of that, a properly conducted time series design can yield quite credible results.

2. Maturation. Although a very serious threat in the one group pretest/post-test design, maturation is not especially problematic in the time series design. There is no conceivable reason why Ss should differentially mature during the intervals in which the experimental manipulations are introduced and not at other times. Suppose, for example, that Ss were growing increasingly weaker as a function of the natural history of their disease. Completely disregarding the existence of experimental treatments, this situation might be graphed as shown in Figure 9-11.

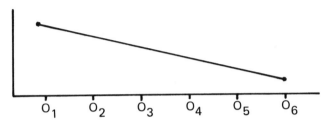

FIGURE 9-11. Example of possible effect of maturation in a time series design (see text for discussion).

If the treatment were viable, however, its introduction might alter the situation as shown in Figure 9-12.

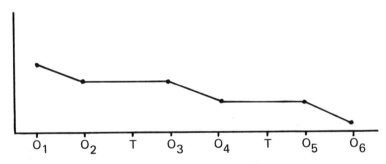

FIGURE 9-12. Example of possible effect of viable treatment on maturation in a time series design (see text for discussion).

In other words, the introduction of the independent variable arrested the decline (maturation) each time it was introduced.

3. Testing. This should not be operative in this design since one of the criteria for its use in the first place was the utilization of a dependent measure immune to the artifact's effect. If a miscalculation occurred, however, most time series designs should be impervious to its effect (as long as a ceiling effect did not occur) for the same reason that maturation was "controlled" (that is, there is no reason why the testing artifact should operate more strongly immediately following an experimental manipulation than before).

4. Instrumentation. This is not normally a problem in a time series design with respect to false positive results as long as the observer does not know when the treatment has occurred. (For example, why should the

problem surface each time the treatment is introduced and not at other times?) Given the number of measurements necessary in this design, however, the probability that an instrumentation problem may occur is greater than in other designs and, as in all research, unreliability in the manner in which scores are assigned Ss can completely invalidate even the most carefully conceived study.

5. Regression. This is essentially not a relevant consideration even if the intact group were selected on the basis of extreme scores on the dependent variable because the bulk of the regression effect would occur between O_1 and O_2, hence dissipating itself before the introduction of the treatment. The chief problem with regression in this particular design is the possibility that it could mask a real treatment effect (Fig. 9-13).

POSITIVE REGRESSION EFFECT PRESENT – VIABLE TREATMENT

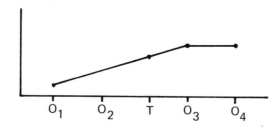

POSITIVE REGRESSION EFFECT PRESENT – IMPOTENT TREATMENT

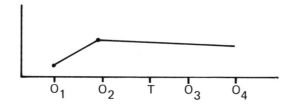

NEGATIVE REGRESSION EFFECT PRESENT – VIABLE TREATMENT

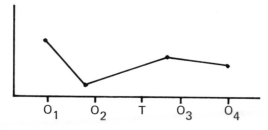

FIGURE 9-13. Examples of ways in which regression could mask the treatment effect in a time series design (see text for discussion).

6. Selection. As a threat to internal validity, selection usually refers to systematic biases between groups. In the present case, only one group is present.
7. Mortality. This is potentially a more serious concern in this design than in the single group pretest/post-test design simply because Ss are normally followed for longer periods of time. The introduction of multiple testing sessions and multiple interventions makes it more feasible to separate out the specific effects of experimental mortality in a time series design than its simpler counterpart.

All in all, time series designs constitute vast improvements over all the preexperimental designs discussed with respect to controls for internal validity. Unfortunately though, like their true experimental counterparts, they do very little to insure external generalizability and, in fact, even contribute some special problems of their own. No designs, for example, are more susceptible to the reactive effects of both testing *and* experimental settings, simply because none utilize more frequent testing schedules or administrations of the experimental treatment. If time series designs are appropriately employed, however, these effects are largely mitigated (that is, if both the dependent variable and the independent variable are relatively unobtrusive).

As stated before, time series designs can be modified to fit the individual circumstances surrounding each research setting. Also, like the one group pretest/post-test analog, it can be strengthened by the addition of either a nonequivalent control group (Fig. 9-14) or a randomly assigned control group (in the latter case, making the design truly experimental in nature).

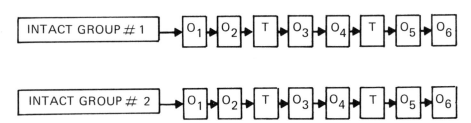

FIGURE 9-14. Two group time series design (nonequivalent groups).

Time series designs, as illustrated in Example 9-10, are further sometimes employed using a single S instead of an entire group in certain types of educational and behavioral research making them quite similar to the classical medical model in which a physician observes a patient's symptoms, prescribes a treatment, measures the resulting effect upon those same symptoms and either continues, discontinues, or initiates a different treatment. The chief distinction between the two models, in fact, lies only in the fact that the physician is not constrained to make an inference while the researcher must. The physician is only interested in the control of the patient's symptoms and is quite satisfied with their disappearance regardless of whether it is a result of the treatment or a fortuitous extraneous variable. To the extent that the physician does care about the *why* of the situation, the physician has become a researcher, for a researcher is chiefly interested in identifying the *cause* of a manipulated change in order to predict the conditions under which it will occur again.

COUNTERBALANCED DESIGN

There are occasions when two intact groups are available to a researcher and the prerequisites for using a time series design are present (see above), but the multiple introduction of the experimental treatment is not feasible. Two options relevant to such a setting have already been discussed, the pretest/post-test and the post-test only nonequivalent control group designs. Both of these strategies, however, have decided limitations that in large part are correctable if each group of Ss is allowed to serve in both the experimental and the control group.

Suppose, for example, that a nurse researcher wished to contrast two types of medications with regard to the maintenance of normal blood pressure but, for some reason, was not at liberty to randomly assign Ss to groups. If two intact groups were available, however, this researcher might prescribe Drug A to the first group and Drug B to the second for a certain interval and compare the two groups (hence drugs) with respect to blood pressure at the end of the interval. As with the nonequivalent control group designs already discussed, however, it is difficult to ascertain exactly what contributed to obtained differences (or lack thereof). Was it differences in the two drugs or simply initial differences between the two groups?

If the experiment could be carried one step further this question could in large part be answered. If Group 1 received Drug A for a week and Group 2 received Drug B during the same period, then the process could be switched with Group 1 now receiving Drug B for a week and Group 2 receiving Drug A.

Now suppose that during the first part of the study, Group 1 (taking Drug A) was found to be superior. If this superiority is a function of the drug and not a differential propensity of Group 1 Ss to register lower blood pressures across time (for example, via statistical regression), then the effect should be reversed during the second half of the study with Group 2 registering lower blood pressures than Group 1 (or at least registering a decrease therein comparable to Group 1's initial decrease). This is called a *counterbalanced* design and is schematically presented in Figure 9-15.

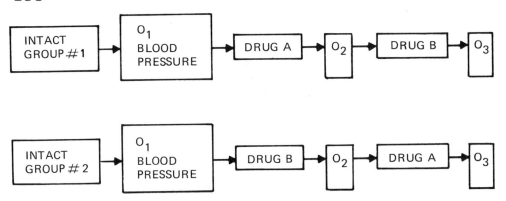

FIGURE 9-15. Counterbalanced design. If Drug A is superior to Drug B, then:

1. Changes from O_1 to O_2 should be greater for Group 1 than Group 2.
2. Changes from O_2 to O_3 should either be greater in Group 2 than Group 1 (if the effects for Drug A do not "wear off") or in the opposite direction (if Group 1 Ss begin registering higher blood pressures after Drug B is withdrawn).
3. For Group 1, changes from O_1 to O_2 should be greater than, or in the opposite direction from, O_2 to O_3 changes.
4. The reverse should be true for Group 2.

Ideally this design should be used for treatments whose effects are relatively transitory and dependent measures that are relatively unobtrusive (and hence not subject to the testing artifact). A creative researcher, however, can often find ways around even these restrictions. In a nursing research project conducted by students in one of the author's classes,[8] the student researchers wished to ascertain the relative effects of two modes of presenting content relevant to infection control. They had two intact classes of undergraduate nursing students with which to work, but since learning was to be the dependent variable they obviously could not present the same material twice to each group. They solved the problem by constructing two different passages and two different tests, presenting the first to Group 1 via Mode A and to Group 2 via Mode B (Fig. 9-16), contrasting the two groups with respect to retention of the contents of the first passage, then repeating the process with the second passage but reversing the mode of presentation (that is, by allowing Group 1 to receive Mode B and Group 2 getting Mode A). If Mode A were superior to Mode B and the groups equivalent, then Group 1 should have learned more than Group 2 the first time, Group 2 more than Group 1 the second time. If this outcome were to be observed, no interpretative problems would accrue, making the design as powerful as a true experimental one.

Unfortunately, however, as with all quasi-experimental designs something is potentially lost in comparison to a true experiment when the results do not

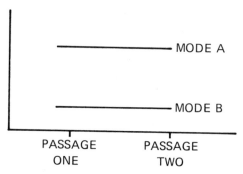

FIGURE 9-16. Counterbalanced design for a study involving two passages of instructional material, two modes of presentation, two presentation times, and two groups of subjects.

come back completely straightforwardly. What conclusions, for example, would the researcher draw if the results shown in Figure 9-17 were obtained?

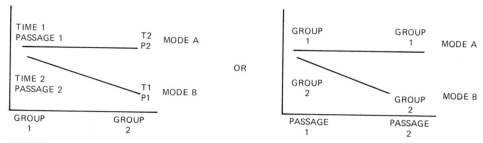

FIGURE 9-17. Results of a study involving two passages of instructional material, two modes of presentation, two presentation times, and two groups of subjects (see text for discussion).

What this figure represents is a situation in which Mode A is superior to Mode B under certain conditions and not others, and represents the actual outcome of the study in question. The question becomes: why did this occur? Since three variables exist in addition to the mode of presentation and they are confounded to various degrees, the explanation might include any of the following (or even any combination thereof):

1. Passage 1 differed from Passage 2 according to some relevant parameter (for example, might have been more interesting), hence causing all Ss to

attend to the former more closely "wiping out" a potential superiority of Mode B on Passage 1. This rival hypothesis could be partly mitigated by careful pilot testing of the passages.

2. The Ss in Group 1 differ from those in Group 2 in such a way that they do equally well under any mode of presentation, whereas the type of Ss in Group 2 do much better under Mode A condition (or worse with Mode B). This is sometimes referred to as an aptitude by treatment interaction, and although rare, has been demonstrated to exist under certain specialized circumstances.

3. Some historical variable intervened at Time 2, either differentially (for example, Ss in Group 2 were worried about an impending exam while those in Group 1 had already taken theirs) or to interact with the treatment (for example, Mode B requires more concentration than A, hence would produce inferior results during times of stress). A threat such as this is best averted by awareness on the part of the researcher concerning the experimental environment.

4. The measure used to test learning of Passage 1 was not sufficiently sensitive (for example, not reliable enough, too easy, too difficult, and so forth) to measure a real superiority while the second measure was. This, too, could be averted by employing a pilot test to refine the dependent measure.

Although not exhaustive, this list should give some indication of the interpretive problems which can accrue from the use of quasi-experimental designs. As stated earlier, there is an almost infinite variety of these designs that can be efficaciously employed in various settings that are not amenable to randomization. The degree to which each is capable of producing acceptable scientific evidence must, in the final analysis, be evaluated in light of the specific research environment in which its use is proposed. In the example above, a counterbalanced design would not be employed until the characteristics of the Ss comprising the two groups had been carefully studied and the possibility of an aptitude by treatment interaction discounted ahead of time. Similarly, care would also be taken that the two tests (and the corresponding passages) would have been piloted and psychometric data gathered to insure their comparability. The moral, in other words, is that as meticulous and careful as a researcher must always be, it is necessary to be even more so when employing quasi-experimental designs.

DESIGN SELECTION

The design that a researcher selects for a study is so dependent upon the purpose, hypotheses, setting, and resources that very few generalizations can be made concerning which designs are most efficacious for which circumstances. Situations differ so greatly in fact, and the permutations of design possibilities are so great, that many studies can best be addressed by designs or combinations of designs not even mentioned in this chapter.

One generalization does stand out, however, and that is that everything being equal the *quality* of knowledge accruing from experimental studies is higher than from any other type of research if quality be defined on a causal continuum. A well executed experimental study (that is, one that adequately controls all threats to internal validity) allows the researcher much greater confidence in inferring that X *caused* Y, or more properly that *changing* X resulted in a change in Y. Other types of research do not result in this type of knowledge. They may document a relationship between X and Y, as will be discussed with correlational research in Chapter 10, but they do not assure that changing one variable will change the other.

For this reason, therefore, it is safe to counsel the researcher interested in causality to select an experimental design over a pre- or quasi-experimental one whenever feasible. It is further safe to suggest that when possible, the researcher select an experimental design that permits maximal control over threats to internal validity. Thus, everything else being equal, the researcher will select a randomized block post-test design, a post-test with covariate design, a factorial model, or some combination of these over a simple post-test only design when circumstances conspire to make this feasible. When they do not, there is absolutely nothing wrong with employing the latter or its variations, which are considerably more powerful than the quasi-experimental designs (normally the next choice) or the pre-experimental designs (which are always the last choice).

ANALYZING THE RESULTS OF EXPERIMENTAL STUDIES

The type of design chosen for a study directly dictates the type of analysis that will be used to test its hypotheses. Those designs that permit greater control of extraneous variables also permit statistical tests that employ greater control of that basic element of all parametric inferential statistics: *variance.*

Appropriately enough, therefore, the statistical procedure used to analyze the results of experimental studies is itself called *analysis of variance* or *ANOVA.* Basically, it allows the researcher to compare the *systematic* variance in the study with the *nonsystematic* variance. If the ratio between the two is great enough, then the researcher concludes that the results are *statistically significant* and rejects the null hypothesis, which is another way of saying that a difference exists between the treatment groups (for example, experimental and control groups) since the experiment is designed to ascertain such a difference.

The purpose of all analyses of variance, therefore, is to test the significance of *differences between groups.* The various ANOVA genre differ primarily with respect to the degree to which nonsystematic variation can be reduced and their choice is dictated by the design that the experimenter was able to employ.

Analysis of variance itself is the brainchild of a nineteenth century agronomist, R. A. Fisher, who adapted it from the more general regression procedures that will be discussed in Chapter 10. Although any experimental study could be analyzed via regression procedures, most researchers find ANOVA conceptually simpler because it formulates its tests in terms of differences between arithmetic means, or more properly, in terms of *a ratio of differences between means* (systematic variance) *to differences between the numbers making up each of these means* (nonsystematic variance).

Analysis of Variance (ANOVA)

Analysis of variance, the statistical technique used to arrive at this ratio (called an F-ratio after its inventer), is a very general procedure that can be used to test whether or not any number of group means differ from one another. Before discussing the statistic in any detail, however, the reader should be aware of some of the assumptions governing its use. Analysis of variance may be used to test differences between two or more means when:

1. *The dependent variable is measured at the interval level or higher.*

   As discussed in Chapter 4, researchers are no longer greatly concerned about strict, absolute interpretations of what is truly interval and what is purely ordinal or nominal. ANOVA should probably not be used with purely ordinal data, however, such as rank orders, in which distortions are sometimes possible. By the same token, ANOVA would make no sense whatever applied to nominal data (other than dichotomies) simply because means involving nominal data make no sense. (For example, what would the mean diagnosis be of 10 diabetics, 5 potential cardiac patients, and 7 Ss believed to be suffering from influenza?) ANOVA is appropriate, however, for any data for which a mean is appropriate, and that includes most data used in nursing research.

2. *The values of at least one of the independent variables are discrete (that is, not continuous).*

   The reader should note that this assumption applies to the independent variable(s), not the dependent variable. The dependent variable, being measured at the interval level is usually continuous, whereas the independent variables in an ANOVA are usually assumed to be nominal (although the only real requirement is that its values can be used to define groups containing a reasonable number of Ss). Experimental and control treatments are examples of independent variables measured at the nominal level; children, adolescents, and adults might be an example of a discrete variable measured at the ordinal level.

   It would, of course, be possible to dichotomize or trichotomize an independent variable measured at the interval level (for example, younger versus older nurses), but generally speaking it is better to use regression techniques (see Chapter 10) in such cases since ANOVA tends to throw away valuable information through the categorizing process.

3. *The variances on the dependent variable do not differ significantly from one group to another.*

   If two group means are to be compared with respect to attitudinal scores, for example, the researcher should first ascertain whether the variances of the scores making up each mean differ from one another. This is done by directly comparing the variances via an F-max[17] or Bartlett's-Box test (which is computed as part of the ANOVA output by SPSS).

Fortunately, it has been demonstrated that ANOVA is quite robust to violations of this assumption *if* the number of Ss is the same in each group. For this reason, the homogeneity of variance assumption is no longer considered of particular importance unless group sizes are quite divergent.

4. *Respondents should be randomly selected from a normally distributed population and randomly assigned to groups.*

This assumption deals more with the interpretation of the F-ratio once computed than with whether or not it should be computed at all.

No other assumption is more commonly violated, simply because the researcher seldom knows a great deal about the population and almost never has the luxury of randomly selecting Ss from that population even when it is defined. Fortunately, most populations are normally distributed on most attributes, so it usually suffices for the experimenter to simply use common sense and

A. Make sure the Ss in each treatment group are relatively representative of the relevant population (for example, if a male versus female student comparison is of interest, the researcher should insure that the males in the study are no less representative of all students than the females are—male graduate students versus female undergraduates would be a negative example).

B. Randomly assign Ss to all treatment groups, which should insure that the distribution of attributes within each group is similar. This is not to say that ANOVA can only be used in experimental studies; it can be used in purely correlational research as will be indicated in the application section. Ss *must* be randomly assigned in experimental research, however, to assure any kind of causal interpretability.

C. Insure that error variance (which is always going to be present) is not introduced *differentially* between groups by artificial means, such as having different experimenters in charge of different groups, and so forth.

These, then, are some of the most important assumptions governing the use and interpretation of analysis of variance. To reiterate, the end product of an ANOVA is an F-ratio that can be compared with a hypothetical distribution of F-ratios representing mean differences occurring by chance. If this calculated F-ratio is larger than 95 percent of the F-ratios in the theoretical distribution, then the experimenter may conclude that the means differ significantly from one another (if the alpha level had been set at 0.05).

The beauty of the procedure lies in its generality. Instead of separate distributions for every conceivable set of data, such as the one used for illustrative purposes in Chapter 2, ANOVA procedures necessitate separate distributions only for every conceivable number of Ss in the total sample and for every conceivable number of groups involved (which is usually four or fewer). The fact that the F-ratio is a ratio of the variation between groups (which really translates to differences between the means of the groups involved) to the variation within groups allows the same statistic to represent experiments involving different types of Ss being measured on different types of tests.

One-Way ANOVA

To understand how this procedure works, consider the simplest possible experimental study in which a dozen Ss have been randomly assigned to two groups, six in each. Ss 1 to 6 were assigned to the experimental treatment (group E) which consisted of instruction regarding alcoholism as a chronic disease, while Ss 7 to 12 were assigned to the control treatment (group C) consisting of instruction regarding an irrelevant topic. At some specified interval following instruction, all Ss were administered an instrument designed to measure attitudes toward alcoholics. The six Ss in group E recorded attitudinal scores of 15, 16, 17, 18, 19, and 20 while the six Ss in group C scored 7, 8, 9, 10, 11, and 12 (Table 9-1).

It will be assumed that the attitudinal measure constituting the dependent variable is measured at some level above straight rank ordering (for example, a composite of several Likert scales). Obviously the independent variable is discrete, dichotomous in this case, the variances within each group do not differ significantly, and Ss have been randomly assigned, hence the basic assumptions regarding ANOVA have been met.

The purpose of doing the experiment was to see whether or not instruction regarding alcoholism (the independent variable represented by two groups, those receiving and not receiving instruction) would result in differences in attitudes regarding alcoholics (the dependent variable represented by the 12 attitudinal scores). The null hypothesis representing this experimental study would therefore be: *There is no significant difference in attitudes toward alcoholics between Ss receiving instruction regarding alcoholism and those not receiving instruction.* Although there are many alternate ways to state this

TABLE 9-1. Scores of Experimental Subjects (S-1 to S-6) and Control Subjects (S-7 to S-12) (See Text for Discussion)

S-1	15	S-7	7
S-2	16	S-8	8
S-3	17	S-9	9
S-4	18	S-10	10
S-5	19	S-11	11
S-6	<u>20</u>	S-12	<u>12</u>

$$\Sigma X = 105 \qquad \Sigma X = 57$$
$$n = 6 \qquad n = 6$$
$$\overline{X} = 17.5 \qquad \overline{X} = 9.5$$
$$\text{Var} = 3.5 \qquad \text{Var} = 3.5$$

hypothesis (for example, *attitudes toward alcoholics are not influenced by instruction*), the question to be answered is always the same: does the mean attitudinal score for the E group differ significantly from that of the C group?

By examination alone it is obvious that E Ss registered higher attitudes following instruction than did Ss in the control group. By examination alone, however, there is no way to ascertain how likely these differences would be to occur by chance alone and it is this question that will dictate the acceptance or rejection of the null hypothesis.

As discussed earlier, the experimenter could throw the 12 scores into a hat and begin to construct an actual distribution of chance results, could tediously compute the exact probability of a difference as large as 8.0 (17.5 − 9.5) occurring by chance alone, or could compute a statistic representing the ratio of between-group to within-group variance and then compare the statistic to an already prepared distribution. For obvious reasons, researchers always choose the latter course.

The specific statistical procedure that would be used with the data in Table 9-1 is called a one-way ANOVA (or single factor ANOVA), which indicates that the experiment contains only *one* independent variable; a fact that says nothing about the number of treatments, which in the present case happens to be two (that is, experimental and control). A one-way ANOVA can be used with *any* number of treatments, as long as all Ss are measured on the same dependent variables, although the interpretation of the F-ratio does change somewhat.

Even though the time has long past when researchers need to compute their ANOVAs by hand, working through the above data step-by-step should enable the reader to get an intuitive "feel" for exactly what the computer is doing when it performs an ANOVA and exactly what the different constituents and labels on the output represent.

The first step is to examine the study's design to ascertain how many possible sources of variation exist. The first and most obvious source is common to all designs regardless of their complexity. It is simply the total variance in all of the scores irrespective of group membership, and is calculated the same way that the variance is always calculated:

$$\text{Var} = \frac{\Sigma X^2 - \frac{(\Sigma X)^2}{n}}{n - 1} \qquad \text{or} \qquad \text{Var} = \frac{SS}{df}$$

$$\text{since } SS = \Sigma X^2 - \frac{(\Sigma X)^2}{n}$$

$$\text{and } df = n - 1.$$

Using the values in Table 9-1:

$$\Sigma X = 15 + 16 + 17 + \ldots + 11 + 12 = 162$$
$$(\Sigma X)^2 = 162^2 = 26244$$
$$\Sigma X^2 = 15^2 + 16^2 + 17^2 \ldots + 11^2 + 12^2 = 2414$$
$$n = 12$$

$$\text{Hence } SS_{total} = 2414 - \frac{26244}{12} = 227$$

$$\text{And } Var_{total} = \frac{227}{11} = 20.64$$

By convention, sums of squares are reported in ANOVA summary tables because they are additive (variances are not) and allow the researcher to check the work (since sums of squares from all sources must ultimately always add up to the total sum of squares, which is 227 in the present case).

Once this total variation has been described, it is necessary to compute the different sources of variation making up this total. The first, and the one that the researcher always hopes will be the most important, is the between-groups or treatment variation. This is the variation that the researcher has "caused" by doing different things to the Ss in the different groups. It is computed by simply substituting each group's total score divided by the number of Ss in each group for the first X in the general SS formula:

$$SS_{\substack{between \\ groups}} = \Sigma X^2 - \frac{(\Sigma X)^2}{n}$$

$$\text{Where } \Sigma X^2 \text{ now becomes } \frac{105^2}{6} + \frac{57^2}{6} = 2379$$

$$\text{And } \frac{(\Sigma X)^2}{n} \text{ remains } \frac{162^2}{12} = 2187$$

$$\text{Thus } SS_{\substack{between \\ groups}} = 2379 - 2187 = 192$$

The final source of variation is comprised of the different scores *within* each group. This is the researcher's nemesis because the researcher did not "cause" S_6 scoring higher than S_1, for example, or S_{10} scoring higher than S_9. This variation was not predicted by any hypothesis and hence must be assumed to be experimental error. Its computation is quite simple (in fact it could be obtained by simply subtracting $SS_{between}$ from SS_{total} since sums of squares are additive and there are only three in this data) and is effected by simply computing the sum of squares *within* E and adding it to the sum of squares *within* C:

$$SS_{within\ E} = \Sigma X_E^2 - \frac{(\Sigma X_E)^2}{n_E} = 15^2 + 16^2 + \ldots + 20^2 - \frac{(105)^2}{6} = 17.5$$

$$SS_{within\ C} = \Sigma X_C^2 - \frac{(\Sigma X_C)^2}{n_C} = 7^2 + 8^2 + \ldots + 12^2 - \frac{(57)^2}{6} = 17.5$$

$$\text{Hence } SS_{within} = SS_{within\ E} + SS_{within\ C} = 17.5 + 17.5 = 35.0$$

Basically, this is all there is to the analysis of variance. These sum of squares can quite easily be converted to variance by dividing them by their appropriate degrees of freedom $\left(Var = \frac{SS}{df} \right)$, and the F-ratio is computed by dividing the between group variance by the within group variance $\left(F = \dfrac{\sigma^2_{between}}{\sigma^2_{within}}\right)$. The final step usually consists of reporting these constituent parts in what is called an analysis of variance summary table. By convention, sum of squares, degrees of freedom, variances (called, also by convention, *mean squares*), and F-ratios are labeled and reported. The summary table for the hypothetical analysis above would be reported as shown in Table 9-2.

TABLE 9-2. Example of an ANOVA Summary Table (See Text for Discussion)

Source of variation	SS	df	MS	F
Treatments[a]	192	1[c]	192[f]	54.86* [i, j]
Error[b]	35	10[d]	3.5[g]	
Total	227	11[e]	[h]	

*$p < 0.05$.[k]

[a]Also sometimes called "between groups," or labeled more specifically, such as "instruction" or a reasonably good description of the independent variable.
[b]Also called "residual" or "within groups."
[c]Determined by subtracting one from the number of groups (i.e., $df_{treatments}$ = number of groups − 1 = 2 − 1 = 1).
[d]Determined by subtracting the number of groups from the total number of Ss (i.e., df_{error} = n − #groups = 12 − 2 = 10).
[e]Determined by subtracting one from the total number of Ss (i.e., df_{total} = n − 1 = 12 − 1 = 11).
[f]$MS_{treatment} = \dfrac{SS_{treatment}}{df_{treatment}} = \dfrac{192}{1} = 192$
[g]$MS_{error} = \dfrac{SS_{error}}{df_{error}} = \dfrac{35}{10} = 3.5$
[h]The total variance or MS is not computed since it is not necessary for computing the F-ratio.
[i]$F_{treatment} = \dfrac{MS_{treatment}}{MS_{error}} = \dfrac{192}{3.5} = 54.86$
[j]Degrees of freedom for the F-ratio consist of the degrees of freedom for treatments (1) *and* the degrees of freedom for error (10).
[k]Significance is determined by looking up the critical value for an F-ratio with 1 df in the numerator (treatments) and 10 in the denominator (error) at the 0.05 level (4.96). If the obtained value (54.86) is larger than the critical value, then the results are statistically significant.

An ANOVA summary table efficiently communicates a good deal of information. It tells at a glance, for example, how many groups were involved in the study ($df_{treatment}$ + 1), how many Ss participated all together (df_{total} + 1), and whether or not the results were significant. Research journals, however, are increasingly discouraging the routine use of ANOVA tables for simple analyses, partly because of space limitations, partly because many readers are unconcerned about sums of squares. When space is not a consideration, ANOVA summary tables are still the rule.

When tables such as the one above are not reported, the text of the article or report must convey the most essential information. For example, "Instruction regarding alcoholism was found to significantly increase attitudes toward alcoholics (F = 54.86 [1, 10] p < 0.05) among . . ." probably communicates all that most readers care to know concerning the ANOVA, but it does not give the reader any real indication of what the data "look like," or of the relative size of the effect. What is needed, regardless of how the inferential results are reported, are descriptive statistics such as treatment means, standard deviations, and numbers of subjects, possibly reported in a format similar to Table 9-3.

TABLE 9-3. Treatment Means and Standard Deviations

	$\overline{X}$	s	n
Experimental Group	17.5	1.87	6
Control Group	9.5	1.87	6

Relationship between F and t

In order to facilitate the introduction of analysis of variance, a simple two group example was used. ANOVA is a much more general procedure than this, capable of being used with any number of groups and with any number of independent variables. It is rare, in fact, to see an F-ratio reported to test a null hypothesis involving only two groups although there is no reason why researchers should adhere to this convention.

It is much more common for a statistic called a *t-test* to be used to ascertain the probability of one given mean difference occurring by chance alone. At first glance the formula for the t bears no immediately apparent relationship to ANOVA computational procedures:

$$t = \frac{\overline{X}_{treatment} - \overline{X}_{control}}{\sqrt{\dfrac{Var_{treatment}}{n_{treatment}} + \dfrac{Var_{control}}{n_{control}}}}$$

but careful examination reveals some interesting simularities. First, the t obviously represents a mean difference ($\overline{X}_{treatment} - \overline{X}_{control}$) in such a way that the larger that difference, the greater the size of the statistic (that is, the t). Second, just as with ANOVA, the larger the number of Ss and the smaller the variances *within* each group, the larger the t, and like all statistics, the larger the more likely the null hypothesis will be rejected. The final similarity is best illustrated by performing a t-test on the hypothetical data from Table 9-1. Substituting these values into the t-test formula:

$$t = \frac{17.5 - 9.5}{\sqrt{\dfrac{3.5}{6} + \dfrac{3.5}{6}}} = \frac{8}{108} = 7.407$$

yields a t of 7.407, which happens to be equal to the square root of the F-ratio obtained in Table 9-2. In other words, $\sqrt{F} = t$ (or $t^2 = F$), a relationship that can be rather simply proved algebraically.

It should follow that ANOVA and the t-test are basically the same statistic when two groups are involved (the t-test can *only* be used to contrast two group means), therefore it makes little difference which statistic is employed. It should further follow that all the assumptions governing ANOVA also hold for the t-test (that is, interval level data, homogeneity of variance, and so forth).

Relationship between F and Other Statistics

Although it probably will not mean a great deal to most readers until Chapter 10 is read and digested, it can be easily demonstrated that an F-ratio bears an equally straightforward relationship to other statistics as well. It would have been possible, for example, to have analyzed the data in Table 9-1 via a correlation coefficient. Suppose the independent variable had been coded as 1 = membership in the experimental group, 0 = membership in control. In that case, two scores would have been available on each S and the data could have been presented as shown in Table 9-4.

TABLE 9-4. Analysis of Data in Table 9-1 by Means of a Correlation Coefficient (See Text for Discussion)

	X (E vs. C)	Y (Attitudes)
S-1	1	15
S-2	1	16
S-3	1	17
S-4	1	18
S-5	1	19
S-6	1	20
S-7	0	7
S-8	0	8
S-9	0	9
S-10	0	10
S-11	0	11
S-12	0	12

A Pearson r calculated on these two sets of numbers would produce a coefficient of 0.92, which when squared would equal 0.85. This latter number (r^2), as will be explained in the next chapter, indicates that 85 percent of the variation between X and Y is shared, or said another way, that 85 percent of the variation between individual attitude scores can be explained by knowing whether or not a S was in the E (or C) group.

Not coincidentally, if the $SS_{treatment}$ has been divided by the SS_{total} in Table 9-2 $\left(\frac{192}{229}\right)$ a coefficient of 0.85 would have been obtained. This quantity, also called eta², assesses the strength of an F (as opposed to its significance), and is equivalent to r^2 (or R^2 when more than two groups are involved). Suffice it to say that all of the common parametric inferential statistics are blood relatives and that the same data can be analyzed via many different statistical procedures.

One-Way ANOVA with Three or More Groups

Analyses of variance performed upon experiments involving three or more levels of the same independent variable are conceptually and computationally identical to the example presented in Table 9-2. The interpretation of the F-ratios yielded by such analyses are slightly different, however.

Suppose a researcher wished to contrast three instructional methods for young surgery patients to see which produced the greatest amount of learning. Suppose further that the data were as presented in Table 9-5.

TABLE 9-5. Sample Data on Three Instrumental Methods (See Text for Discussion)

Treatment 1 (verbal instruction)		Treatment 2 (instruction with pictures)		Treatment 3 (instruction with 3-D models)	
S-1	7	S-8	15	S-15	16
S-2	5	S-9	14	S-16	15
S-3	7	S-10	15	S-17	16
S-4	9	S-11	16	S-18	17
S-5	10	S-12	15	S-19	16
S-6	10	S-13	17	S-20	18
S-7	8	S-14	18	S-21	18
$\Sigma X = 56$		$\Sigma X = 110$		$\Sigma X = 116$	
$n = 7$		$n = 7$		$n = 7$	
$\overline{X} = 8.0$		$\overline{X} = 15.7$		$\overline{X} = 16.6$	
$\sigma^2 = 3.33$		$\sigma^2 = 1.91$		$\sigma^2 = 1.29$	

A one-way ANOVA computed on these data via the SPSS program called ONE-WAY would produce the significant F-ratio indicated in Table 9-6. The reader will note, however, that there are three possible mean differences (that is, T_1 vs. T_2, T_1 vs. T_3, and T_2 vs. T_3) and only one F. The reason for this is that the ANOVA presented in Table 9-6 only tests the hypothesis that a significant difference exists between at least one of the three mean differences; it does not specify which means differ from which. The above ANOVA, in other words, tests the hypothesis that a significant difference exists between at least two of the three instructional methods. It does not indicate which specific methods differ from one another.

Obviously, any researcher would want to know which groups differed significantly from which other groups. In the past, many investigators solved this

TABLE 9-6. One-Way ANOVA for Data in Table 9-5 Computed Via SPSS Program[a]

Source	df	SS	MS	F ratio	F prob.[b]
Between groups	2	312.000	156.000	71.737	0.000
Within groups	18	39.143	2.175		
Total	20	351.143			

Group	Count[c]	Mean[d]	Standard deviation	Minimum[f]	Maximum[g]
Grp 01	7	8.000	1.826	5.000	10.000
Grp 02	7	15.714	1.380	14.000	18.000
Grp 03	7	16.570	1.134	15.000	18.000
Total	21	13.429	4.190	5.000	18.000

[a]The analysis of variance summary table is interpreted in exactly the same way as in Table 9-2.

[b]The actual probability of the F of 71.737 occurring by chance alone. Since SPSS and many other ANOVA programs round off to three decimal points this 0.000 value indicates that overall differences between three means as large as those observed in this study would occur by chance alone less than one time in 5000.

[c]The number in each group and the total for the study.

[d]Learning means of each group and the total.

[e]Standard deviations of each group and the total.

[f]Lowest score in each group and total.

[g]Highest score in each group and total.

problem by simply computing t-tests between all the possible combinations of treatments. Unfortunately, this practice artifactually increased the chances of obtaining significant differences because the F distribution was constructed on the assumption that each F represents a differing, *independent* set of data. Performing multiple t-tests is analogous to performing multiple F-ratios (since $t^2 = F$) on the same experiment.

To veridically compare multiple treatment means in the same experiment, a researcher must protect the alpha level. This may be done by changing the alpha level to reflect the number of constrasts to be performed and then computing t-tests to see if the groups differ (for example, corrected alpha = $\frac{alpha}{\# comparisons}$ or in the present study $\frac{0.05}{3} = 0.017$) or conducting post hoc or a posteriori tests following a significant F-ratio.

This latter option is most commonly employed and is made extremely simple by computer packages such as SPSS that compute them automatically upon request. The most commonly used of these procedures are probably Newman-Keuls (which is the most liberal that knowledgeable journal editors will allow), the Duncan Multiple Range Test, and Scheffe's Test (which is the most conservative and defendable). Winer[17] and Nie and associates[12] have excellent discussions of these tests with Winer being especially easy to follow should the researcher wish to compute the tests personally. Table 9-7 illustrates the type of

TABLE 9-7. Type of Information Obtained from Computer-Performed Newman-Keuls Procedure on Data in Table 9-5

Variable: Preoperative Learning

Multiple Range Test

Student-Newman-Keuls Procedure
Ranges for the 0.05 Level —

2.97   3.60

HOMOGENEOUS SUBSETS   (Subsets of groups, no pair of
which has means that differ by
more than the shortest significance
range for subset of that size)

Subset 1[a]		
Group Mean	Grp 01	
	8.0000	

Subset 2[b]		
Group Mean	Grp 02	Grp 03
	15.7143	16.5714

[a]Since only one mean, that of T_1 is found in Subset 1, this indicates that T_1 does differ significantly from both T_2 and T_3.
[b]Since the means of T_2 and T_3 are presented in this subset, the researcher knows that they do not differ significantly from one another. If there had been no significant differences between means the output would have looked like this:

Subset 1			
Group Mean	Grp 01	Grp 02	Grp 03
	8.0000	15.7143	16.5714

In other words, any means appearing in any given subset do not differ significantly from one another.

information obtained should the researcher opt for allowing the computer to perform a Newman-Keuls procedure on the data presented in Table 9-5.

In addition to a posteriori tests there exist a priori statistical procedures that can advantageously be employed under certain circumstances. They are especially attractive when those conditions apply, both because of their sizeable advantage over a posteriori procedures with respect to statistical power (no protection of alpha is required) and the fact that they can be performed even if a significant F-ratio is not obtained. Basically, the researcher must meet three requirements before employing them: (1) the number of comparisons is limited to the number of groups minus 1 (this is a heavy price in some settings because if five groups were involved in the ANOVA only four out of the dozens of possible contrasts could be made), (2) the comparisons must be specified in advance (thus, to convince critics that they were, the researcher must have very good reasons for the choices made), and (3) they must be independent (orthogonal) of one another. This latter requirement probably deserves some amplification.

In the three group experiment in which three instructional methods were administered to young surgery patients, if the researcher wished to maximize the chances of documenting differences among individual treatments and was more interested in some combinations than others, the researcher might well decide to plan a priori contrasts before conducting the experiment. If the researcher could be satisfied with making only two contrasts (that is, number of groups − 1), the first two requirements mentioned above would be met. If the researcher was not satisfied, it would probably be better to employ, say, the Newman-Keuls procedure to test all possible differences between group means.

Even if the first two conditions had been met, the researcher would unfortunately not be free to choose any two comparisons desired. The researcher would have to insure that the same set of numbers was not employed in both contrasts to insure orthogonality. If, for example, the experimenter decided to contrast treatment #3 vs. treatment #2, neither group could then be compared to verbal instruction since the same set of numbers would have to be employed twice. Verbal instruction (treatment #1) could, however, be contrasted with treatments #2 and #3 combined, since this would involve the comparison of new means. (Again, see Winer[17] or Nie and associates[12] for discussions of the techniques plus algorithms for determining orthogonality.) A priori orthogonal contrasts are quite easy to compute once the original ANOVA has been per-

TABLE 9-8. A Priori Contrasts Involving T_1 vs. $T_2 + T_3$ and T_2 vs. T_3

Variable: Preoperative Learning

CONTRAST COEFFICIENT MATRIX

	Gr 01	Gr 02	Gr 03
Contrast 1	1.0	−0.5	−0.5[a]
Contrast 2	0.0	1.0	−1.0[b]

	VALUE	POOLED VARIANCE T VALUE	T PROB.
Contrast 1	−8.1429[c]	−11.929[d]	0.000[e]
Contrast 2	−0.8571[f]	−1.087[g]	0.291[h]

[a]The 1 under T_1 and the −0.5s under T_2 and T_3 indicate that the former's mean will be compared directly to the latter two. These coefficients must add up to 0 [1.0 + (−0.5) + (−0.5) = 0]. The magnitudes of the numbers themselves indicate the relative weights assigned to each mean in the contrast.
[b]The 0 under T_1 (Gr 01) indicates that this mean will not be considered in the second contrast. The 1 under T_2 and the −1 under T_3 indicate that these two means will be directly compared to one another.
[c]The mean difference between T_1 and the combination of $T_2 + T_3$.
[d]The t statistic computed between the means of T_1 and the combination of $T_2 + T_3$.
[e]The significance level of the t of −11.929, indicating that the means of T_2 and T_3 combined do differ significantly from T_1.
[f]The mean of $T_2 − T_3$.
[g]The t statistic computed between the means of $T_2 − T_3$.
[h]The significance level of the t of −1.087, indicating that the means of T_2 and T_3 do not differ significantly from one another.

formed because all they require is knowledge of the MS_{error} and the group means upon which they are to be performed. It is not even necessary to perform an overall ANOVA since the above study employing a priori contrasts would not really hypothesize that a difference exists between several means but rather that two *specified* differences exist. Table 9-8 is illustrative of the type of information which would be obtained if the above two contrasts were requested of SPSS.

Factorial ANOVA

From a semantic viewpoint it is probably obvious that if a one-way ANOVA exists, so must a more-than-one-way ANOVA. From a logical viewpoint, it is probably equally obvious that if a procedure exists for one independent variable it should probably be generalizable to more than one independent variable. Such is indeed the case, and the very existence of the procedure greatly expands the options open to researchers. It is called two-way, three-way, or four-way ANOVA (depending upon the number of independent variables), or simply factorial ANOVA.

Factorial ANOVA is capable of serving two purposes simultaneously. It allows the researcher to investigate two or more variables at the same time, thereby observing their effect in conjunction with one another, and it allows the researcher to *decrease* within-group error variance, thereby greatly increasing the probability of obtaining significance (that is, rejecting the null hypothesis). These advantages can perhaps best be illustrated by returning to the study represented in Table 9-2.

As previously discussed, it is the variation between Ss in the E and C groups that the experimenter "understands" because it is this variable that has been "caused" by the experimental manipulation. The variation within each group, on the other hand, represents something that the researcher does not understand, something neither predicted, wanted, nor caused. This unexplained variance is the bane of all researchers because, unexplained, it must be considered error, and the greater the error present in an experiment the smaller are its chances of success.

It follows, however, that if the experimenter had been able to predict which Ss in both the E and C groups would be most likely to register high attitudes, then this within-group variation could no longer be considered error. It would no longer be unexplained and the MS_{error} would therefore be reduced to the direct extent that the researcher was able to predict which Ss would register the highest (or lowest) attitudes. Since $F = \dfrac{MS_{treatment}}{MS_{error}}$ any substantive decrease in MS_{error} is capable of drastically affecting a hypothesis test.

There are several strategies that the researcher might employ to predict which Ss would register high or low attitudes toward alcoholics. The most direct way might well be to administer an attitudinal premeasure on the assumptions that Ss' relative positionings on the attribute would remain constant and that the premeasure would not interact with the instruction. Since this strategy would result in a continuous, interval measure however, it would be better handled via analysis of covariance procedures discussed later. Suppose, however, that the experimental sample were about equally divided in terms of those having had some experience with alcoholics and those not having had any previous contact. Suppose further that there was good reason to believe that familiarity resulted in a more tolerant outlook toward these patients. If there was indeed some good reason to hypothesize such a relationship (such as previous research findings or a theory predicting same), then the researcher would have been wise to have employed two independent variables rather than one (that is, instruction vs. no instruction, and previous exposure to alcoholics vs. none) and to have randomly assigned half of the Ss with previous exposure to the E group, half to C—repeating the process with Ss with no previous experience with alcoholics. (Note that this corresponds to the fifth experimental design discussed before, the factorial post-test design.) Suppose that Ss 1 to 3 were thus randomly assigned to Group 1, Ss 4 to 6 to Group 2, Ss 7 to 9 to Group 3, and Ss 10 to 12 to Group 4 (Table 9-9).

TABLE 9-9. Assignment of Subjects Using Two Independent Variables

	E		C	
PREVIOUS EXPOSURE	S—1 S—2 S—3	1	S—7 S—8 S—9	3
NO PREVIOUS EXPOSURE	S—4 S—5 S—6	2	S—10 S—11 S—12	4

GROUP 1 = Ss WITH PREVIOUS EXPOSURE RECEIVING INSTRUCTION.
GROUP 2 = Ss WITH NO PREVIOUS EXPOSURE RECEIVING INSTRUCTION.
GROUP 3 = Ss WITH PREVIOUS EXPOSURE NOT RECEIVING INSTRUCTION.
GROUP 4 = Ss WITH NO PREVIOUS EXPOSURE NOT RECEIVING INSTRUCTION.

Once the Ss had been assigned, the experiment would proceed as before with half the sample receiving the experimental manipulation and half not. The reader should be reminded, however, that in an experimental study this assignment should be done *prior* to the experimental manipulation to avoid the possibility that all Ss with previous exposure might be assigned to the E group.

Strictly speaking, the above design contains only one truly experimental variable since the previous exposure variable serves in a correlational posture. This mixing of experimental and correlational variables is the rule rather than the exception in factorial ANOVA applications, although there are some instances in which both independent variables have been either experimental or correlational. The present study could have been completely experimental, for example, if all Ss had started out with no exposure to alcoholism and had been randomly assigned to four groups, two of which consisted of, say, spending a day in an alcohol rehabilitation center. The computation of this factorial ANOVA would be identical to the first model, the only difference being in the causative implications of the latter (since exposure was experimentally manipulated) as opposed to the correlational interpretation necessitated by the former procedure.

Computationally, factorial ANOVA is almost as simple as the one-way model. Conceptually, however, the user must take into account the additional sources of variation introduced by the second independent variable. In a one-way model the reader will recall that there are only three sources of variation:

$$SS_{total} = SS_{treatment} + SS_{error}$$

which could be rephrased as:

$$SS_{total} = SS_{independent\ variable} + SS_{within}$$

In a factorial model there are other sources. Consider the data from Table 9-1 as it now applies to the present design shown in Table 9-10.

TABLE 9-10. Four Groups of Subjects from Table 9-9 plus Attitudinal Scores

	E		C	
PREVIOUS EXPOSURE	S—1	15	S—7	7
	S—2	16	S—8	8
	S—3	17	S—9	9
NO PREVIOUS EXPOSURE	S—4	18	S—10	10
	S—5	19	S—11	11
	S—6	20	S—12	12

Obviously, the total variation will remain the same since an identical number of Ss possessing identical scores are involved. Similarly, the variation between E and C groups also remains the same, thus it follows that any additional sources must be subtracted from SS_{within}. All that remains is to ascertain exactly what these sources are.

Consider the information in Table 9-11 in which Ss scores have been summed.

TABLE 9-11. Sums of Subjects' Scores from Table 9-10

	E	C	TOTAL
EXPOSURE	48	24	72
NONE	57	33	90
	105	57	162

One new component is the comparison between the overall means of the two groups representing the second independent variable (previous exposure to alcoholics). The sum of squares for this source is computed in the same way as was the sum of squares for the instructional variable:

$$SS_{exposure} = \Sigma X^2 - \frac{(\Sigma X)^2}{n}$$

Where ΣX^2 becomes $\dfrac{72^2}{6} + \dfrac{90^2}{6} = 2214$

And $\dfrac{(\Sigma X)^2}{n}$ remains $\dfrac{162^2}{12} = 2187$

Hence $SS_{exposure} = 2214 - 2187 = 27$

There is one additional way in which the scores in this little experiment can systematically vary which, unfortunately, is not quite as obvious as its counterparts. The use of additional tables of the genre of Table 9-11 should expose this source, however. Table 9-12 shows three of the many possible ways that a hypothetical set of data could be distributed in a two-way ANOVA with independent variables A and B, each of which are represented by two groups.

TABLE 9-12. Three Possible Data Distributions for a Two-Way ANOVA with Independent Variables A and B

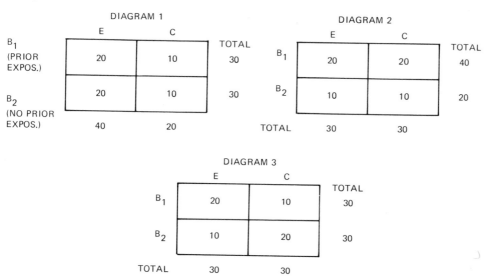

Diagram 1 represents a situation in which the two A groups differ from one another, but in which there are no real differences between B₁ and B₂. Diagram 2 represents the opposite. Diagram 3 presents an unusual situation, however. Although there are absolutely no differences between the four groups with respect to the two independent variables, closer examination does reveal that another relationship exists. For this to be true there must therefore be another source of variation over and above those identified so far, since this relationship is obviously not within-group variance.

This particular genre of relationship, in which different treatments are differentially effective within different levels of another independent variable, is called an *interaction*. In Diagram 3, A_1 is superior to A_2 for Ss in B_1, but the opposite is true for B_2, that is, A_2 is superior to A_1. In other words, such a relationship could have occurred if instruction (E) resulted in superior attitudes among Ss with no previous exposure while at the same time having a negative effect for Ss with previous exposure. Diagrams 1 and 2 have no comparable situation, and thus would not have a significant interaction.

Many researchers find that the easiest way to interpret an interaction is to graph it. Consider another possible outcome for the alcoholism study in which Ss with previous exposure generally had more positive attitudes toward alcoholics when no instruction was administered. If these attitudes were impervious to instruction, however, and if Ss with no exposure *were* radically affected by instruction, then an interaction would exist because the treatment variable (instruction) was differentially effective within the two levels of the second independent variable. Diagrammed, this situation might resemble Table 9-13.

TABLE 9-13. Diagram of Data from Study in which Treatment Was Differentially Effective and Interaction Exists

	E	C	TOTAL
EXPOSURE	40	40	80
NONE	40	20	60
TOTAL	80	60	

Graphed (Fig. 9-18, top), it will be noticed that the treatment lines converge and are not parallel, which is the geometric cue that an interaction exists. To illustrate, compare the graph of the data presented in Table 9-13 to that of Table 9-14 in which both prior exposure and instruction resulted in superior, but not differentially superior, attitudes. Note that the latter example does not contain a significant interaction as illustrated by the fact that the treatment lines are relatively parallel. This is in direct contrast to the data in Table 9-13 in which Ss having previous exposure still tended to have higher attitudes as a group toward alcoholics than those having no such exposure and, overall, instruction also still tended to be effective. These two relationships do not tell the entire story, however, because closer examination reveals that instruction was *only effective if Ss had no prior exposure to alcoholics; it had no effect for Ss with prior exposure.* In a factorial ANOVA, no interpretation of the F-ratios for main effects (exposure vs. no exposure and E vs. C in the above sample) can verdically be made until the significant interactions are interpreted.

Although interactions such as these, once graphed, are relatively easy to interpret in simple studies (since if the lines are relatively parallel, then the treat-

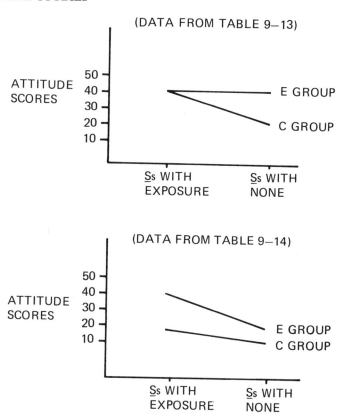

FIGURE 9-18. Treatment lines based on data in Tables 9-13 and 9-14.

ments are not differentially effective and no interaction exists, but if the lines diverge radically from the parallel, then said treatments are differentially effective), the same is unfortunately not true if there are more than two levels of either independent variable. Graphing a significant interaction in such situations will no more reveal where the true differences lie than will simple examination of the means in a three group ANOVA. Interactions can, in fact, be exceedingly complex if several levels of each independent variable exist (Fig. 9-19).

The interaction in Figure 9-19 would be exceedingly difficult to describe, much less to ascertain exactly where significant differences existed. Techniques, sometimes called simple effects tests[17] do exist (analogous to the a pos-

TABLE 9-14. Diagram of Data from Study in which Treatment Was Not Differentially Effective and No Interaction Exists

	E	C	TOTAL
EXPOSURE	40	20	60
NONE	20	10	30
TOTAL	60	30	

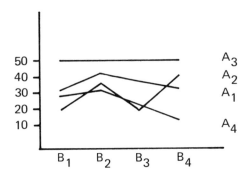

FIGURE 9-19. Graph of interactions when several levels of each independent variable exist.

teriori strategies mentioned above) however, to unravel interactions with more than two levels in any given variable. The average researcher might still be well advised to avoid situations such as the one represented in Figure 9-19 by using as few levels of the independent variables as possible.

Returning to the factorial example represented by the data in Table 9-6, the final source of variation therefore belongs to the interaction between the two independent variables. It is denoted $SS_{interaction}$ and its computation is fairly straightforward, necessitating only the substitution of each cell's summed score divided by the number of Ss in each cell for ΣX^2 in the general sum of squares equation below (since the interaction takes into account variation between each cell minus the variation already explained by the two independent variables). In other words:

$$SS_{interaction} = \left[\Sigma X^2 - \frac{(\Sigma X)^2}{n}\right] - SS_{treatment} - SS_{exposure}$$

$$\text{Where } \Sigma X^2 \text{ becomes } \frac{48^2}{3} + \frac{57^2}{3} + \frac{24^2}{3} + \frac{33^2}{3} = 2406$$

$$\text{And } \frac{(\Sigma X)^2}{n} \text{ remains } \frac{162^2}{12} = 2187$$

$$SS_{treatment} = 192$$
$$SS_{exposure} = 27$$

$$\text{Hence } SS_{interaction} = (2406 - 2187) - 192 - 27 = 0$$

The final source of variation has now been identified and computed, hence all that remains is to observe the effect of these new sources upon the within-group variance. Since $SS_{total} = SS_{1st\ IV} + SS_{2nd\ IV} + SS_{interaction} + SS_{within}$ it follows that $SS_{within} = SS_{total} - SS_{1st\ IV} - SS_{2nd\ IV} - SS_{interaction}$ or $SS_{within} = 227 - 192 - 27 - 0 = 8$, which, when compared with SS_{within} of 35 in Table 9-2, represents a drastic reduction in error variance from the one-way model.

Certainly this contrived example greatly exaggerates the ability of factorial ANOVA to reduce within-group variance, but perhaps it does help to underscore a fundamental advantage of studying more than one variable at a time. A second very considerable advantage illustrated by the ANOVA summary table in Table 9-15 resides in the fact that the interaction F-ratio is a pure bonus. It represents a hypothesis that could not be tested if two separate analyses had been performed: one to ascertain the effect of instruction; the second to determine if attitudes were indeed related to prior knowledge. Actually there are now three hypotheses, two for the independent variables and one for their interactions with one another.

TABLE 9-15. Example of a Factorial ANOVA Summary Table (See Text for Discussion)

Source of Variation	SS[c]	df	MS	F
A (Treatment)[a]	192	1	192	192.0*
B (Exposure)	27	1	27	27.0*[f]
AB[b]	0	1[d]	0	0.0[g]
Error	8	8[e]	1	
Total	227	11		

*$p < 0.01$

[a]Letters followed by a descriptive label are usually used to designate main effects (i.e., effects due to the independent variable) in factorial summary tables.
[b]Represents the interaction (A × B) of the treatment and prior exposure.
[c]Note that treatment and total SS, df, and MS remain the same from Table 9-2.
[d]Computed by multiplying $df_{treat.}$ by those of exposure (1 × 1 = 1).
[e]Note that the df_{error} have been reduced by exactly the same number of df which were added to the table by the new sources of variation. If the experimenter had guessed incorrectly and had not predicted which Ss would score higher or lower on the attitudinal variable, then chances of obtaining significance would have been *decreased* because the MS_{error} would have been increased.

[f]$F_{exposure} = \dfrac{MS_{exposure}}{MS_{error}}$

[g]$F_{AB} = \dfrac{MS_{AB}}{MS_{error}}$

The SPSS printout, as illustrated in Table 9-16, is a little more complicated than Table 9-10, chiefly because of the amount of redundant information supplied.

Although there is no theoretical limit upon the number of independent variables that can be handled by a factorial design, there are some very real practical constraints. The first concerns the problem of having sufficient Ss to fill all the generated cells. The simple 2 × 2 design employed above (that is, two levels of the first variable and two levels of the second) employed only four cells. If each variable had had three groups associated with it there would have been nine cells (3 × 3). The addition of a third independent variable would have yielded 27, and so forth.

The second problem with using any sizeable number of independent variables lies in the resulting proliferation of interaction terms. With two factors (that is, two independent variables) there is only one possible interaction be-

TABLE 9-16. Example of SPSS Printout

SOURCE OF VARIATION	SUM OF SQUARES	DF	MEAN SQUARE	F	SIGNIF.[i] OF F
Main effects[a]	219.000	2	109.500	109.50	0.001
Treatment[b]	27.000	1	27.000	27.00	0.001
Exposure[c]	192.000	1	192.000	192.00	0.001
2-way interactions[d]	0.000	1	0.000	0.00	0.999
Treatment Exposure[e]	0.000	1	0.000	0.00	0.999
Explained[f]	219.000	3	73.000	73.00	0.001
Residual[g]	8.000	8	1.000		
Total[h]	227.000	11	20.636		

Grand Mean = 13.50[j]

Variable + Category	N	Unadjusted[k]. . . . .
		Dev'n Eta
Exposure		
None	6	−1.50
Prior	6	1.50
		0.34[l]
Treatment		
Experimental	6	4.00
Control	6	−4.00
		0.92[m]

Multiple R squared[n]	0.965
Multiple R	0.982

[a]This is a combination of the effects of both independent variables. The F of 109.50 at the 0.001 significance level indicates that both variables in conjunction are significantly related to attitudes toward alcoholics (note that $SS_{main\ effects} = SS_{exposure} + SS_{treatments}$). This is usually not reported in the study itself.

[b, c]See Table 9-15.

[d]Similar to (a) above applied to interactions. Since there is only one interaction term in this study, its values are the same as the treatment × exposure interaction (e).

[e]See Table 9-15.

[f]This, like (a) and (d) above, is not normally reported. It is a combination of all systematic sources of variation in the study (e.g., note that $SS_{explained} = SS_{treat.} + SS_{exposure} + SS_{interaction}$).

[g]Same as error or within group variation.

[h]See Table 9-15.

[i]Actual significance level of each F-ratio.

[j]This number is the mean of all Ss in the study on the dependent variable (attitudes toward alcoholism). Its only function is to permit the researcher to ascertain means for each of its groups. A definite limitation of this program is that the computer does not print out these means directly as well as individual cell means, which must be computed separately.

[k]These numbers represent each group's deviation from the grand mean. To ascertain the six Ss' mean attitude score with no prior exposure to alcoholics, for example, the

TABLE 9-16. *Continued*

researcher would subtract 1.50 from the grand mean of 13.50. The mean attitudinal score for E Ss would thus be 13.50 + 4.00 = 17.50, for control Ss 13.50 − 4.00 = 9.50. ^lThis is simply the correlation between the independent variable prior exposure and the dependent variable, attitudes toward alcoholism.

^mThe correlation between treatment (E vs. C) and attitudes.

ⁿThis value indicates that 96.5 percent of individual variations in attitudes toward alcoholics can be explained by the two independent variables and the interaction between them.

tween them: AB. With three factors there are four: AB, AC, BC, and ABC; with four, there are ten: AB, AC, AD, BC, BD, CD, ABC, ACD, BCD, and ABCD. Each interaction represents a hypothesis and very few studies really merit this many. Furthermore, the three-way interactions (for example, ABC) are often quite difficult to interpret, the four-way one almost impossible. For these reasons, therefore, factorial ANOVAs employing more than three factors are very rare and usually result in the ignoring of higher level interactions. SPSS, in fact, has an option that permits the researcher to specify which interactions need not be calculated.

It is wise to plan a factorial ANOVA in such a way that each cell contains the same number of scores since unequal numbers can result in non-orthogonality or non-independence. If Ss are randomly assigned to cells, then there is normally no problem with unequal frequencies. If *slight* discrepancies exist, then Ss can be randomly dropped to insure equality. If more serious inequities exist, however, this strategy is not feasible, so other strategies must be employed. The best option is probably to employ regression procedures to partial out dependence between variables caused by unequal cell sizes. A few statistical packages, such as SPSS, allow the researcher this option.

Pretest/Post-Test Repeated Measures and Randomized Block ANOVA

As valuable as factorial ANOVA can be with respect to reducing within-group variation, far more powerful procedures exist. The most useful are those employed with designs that permit the same Ss to be represented in more than one treatment or permit similar Ss to be assigned to the different treatments in an experiment.

It is usually not feasible to allow the same Ss to participate in two treatments. Besides practical constraints, such as requiring far more participant time (hence making it more difficult to secure cooperation), serious threats to internal validity often accrue as discussed earlier. In circumstances in which participation in one treatment cannot contaminate participation in another or in which the effects of an intervention need to be studied over time, *repeated measures ANOVA* can result in a great deal more statistical power than analyses that presuppose different Ss in all cells.

The reason for this is quite straightforward. The main element of within-group variance is individual differences between Ss. Even after the successful introduction of a second independent variable in the factorial design represented in Table 9-10, for example, unexplained within-group variance still existed: S_3 possessed a more positive attitude than S_1 even though they were in the same group; S_6 was similarly different from S_4. A very probable reason for this phenomenon is that S_3 and S_6 simply started out with higher attitudes toward alcoholics, toward people in general, or possibly simply preferred to mark higher numbers on scales than did S_1 and S_4. They were different, in other words, and these differences would have been operative regardless of the treatments to which they were assigned.

If these particular Ss had been assigned to *both* E and C groups, however, and if S_3 did indeed retain the propensity for exhibiting relatively high attitudes in both conditions, then this individual difference would no longer need be considered error variance since it had been controlled (explained). It could therefore be *subtracted from* the study's error variance, resulting in a sizeable increase in the resulting F-ratio.

To clarify how this process works, consider the following example in which the efficacity of two drugs was tested on patients with chronic pain. Suppose each drug were tried on each patient for two days with one half being assigned to try Drug 1 first followed by Drug 2, half being assigned the opposite order. The number of times patients requested additional medication during each 2-day period served as the dependent variable (Table 9-17).

TABLE 9-17. Data in Study of Medication Requests (See Text for Discussion)

	Drug 1	Drug 2
S-1	4	10
S-2	2	8
S-3	1	6
S-4	8	16
S-5	12	25
S-6	<u>16</u>	<u>24</u>
	$\overline{X} = 7.17$	$\overline{X} = 14.83$
	Var = 29.47	Var = 56.14
	n = 6	n = 6

If these data were analyzed as though different Ss were assigned to the two drug treatments, the resulting ANOVA summary table would appear as shown in Table 9-18.

Even though all six Ss required more medication in the second condition than the first, and even though the mean number of requests was twice as great, the resulting F was not significant. This is due mainly to the very large within group variance shown in Table 9-18 (plus, of course, the extremely small sample used for demonstration purposes). Examination of the data, however, reveals an interesting phenomenon. Even though Ss differed greatly from one another in each condition, their relative differences between one another

TABLE 9-18. ANOVA Summary Table for Data in Table 9-17

Source	SS	df	MS	F
Drugs	176.33	1	176.33	3.43
Error	513.67	10	51.37	
Total	690	11		

changed very little. S_3 requested medication fewer times than the five other Ss when using both Drug 1 and Drug 2. S_2 registered the next fewest number of demands in both conditions; in fact, only S_5 and S_6 changed their relative ordering and then only barely. Apparently, therefore, variation exists in these data due to individual differences that are constant across treatments. All that remains for the researcher to do is to identify this variance and *subtract* it from within-group error variance.

Since it is individual differences irrespective of treatments that are of interest, it is each S's combined score divided by the number of treatments (2) that is substituted into the general sum of squares formula:

$$SS_{\substack{individual \\ differences}} = \Sigma X^2 - \frac{(\Sigma X)^2}{n}$$

$$\text{Where } \Sigma X^2 = \overset{S_1}{\frac{(4 + 10)^2}{2}} + \overset{S_2}{\frac{(2 + 8)^2}{2}} + \overset{S_3}{\frac{(1 + 6)^2}{2}} + \overset{S_4}{\frac{(8 + 16)^2}{2}} + \overset{S_5}{\frac{(12 + 25)^2}{2}}$$

$$+ \overset{S_6}{\frac{(16 + 24)^2}{2}} = 1945$$

$$\text{And } \frac{(\Sigma X)^2}{n} = (4 + 2 + 1 + \ldots + 25 + 24)^2 = \frac{132^2}{12} = 1452$$

$$\text{Thus } SS_{\substack{individual \\ differences}} = 1945 - 1452 = 493$$

SS_{drugs} and SS_{total} will remain constant from Table 9-17 (since the scores did not change), thus the only place the new individual differences variation can be subtracted from is SS_{error}. The new SS_{error} thus becomes $513.67 - 493 = 20.67$, a drastic reduction indeed. The repeated measures summary table indicates the effect that subtracting out individual difference (also called between-people difference) variation can exert on the F-ratio (Table 9-19).

Certainly this, as well as the factorial example, is a contrived situation. In real life, the scores would not have remained constant when switching from the design represented in Table 9-18 to the one represented in Table 9-19. In real life, the effect on the F-ratio would also not have been so great, but the increased power associated with repeated measures analysis does very often spell the differences between a significant and a nonsignificant F-ratio. Furthermore, it should be noted that most researchers would have computed a de-

TABLE 9-19. Repeated Measures Summary Table for Data in Table 9-17

Source	SS	df	MS	F
Between people	493	5		
Drugs	176.33	1	176.33	42.69*
Error	20.67	5[a]	4.13	
Total	690	11		

*p < 0.01

[a]Calculated by subtracting one from the number of different Ss. Note the drastic reduction in degrees of freedom for the error term from Table 9-18 to Table 9-19. If there are not substantive individual differences in an experiment (that is, if Ss' scores are not similar from treatment to treatment), then a repeated measures design can have disastrous results.

pendent group t-test for this two group design. Since the relationship between t and F holds for repeated measures and randomized block designs as well as for independently grouped designs, either practice is acceptable.

Although repeated measures ANOVAs are not uncommon in nursing research, especially in those studies using pre- and post-tests, many experimental settings, though sadly in need of the added precision offered by repeated measures analysis, simply do not lend themselves to having the same Ss in different treatments. Fortunately, there is a very effective way to simulate that situation and this is by randomly assigning matched Ss to the various treatments. These randomized block designs have already been discussed; their analysis, aptly enough termed *randomized block ANOVA*, is identical to repeated measures ANOVA. Randomized block ANOVAs furthermore often result in practically as much added statistical power as their repeated measures counterparts, depending completely upon the success of the blocking variable. If there is more similarity in scores between matched than unmatched Ss across treatments, then the randomized block ANOVA will prove profitable. Since this is usually the case, researchers would be well advised to use these procedures whenever possible.

As with factorial ANOVA, there is no limit upon the number of independent variables that can be used in repeated measures and randomized block ANOVAs. Factorial ANOVA, in fact, is a generic term applied to between-subjects designs (that is, experiments in which different Ss are assigned to different groups), multifactor repeated measures designs, and analyses in which some independent variables are represented as repeated measures (or blocked variables) and some contain independent scores. The more complex of these can become rather laborious to compute, having complicated, multiple sources of error variance. The average researcher is well advised to rely on the computer in these situations and although SPSS is not particularly helpful, many excellent programs do exist.

Analysis of Covariance (ANCOVA)

There is one remaining statistical procedure for decreasing error variance that must be discussed because of its wide applicability for all types of research. It is called analysis of covariance (ANCOVA), and it is used when the researcher has a nonmanipulated, nonexperimental independent variable (called a covariate) that is capable of predicting Ss' performance on the dependent variable. The assumptions governing its use are identical to those applying to ANOVA with the addition of some unique to the covariate itself. In ANCOVA, the covariate must:

1. *be measured at the interval level.*

    This is not an assumption for independent variables used in factorial ANOVA, in which normally independent variables are no more than nominal.

2. *be correlated at least 0.30 with the dependent variable.*

    If it is not, then nothing is gained by using ANCOVA and something is lost in the form of one degree of freedom per covariate.

3. *be obtained prior to the experiment or at least be totally noninfluenced by the experimental treatment (that is, its values are immutable across time.)*

4. *not be related to the purposes of the study.*

    The reason for this requirement will become more obvious during the discussion that follows.

5. *be similarly related to the dependent variable within each treatment group.*

    This assumption is all too often ignored. What it basically means is that a covariate could not be used that was highly related to, say, E group Ss dependent variable measures but had a different relationship with C Ss. Careful researchers test this assumption, which is basically a matter of determining the homogeneity of the different regression effects within a given design (as well as their linearity). Most statistical packages contain procedures for testing these assumptions, although some (such as SPSS) require an extra step on the part of the investigator, one that would be wise to take.

The chief purpose of ANCOVA, as in factorial ANOVA, is to lend more precision to the analysis and thereby reduce error variance. There are important differences between the two procedures. One is that the independent variable selected as the covariate can be measured on a continuous scale (for example, age in years or months) rather than discretely as in factorial ANOVA (for example, children, adolescents, young adults, and adults, or E vs. C). The reason for this lies in the fact that the different values associated with the covariate are not used to determine groups as are different independent variable values in factorial ANOVA and thus need not and should not be collapsed into categories (because of the concomitant loss of information).

The second and most important distinction lies in the relative emphasis or importance placed upon the covariate as opposed to a second independent variable in a factorial ANOVA. The independent variable selected as the covariate is not of primary interest; the experimenter has little interest in its significance level and assumes that it does not interact with other independent variables. Factorial ANOVA treats its independent variables as equals, assessing the effect of each separately and in combination. ANCOVA treats its covariate(s) as a sort of nuisance or source of contamination. It asks the question: "Did the treatments differ from one another *after* the effects of the covariate had been considered?" or said another way, "Were treatment means significantly different after initial differences on the covariate had been partialled out?" Implicit in the answering of these questions is the fact that the relationship between the covariate and the dependent variable must be accounted for and set aside *before* the effects of other independent variables can be studied. This is accomplished by measuring the relationship between the covariate and the dependent variable *within* each level of the other independent variables and *between* each level. These values are then used to statistically adjust each S's score on the dependent variable with respect to that S's score on the covariate. Once these adjusted scores are computed for each S, an ANOVA is then performed on the adjusted scores, and is identical to standard ANOVAs except (1) one degree of freedom is subtracted from MS_{error} for each covariate used, (2) the resulting F-ratios test ANCOVA rather than ANOVA hypotheses, and (3) the means, differences between which these F-ratios test, are means of adjusted scores rather than the raw means of ANOVA procedures.

This third point regarding adjusted means is crucial to understanding ANCOVA, because an adjusted mean can be very different indeed from an unadjusted one. In the example used for one-way ANOVA, Ss were randomly assigned to two groups and measured with respect to their attitudes toward alcoholics following an experimental manipulation. If the experimenter had access to, or could administer, another measure that the researcher had good reason to believe would be related to such attitudes, then it would be possible to use this measure as a covariate and predict which Ss in both the E and C groups would have high and low attitudes, thus reducing the error variance. The method by which this prediction occurs is what is unique about analysis of covariance.

Choosing a reasonable covariate is the first and most important step in the process. The covariate, to be successful, must be measured at the interval level* and must have a reasonably strong linear relationship with the dependent variable. Since the actual relationship cannot be measured until the completion of the experiment, a certain degree of risk is involved but usually researchers

---

*In ANOVA, it is usually assumed that the independent variable will be measured at the nominal level (although it does not have to be). This cannot occur in ANCOVA, however. Religious preferences, for example, might well be related to attitudes toward alcoholics, but could not be used in classical ANCOVA procedures unless dichotomized (such as christians vs. nonchristians or protestants vs. nonprotestants), although it could be considered via certain regression techniques as will be discussed in Chapter 10.

have a good idea of what is and is not related to their dependent variables from previous research or pilot work. The covariate may be anything meeting these requirements that exists as a measure prior to the experimental manipulation and does *not* run counter to the purposes of the experiment.* For present purposes it will be assumed that the experimenter was in a position to administer the attitudes toward alcoholics instrument prior to the beginning of the experiment (usually a premeasure of this sort is related adequately with a similar or identical postmeasure).

Since there are only two groups (E and C), there are three possible outcomes of this preadministration of the attitudinal measure: (1) Ss in E and C started the experiment with identical or nearly identical attitudes toward alcoholics, (2) Ss in E started with more favorable attitudes, and (3) Ss in C started with superior attitude scores. The first possibility is by far the more likely in a true experiment containing randomization. In this situation, the adjusted means will be identical (or nearly so) to the raw score means, but the MS_{error} will be reduced proportionate to the relationship between the pre- (covariate) and postattitudinal measures.

Suppose the experiment represented by the data in Table 9-1 had included a premeasure designed as a covariate, and suppose the randomization process had resulted in identical E and C preattitudinal means. If Ss' scores on the covariate are designated X and their dependent variable scores as Y, the data might have looked similar to Table 9-20.

The ANCOVA summary table, in which ′ indicates an adjusted value, might resemble Table 9-21.

In Table 9-21, in comparison with Table 9-2, $SS_{between}$ is not affected because the treatment covariate means were identical, hence the adjusted post-test means were the same as the raw score means. SS'_{total} and SS'_{error} are by no means the same as their unadjusted counterparts in Table 9-5. They are both considerably lower because of the relationship between X and Y, which was simply subtracted or partialled out of the SS_{error}. This of course resulted in a huge decrease in the MS_{error} followed by a concomitant increase in the ANCOVA F-ratio. In other words, there were no initial differences between groups on the covariate, but this same covariate did substantially reduce within-group variation by predicting which Ss would score high and which low within each

---

*An example of this requirement might be the use of age as a covariate in the factorial experiment discussed above involving the previous exposure variable. If the experimenter were truly interested in ascertaining the relationship between previous exposure to alcoholics and attitudes, both alone and as the relationship interacts with instruction, then age employed as a covariate might run counter to these objectives. It would probably be found that persons with prior exposure to alcoholics tended to be older than persons without such experiences, simply because they had had more time to be involved. Age as a covariate would tend to statistically equate Ss in the two exposure groups by adjusting their attitudinal scores as though everyone started the experiment with the same age, hence also adjusting attitudinal scores as though everyone started the experiment with the same degree of previous exposure and completely negating one of the primary purposes of the study.

TABLE 9-20. Addition of a Premeasure to Data in Table 9-1

	E			C	
	X	Y		X	Y
S-1	7	15	S-7	8	7
S-2	9	16	S-8	7	8
S-3	8	17	S-9	9	9
S-4	10	18	S-10	11	10
S-5	12	19	S-11	10	11
S-6	11	20	S-12	12	12
	$\overline{X} = 9.5$	$\overline{X} = 17.5$		$\overline{X} = 9.5$	$\overline{X} = 9.5$

X = score on covariate.
Y = score on dependent variable.

TABLE 9-21. ANCOVA Summary Table for Data in Table 9-20

Source	SS'	df	MS'	F'
Treatment'	192.00	1	192.00	229.09*
Error'	7.54	9	0.84	
Total'	199.54	10		

*p < 0.01.
'indicates an adjusted value.

group. The F-ratio, though considerably more significant than the ANOVA F, is still interpreted as indicative of the superiority of the E treatment over the C, only now with the added precision of having taken Ss attitudinal predispositions into account.

Most certainly, the data presented in Table 9-20 are contrived with regard to both the strength of the relationship between X and Y and the highly improbable absolute equality of the two groups' covariate means. Still, the data should illustrate the potential utility of ANCOVA in reducing the error variance irrespective of its added potential to adjust between-group differences on the dependent variable by taking into account between-group covariate differences.

To illustrate this latter characteristic, consider the situation in which, for some reason, Ss assigned to E began the experiment with superior attitudes toward alcoholics (Tables 9-22 and 9-23).

Note that although E and C Ss' postexperimental attitude scores have not changed at all, the new ANCOVA F-ratio has been reduced drastically. Examination of Table 9-23 reveals that the adjusted SS_{error} has remained constant from Table 9-21 but the $SS'_{treatment}$ has been decimated. The reason for this has been previously given: analysis of covariance procedures use the relationship between the covariate and the dependent variable to adjust each S's score on the dependent variable with respect to that S's covariate score, resulting in a decrease in within-group variance and an adjustment in between-group vari-

TABLE 9-22. Modification of Data in Table 9-20 Such That E Subjects Entered the Experiment with Higher Values on the Dependent Variable

	E			C	
	X	Y		X	Y
S-1	15	15	S-7	8	7
S-2	17	16	S-8	7	8
S-3	16	17	S-9	9	9
S-4	18	18	S-10	11	10
S-5	20	19	S-11	10	11
S-6	19	20	S-12	12	12
$\overline{X} =$	17.5	17.5		9.5	9.5

TABLE 9-23. ANCOVA Summary Table for Data in Table 9-22

Source	SS'	df	MS'	F'
Treatment'	0.39	1	0.39	0.46
Error'	7.54	9	0.84	
Total'	7.93	10		

ance in the form of adjusted means if the original groups initially differed with respect to covariate scores. In this last case, the groups did so differ: E Ss began the experiment with an average attitudinal score of 17.5, while C Ss had a mean of only 9.5. This decrepancy resulted in adjusted postexperimental means (that is, adjusted dependent variable means) of 13.96 and 13.04 respectively. In other words, the E group was "penalized" because of its Ss' initial high scores on the covariate while C Ss were "compensated." The ANCOVA $SS_{treatment}$ was then computed on the basis of this relatively small adjusted mean difference (13.96 − 13.04 = 0.92), as compared with the original ANOVA $SS_{treatment}$ based on the raw score mean difference of 17.5 − 9.5 = 8.0.* This potential to reduce a significant ANOVA F-ratio to an insignificant ANCOVA F is one reason why, especially for nonexperimental variables, the covariate should never be at cross-purposes with the objectives of the study. Before continuing, it would probably be wise to examine the actual output accruing from an SPSS run on the data in Table 9-22 (Table 9-24) since it contains, as does the factorial ANOVA output, several redundant entries.

---

*Some researchers find it conceptually useful to visualize ANCOVA as a process in which:

    A. Each S's score on the covariate is used to determine a *predicted score* on the dependent variable.

    B. Each S's predicted score is subtracted from that S's actual score.

    C. An ANOVA is then performed upon these *difference scores* using an adjusted MS_{error} being reduced proportionately to the magnitude of the correlation between the covariate and the dependent variable. Although this is actually an oversimplication, it does present the gist of ANCOVA.

TABLE 9-24. SPSS Printout for Data in Table 9-22.

SOURCE OF VARIATION	SUM OF SQUARES	DF	MEAN SQUARE	F	SIGNIF. OF F
Covariates[a]	219.070	1	219.070	261.391	0.001
Preattitudes[b]	219.070	1	219.070	261.391	0.001
Main Effects	0.387	1	0.387	0.461	0.999
Treatments[c]	0.387	1	0.387	0.461	0.999
Explained	219.457	2	109.729	130.926	0.001
Residual	7.543	9	0.838		
Total	227.000	11	20.636		

Covariate	Beta
Preattitudes	0.982[d]

Grand Mean = 13.50

Variable + Category	N	Unadjusted Dev'n Eta	. . . .	Adjusted for independents + covariates Dev'n Beta
Treatments				
Experimental	6	4.00		4.00[e]
Control	6	−4.00		−4.00
		0.92		0.92
Multiple R squared				0.967[f]
Multiple R				0.983

[a]The effect of all the covariates. Since there is only one in this study its values are identical to that of (b).

[b]This information simply assesses the relationship between the covariate and the dependent variable. Obviously the researcher hopes that this effect is significant, although this particular information does not normally appear in the research report.

[c]Information concerning the effects of the treatment *after* the effects of the covariate have been partialled out. In other words, the difference between experimental and control group *adjusted* means is tested here, not raw means.

[d]The correlation between the covariate (preattitudes) and the dependent variable (post-treatment attitudes toward alcoholics).

[e]These values are added and subtracted from the grand mean to produce *adjusted means*. In almost all real life situations the adjusted means will differ somewhat from the unadjusted ones.

[f]96.7 percent of the variance in the dependent variable can be explained by the covariate *and* the independent variable.

Consider, finally, the opposite situation in which the C group started the experiment with superior attitudes (Tables 9-25 and 9-26).

Note that although SS'_{error} has remained constant from Tables 9-21 and 9-23, $SS'_{treatment}$ and SS'_{total} have again changed. $SS'_{between}$, hence the F-ratio, for this last example has greatly increased from the previous situation, basically because the C group was "penalized" and E "compensated" for the initial

TABLE 9-25. Modification of Data in Table 9-1 Such That C Subjects Entered the Experiment with Higher Values on the Dependent Variable

	E			C	
	X	Y		X	Y
S-1	8	15	S-7	15	7
S-2	7	16	S-8	17	8
S-3	9	17	S-9	16	9
S-4	11	18	S-10	18	10
S-5	10	19	S-11	20	11
S-6	12	20	S-12	19	12
$\overline{X} =$	9.5	17.5		17.5	9.5

TABLE 9-26. ANCOVA Summary Table for Data in Table 9-25.

Source	SS'	df	MS'	F'
Treatment'	105.27	1	105.27	125.60*
Error'	7.54	9	0.84	
Total'	112.81	10		

*$p < 0.01$.

superiority of the former. This resulted in adjusted means of 21.04 and 5.96 as compared with raw dependent variable means of 17.5 and 9.5 for E and C, respectively. In other words, the original superiority of E Ss was magnified via ANCOVA procedures.

Hopefully, these examples will give the reader some idea of what ANCOVA is all about. Although similar in many respects to ANOVA, it addresses a very distinctly different hypothesis: whether or not significant differences exist *after* the effect of another variable has been accounted for. This difference sometimes results in significance where significance did not exist in ANOVA, or lack of significance where differences were found in ANOVA. While an experiment with only one covariate and one independent variable has been discussed, ANCOVA is generalizable to more than one covariate and more than one factor.

The present discussion will be ended with a warning. ANCOVA cannot substitute for random assignment; it also cannot equate unequal groups. This is not to say that the procedure cannot be used in nonexperimental research with intact groups, it simply means that the same limitations attached to the interpretation of nonexperimental research that exist prior to the use of ANCOVA also exist subsequent to its use. The best ANCOVA can do is to vitiate one rival hypothesis per covariate.

Other Types of Analyses of Variance and Covariance

There are many ANOVA variations, all of which serve the same purpose: allowing the researcher to subtract sources of systematic variation from the within-group variance error term. The reader should remember that these statistical manipulations are made possible by the investigator's design that permits certain possible sources of error (that is, within-group variance) to be controlled in the first place. Nested, latin square, and split plot designs are all examples of other designs that can be employed to increase the precision of an investigation. Since these analyses will not be discussed in detail here (see Winer[17] for further explanation), the best advice that can be offered at this point is for the researcher to design the study to control all extraneous sources of variation possible. The researcher should then choose the ANOVA-ANCOVA combination that will permit the subtraction of all these controlled sources of variation from the error term. To illustrate how this process of careful design and analysis works, the following discussion examines an educational study by one of the authors.

For years, educators had recommended tutoring for children needing more intensive educational help than provided in the classroom on the assumption that children learned more in a tutorial than in a classroom setting. Determined to test the validity of this assumption, an experiment was designed in which some children of varying abilities (high, medium, and low) would be instructed in the same curriculum, for the same length of time, and by the same teachers in both classroom and tutorial settings. Since tutoring by classroom teachers is often impractical, two types of teachers were employed: one involving individuals with some training and experience, one consisting of individuals with neither of these in an attempt to see if paraprofessionals could be efficaciously employed as tutors if tutoring proved as effective as expected. To reduce within-group variance, each student was administered a pretest and students were measured on another variable that was known to be related to learning, matched, and randomly assigned in pairs to the tutoring and classroom instruction treatments.

TABLE 9-27. ANCOVA Summary Table for Data in the Experiment on Teaching Methods (See Text for Discussion)

	Source	df	SS	MS	F
A	(Training)	1	15.80	15.80	1.6
B w. A	(Teachers nested in training)	17	172.23	10.13	
C	(Tutoring)	1	53.33	53.33	4.7*
AC		1	1.41	1.41	0.1
C × (B w. A)		17	192.64	11.33	
D	(Ability level)	2	179.60	89.80	12.8**
AD		2	3.32	1.66	0.2
C × (B w. A)		35	246.30	7.04	
CD		2	6.96	3.48	0.4
ACD		2	21.30	10.65	1.2
C × D × (B w. A)		35	299.24	8.55	

*$p < 0.05$.
**$p < 0.001$.

Since this study was designed in such a way that teacher effects were controlled in the sense that each teacher taught each type of student (high, medium, and low ability) under each treatment (classroom vs. tutorial instruction), then differences between teachers could be subtracted out of the analysis. Since there were two types of teachers with different teachers within each type, the effect for teachers constituted a nested factor (that is, nested within types). Teacher type, treatment, and ability level of the student each constituted separate independent variables with students' prior knowledge serving as a covariate. What resulted, therefore, was a 2 (treatment) × 3 (ability) × 2 (training) × 10 (teachers) randomized block ANCOVA with teachers used as a nested variable. The ANCOVA summary table is presented in Table 9-27.

This example should illustrate the facts that ANOVA and ANCOVA (1) can vary greatly in complexity and (2) can be used to statistically control everything that the investigator took the pains to experimentally control. ANOVA and ANCOVA are truly powerful aids to experimental research and, though not especially easy to learn in their more complicated forms, are certainly worth the effort their study involves.

NONPARAMETRIC ANOVA PROCEDURES

Since nonparametric statistical procedures are primarily designed for data measured at the nominal and ordinal levels, and since variances are not relevant for such data, nonparametric analyses of variance are, strictly speaking, misnomers. There are occasions, however, when a researcher wishes to ascertain whether or not differences exist between groups or treatments whose Ss have been measured on an instrument yielding clearly ordinal scores (for example, ranks). Several procedures exist whereby a probability can be assigned to the likelihood that the observed differences between said groups would have occurred by chance alone. They are analogous to classical ANOVA procedures in that differences between groups can be tested for statistical significance; they differ in that it is differences in ranks rather than differences between means that are tested. The analogy can be carried further in the sense that procedures exist to test differences between groups in which different Ss have been assigned (that is, between-Ss designs), as well as between groups in which the same (or matched) Ss are represented (that is, repeated measures and randomized block designs). One example of each procedural type will be briefly discussed.

Kruskal-Wallis One-Way Analysis of Variance

The Kruskal-Wallis test is an example of a procedure used to determine whether groups containing different Ss differ from one another on a dependent variable measured at the ordinal level. Basically, all that is involved with the procedure is the rank ordering of all Ss in the study irrespective of their group membership. The sum of the ranks in each group is then computed, squared, and converted to an H statistic (synonymous with chi-square for large samples), which can then be compared to a distribution to ascertain whether significant differences exist between the different sets of ranks (or more properly, the probability that Ss within the different groups are representatives of different populations). A significant H is interpreted in much the same way as a significant F in the sense that more than two groups necessitate post hoc (nonparametric) contrasts. The actual computational procedures involved are quite simple for the Kruskal-Wallis test with the H formula obtainable from Siegal[15] among other places.

Friedman Two-Way Analysis of Variance

The Friedman test is doubly misnamed: it does not involve analysis of variance and it does not involve two factors in the usual sense of the word. It is an example, however, of a nonparametric procedure that can be used with repeated measures and randomized block designs involving one independent variable. Like the Kruskal-Wallis test, the Friedman test also involves ranks. The difference is that since each person possesses as many scores as there are treatments, each person's scores are rank ordered by themselves. If there are five groups, for example, S_1's five scores will be rank ordered from 1 for lowest to 5 for highest. The process is repeated for all other Ss and the ranks are then added, squared, and substituted into a formula for a χ_F^2 statistic. The computed χ_F^2 is then compared to its distribution to ascertain whether between-group differences existed for the ranked scores. A significant χ_F^2 is interpreted in the same way that a significant F or H is interpreted.

REFERENCES

1. Brock, A. M.: *Impact of a management-oriented course on knowledge and leadership skills exhibited by baccalaureate nursing students.* Nurs. Res. 27:217, 1978.
2. Campbell, D. T. and Stanley, J. C.: *Experimental and Quasi-Experimental Designs for Research.* Rand McNally, Chicago, 1963.
3. Crosley, M. H.: *Teaching strategies: A microteaching project for nurses in Virginia.* Nurs. Res. 26:144, 1977.
4. Dean, N. R.: *Effect of free time the day prior to mastery testing on nursing students' scores.* Nurs. Res. 28:40, 1979.
5. Diers, D., et al.: *The effect of nursing interaction on patients in pain.* Nurs. Res. 21: 419, 1972.
6. Gerber, R. M. and Van Ort, S. R.: *Topical application of insulin in decubitus ulcers.* Nurs. Res. 28:16, 1979.
7. Glass, G. V. and Bracht, G. H.: *The external validity of experiments.* Am. Ed. Res. J. 5:437, 1966.
8. Hall, K., Irwin, B., and Murphy, K.: *A comparison of audio-visual and written presentations in self-instructed learning.* J. Ed. Res. 71(5):290, 1978.
9. Harrison, O. A.: An experimental study of psychomotor skill learning of a nursing procedure using two methods of critique in instruction. Unpublished doctoral dissertation, University of Colorado, Boulder, Colorado, 1972.

10. Huckabay, L. M.: *Cognitive and affective consequences of formative evaluation in graduate nursing students.* Nurs. Res. 27:190, 1978.
11. Kempthorne, O.: *The design and analysis of experiments, with some reference to educational research.* In Collier, R. O. and Elam, S. M. (eds.): *Research Design and Analysis: The Second Annual Phi Delta Kappa Symposium on Educational Research.* Phi Delta Kappa, Bloomington, Indiana, 1961.
12. Nie, N. H., et al.: *Statistical Package for the Social Sciences.* McGraw-Hill, New York, 1975.
13. O'Neil, S.: *The application and methodological implications of behavior modification in nursing research.* In Batey, M. V. (ed.): *Communicating Nursing Research: The Many Sources of Nursing Knowledge.* Western Interstate Commission for Higher Education, Boulder, Colorado, 1972.
14. Schmitt, F. E. and Wooldridge, P. J.: *Psychological preparation of surgical patients.* Nurs. Res. 22:108, 1973.
15. Siegel, S.: *Nonparametric Statistics.* McGraw-Hill, New York, 1956.
16. Walston, K. A., et al.: *Increasing nurses' person-centeredness.* Nurs. Res. 27:156, 1978.
17. Winer, B. J.: *Statistical Principles in Experimental Design.* McGraw-Hill, New York, 1971.

CHAPTER 10

CORRELATIONAL STUDIES

CORRELATIONAL STUDY DESIGNS

Correlational studies are studies of relationship. That is, when undertaking the conduct of a correlational study, the researcher utilizes correlational procedures and techniques to examine the systematic relationship that does or does not exist between two or more variables. Correlational studies, of which regression studies are a special case, may be designed either to predict or explain this relationship depending upon the researcher's concerns and interests. Thus, in designing correlational research, an important decision needs to be made early in the process: Will the intent be to predict changes in one variable on the basis of what is known of other variables or to explain the nature of the relationship between the variables? Once this conceptual decision is made, the basic analytic techniques and statistical procedures are the same when used to predict or explain and include a variety of both nonparametric and parametric statistical methods.

Instrumentation in correlational studies includes the gamut of those techniques discussed in Chapter 5. Data collection methods are therefore selected by the researcher on the basis of the research questions and/or hypotheses with consideration given to the selection of the most appropriate statistical procedure for the level of measurement of the data obtained.

A variety of computer programs are available for analyzing the data from correlational studies. These are exemplified by the SPSS programs CROSSTABS, PEARSON CORR, SCATTERGRAM, NONPAR CORREL, and REGRESSION.

Descriptive versus Experimental

A correlational study is *descriptive* if it is conducted in a natural setting and no attempt is made to introduce something new or to modify or control the study environment. If designed correctly, a descriptive correlational study can afford a relatively inexpensive approach to the determination of hypotheses worthy of subsequent more precise experimental investigation. Too frequently, however, researchers erroneously use correlational data to imply causation when all they can validly speak to is how two or more variables vary together. For example, a group of subjects who have experienced the variable of interest (X) is compared with one that has not for the purpose of considering the effect of X. This approach is valid only if the intent is simply to construct a picture of what exists and no attempt is made to account for why. This approach is not valid for determining the effect of X. The comparison of two natural units in this manner is limited in that they differ not only in the presence and absence of X, but also in a number of other attributes that are not measured. Each of these attributes could create differences in subjects and each therefore provides a rival hypothesis to the hypothesis that the variable X had an effect. *Correlation does not imply causation* and the results of descriptive correlational studies cannot be correctly used to speak to the effect of one variable on another. Correlational descriptive studies can, however, be employed to describe how variables systematically vary together. Researchers who design correlational descriptive studies should concern themselves with the characteristics of descriptive studies discussed in Chapter 8.

EXAMPLE 10-1. Published Example of a Descriptive Correlational Study

Title: *Clinical signs associated with the amount of tracheobronchial secretions.*

Source: Amborn, Nursing Research, vol. 25, no. 2, March–April, 1976, pp. 121–126.

Purpose: To answer the research question—"What clinical signs are predominately associated with the amount of tracheobronchial secretions obtained by mechanical aspiration?" (p. 122)

Design: 1. Through the literature and on the basis of clinical nursing experience, the problem was defined as a need to investigate the clinical situation of patients on volume cycled respirators for manifestations associated with the amount of tracheobronchial secretions in an effort to identify indicators for tracheobronchial suctioning.
           2. Literature was reviewed in three areas related to the problem, (a) response to tracheobronchial secretion retention, (b) response to the volume cycled ventilator, and (c) effects of tracheal suctioning.
           3. On the basis of the literature review, 22 clinical signs were identified as variables to be investigated in this study (pp. 122–123).
           4. The design selected as most appropriate for answering the research question was a descriptive correlational study. That is, data were to be collected in the natural setting in an attempt to explain the relationship between the study variables and amount of secretion.
           5. The target population was identified and 35 subjects meeting the stated criteria for inclusion in the study were observed over a 1-hour period.
           6. Physiologic measures and observational techniques were combined for the collection of data (p. 123).

EXAMPLE **10-1.** *Continued*

> 7. Data were analyzed utilizing biserial correlation coefficients and chi-square analysis.
> 8. Results were interpreted and disseminated in a nursing research journal.

In correlational studies in which the intent is to obtain evidence for a causal relationship, a *true experimental design* with randomization and a control group is required. These designs, along with their quasi-experimental counterparts when randomization and/or control groups are not feasible, are discussed in Chapter 9 (see also the cross-lagged correlation analysis approach discussed later in this chapter).

Prediction versus Explanation

In *predictive correlational studies* the main emphasis is on practical application. On the basis of knowledge about one or more predictors, the researcher wishes to develop a regression equation to be used for the prediction of the criterion variable that is usually some standard of performance or accomplishment. For example, most graduate schools require applicants to take a battery of tests prior to admission. These tests are believed to predict success in their respective program and thus are used to determine who should or should not be admitted on the basis of their potential for successfully completing the program. The specific tests that comprise the battery are usually determined on the basis of a predictive correlational study in which a number of regression analyses are employed in order to determine the variance in the criterion variable (success) that is predictable on the basis of the test scores. Regression equations resulting from these analyzes are used to identify those tests whose scores contribute the most to the prediction of success and to provide weights for each predictor depending on its correlation with the criterion that are used to weight the scores of students who subsequently apply to the school. The decision to admit or reject is then made in part on the basis of each student's resulting weighted score for the test battery.

The choice of predictor variables in the case of a predictive correlational study is determined primarily by their potential effectiveness in enhancing the prediction of the criterion. Under these circumstances, therefore, the researcher's concern is toward obtaining as high a squared regression coefficient as possible. Methods for conducting predictive studies include general, forward, true stepwise, and backward regression solutions which are discussed in detail later in this chapter.

EXAMPLE **10-2.** Published Example of a Predictive Correlational Study

Title: *Selected National League for Nursing Achievement Test scores as predictors of State Board Examination scores.*

EXAMPLE 10-2. *Continued*

Source: Deardorff, Denner, and Miller, Nursing Research, vol. 25, no. 1, January–February, 1976, pp. 35–38.

Purpose: To formulate regression equations to be used to predict performance on the licensing examinations of graduates of an associate degree nursing program.

Design: 1. Previous studies that investigated the correlations between scores on the National League for Nursing tests (NLN), State Board Examinations (SBE), and other variables were reviewed.
             2. The criterion variable was SBE scores and predictor variables were NLN achievement test scores.
             3. Data were obtained from test score records of graduates from a particular associate degree nursing program over a 5-year period.
             4. Stepwise multiple regression procedures were utilized to analyze the data and to obtain regression equations for the determination of weighted scores.
             5. Results were interpreted and reported in a nursing research journal.

When an *explanatory* framework is employed in a correlational study, the main emphasis is on the explanation of the variability in a criterion variable by using information from one or more predictor variables. The choice of predictor variables is determined by theoretical formulations and considerations. In other words, when the concern is explanation, the emphasis is on formulating or testing theories, conceptual models, or schemes. Within this context, questions regarding the relative importance of predictor variables become particularly meaningful. Explanatory schemes under certain circumstances may be enhanced by inferences about causal relations among the variables under study. Commonality analysis and path analysis are two approaches that exemplify an explanatory correlational study. *Commonality analysis* is a method of analyzing the variance of a criterion variable into common and unique variance to help identify the relative influence of independent variables.[16, 17] *Path analysis*[28] was developed as a method for studying the direct and indirect effects of variables taken as causes of variables taken as effects. It should be noted that path analysis is useful in testing theory. Both commonality and path analyses are very complex, sophisticated procedures. For this reason, only the basic elements of the two approaches are presented later in this chapter and the interested reader is referred to additional sources that address greater detail.

EXAMPLE 10-3. Published Example of an Explanatory Correlational Study

Title: *Orientation of senior nursing students toward access to contraceptives.*

Source: Elder, Nursing Research, vol. 25, no. 5, September–October, 1976, pp. 338–345.

Purpose: To assess attitudes of senior nursing students toward providing contraceptive services to all who want them.

EXAMPLE 10-3. *Continued*

Design: 1. Literature was reviewed in relation to (a) utilization of contraceptive services, (b) sexual practices, (c) unwanted conceptions, (d) changes in the area of fertility control and orientation of health professionals toward these changes.
  2. On the basis of the literature review, a hypothesis regarding the effect of various social and demographic variables on students' orientations was formulated. Criterion variables were permissive attitudes and willingness to participate in providing contraceptives. Predictor variables were age, education, type of school attending, religious orientation, sexual experience, degree of concern re population problems, and nature of sex-role attitudes.
  3. The study was designed as a descriptive correlational study with the intent to explain the variables that may influence the criterion variable.
  4. Subjects were 264 senior nursing students in six schools of nursing who were surveyed by a questionnaire designed to elicit orientations to fertility control. Data were collected by mail and face-to-face in the classroom setting.
  5. Data were analyzed by number and percent and utilizing factor analysis and Pearson r to test the research hypothesis.
  6. Results were interpreted and published in a nursing research journal.

ADVANTAGES AND DISADVANTAGES OF CORRELATIONAL STUDIES

The *advantages* of correlational studies stem from the fact that they:

1. Provide more information (that is, regarding the extent to which variations in one factor correspond with variations in one or more other factors) than is obtained using other descriptive study designs in situations in which variables are very complex and/or do not lend themselves to an experimental design.
2. Provide information regarding the degrees of relationship between two or more variables in addition to the all or none question answered by most experimental designs — "Is an effect present or absent?"
3. Permit the consideration of several variables and their interrelationships simultaneously and in a realistic setting.[10]

Disadvantages, on the other hand, include:

1. The tendency for users to overinterpret results, that is, attribute cause and effect relationships on the basis of purely descriptive findings.
2. The tendency for users to indiscriminately include data from miscellaneous sources precluding any meaningful or useful interpretation.

STEPS IN A CORRELATIONAL STUDY

In designing a correlational study, the researcher:

1. Defines the problem.
2. Reviews the literature in relation to the problem.
3. Identifies relevant variables.
4. Conceptualizes the study as predictive or explanatory.
5. Selects subjects.
6. Selects or constructs measuring instruments.
7. Selects the correlational statistical procedure that fits the problem.
8. Collects data.
9. Analyzes, interprets, and reports results.

STATISTICAL PROCEDURES USED IN CORRELATIONAL STUDIES

Both nonparametric and parametric procedures exist for determining the relationship between two or more variables. *Nonparametric* measures of association are usually employed when data are measured at the nominal or ordinal level or when no assumptions are made regarding an underlying sampling distribution. Nonparametric techniques are also particularly useful for small sample sizes. *Parametric* measures of relationship have more assumptions governing their use than do nonparametric techniques. Parametric procedures are used with interval or ratio level data; assumptions regarding an underlying sampling distribution are made; and sample sizes are generally larger than those required for nonparametic statistics.

Nonparametric Measures of Association

Nonparametric techniques are often called "distribution free" or "ranking tests." They are called "distribution free" because they do not assume that the scores under analysis were drawn from a population distributed in a certain manner, for example, from a normally distributed population. Some nonparametric measures are "ranking tests" in the sense that they may be used with scores that are ordinal, that is, are simply ranks. Nonparametric techniques are simple to compute and are useful with small samples. Thus, the nurse researcher who is collecting pilot data or whose samples must be small because of their nature (for example, samples of patients with a rare form of illness) will find them most useful.

CHI-SQUARE

The researcher who is interested in the number of subjects, objects, or responses that fall in various categories will find chi-square (χ^2) a useful statistical test. For example, a group of patients may be classified according to their compliance with a diabetic nutritional regimen, and the investigator may predict that certain types of patients will comply more frequently than others. Or, students may be categorized according to their preferences for nursing practice after exposure to a particular clinical experience, to test the hypothesis that these preferences will differ in frequency.

When χ^2 is used for analyzing nominal data such as these it is often referred to as a *goodness of fit* test in that it is used to ascertain whether a significant difference exists between an *observed* number of subjects, objects, or responses falling in each category and an *expected* number based on the null hypothesis.

In order to compare an observed with an expected group of frequencies, one needs to be able to specify what frequencies would be expected. The null hypothesis states that an equal number of subjects will fall in each of the categories. In some cases, however, expected frequencies are determined by other considerations, such as prior performances, empirical or theoretical distributions, and so forth. χ^2 then tests whether the observed frequencies are sufficiently close to those expected to occur under the null hypothesis, that is, by chance alone.

(Formula 10-1)[23]
$$\chi^2 = \sum_{i=1}^{K} \frac{(O_i - E_i)^2}{E_i}$$

where:

O_i = observed number of cases categorized in i-th category

E_i = expected number of cases in i-th category under the null hypothesis

$\sum_{i=1}^{K}$ = sum over all categories (K)

Thus, Formula 10-1 directs the researcher to sum over all categories the squared differences between each observed and expected frequency divided by the corresponding expected frequency. If the agreement between the observed and expected frequencies is close, the difference $(O_i - E_i)$ is large, and χ^2 will also be large.

When employing a 2×2 or 1×2 contingency table, many researchers[29] prefer to employ the following, more conservative, formula:

$$\chi^2 = \sum \frac{(|O_i - E_i| - 0.5)^2}{E_i}$$

Example

Patients attending the diabetic ambulatory care clinic at Health Haven Hospital are assigned by the clerk to be seen by Nurse A, B, C, or D. The clinic supervisor notes at the end of a particularly busy week that Nurse B has seen more patients who are not in compliance with their treatment regimens than have the other nurses. She is concerned that some factor may be systematically biasing the assignment of the nurses' caseloads and thus decides to investigate the problem further. She assembles the patient records for the week and records the number of noncomplying patients assigned to each of the four nurses. The data are:

Number of Noncomplying Patients Seen by Each Nurse	
Nurse	Number of Patients
A	22
B	39
C	11
D	28
	n = 100

Intuitively from the data, it appears that Nurse B is seeing the greatest number of patients who are not in compliance with their treatment regimens. But the question remains, is some factor systematically biasing the assignment or is it the result of chance alone? To objectively answer this question, the supervisor employs a χ^2 statistical procedure because it will enable her to estimate the probability that the observed result occurred by chance alone. She decides to test her null hypothesis that there is no statistically significant difference in the assignment of noncomplying patients to the four nurses at the 0.05 level of significance ($\alpha = 0.05$ or $p \leq 0.05$). Under purely chance conditions, the supervisor would expect each of the four nurses to receive an equal number, that is, one fourth or 25 percent of the noncomplying patients. Since there are 100 such patients, she would have expected each nurse to receive 25 patients. She computes the χ^2 statistic in the following manner:

$$\chi^2 = \sum_{i=1}^{K} \frac{(O_i - E_i)^2}{E_i}$$

Nurse	O_i	E_i	$O_i - E_i$	$(O_i - E_i)^2$	$(O_i - E_i)^2/E_i$
A	22	25	−3	9	0.36
B	39	25	14	196	7.84
C	11	25	−14	196	7.84
D	28	25	3	9	0.36
					$\chi^2 = 16.40$

To interpret the meaning of the $\chi^2 = 16.40$, the supervisor must determine the degrees of freedom. The degrees of freedom represent the extent to which the observations are free to vary, that is, in the example the four numbers had to add up to 100, placing one restriction on the data. In other words, while three of the numbers could vary, the fourth frequency count was restricted to a number that would make all four sum to 100. The number of nurses was four and therefore the degrees of freedom equal 4 − 1, or 3.

The supervisor is now ready to consult the Chi-Square Table for 3 degrees of freedom (Appendix—Table 2). A portion of the table is produced here.

df	.99	.98	.95	.90	.80	.70	.50	.30	.20	.10	.05	.02	.01	.001
1	.00016	.00063	.0039	.016	.064	.15	.46	1.07	1.64	2.71	3.84	5.41	6.64	10.83
2	.02	.04	.10	.21	.45	.71	1.39	2.41	3.22	4.60	5.99	7.82	9.21	13.82
3	.12	.18	.35	.58	1.00	1.42	2.37	3.66	4.64	6.25	7.82	9.81	11.34	16.27
4	.30	.43	.71	1.06	1.65	2.20	3.36	4.88	5.99	7.78	9.49	11.67	13.28	18.46
5	.55	.75	1.14	1.61	2.34	3.00	4.35	6.06	7.29	9.24	11.07	13.39	15.09	20.52

Across the top of the table are the levels of significance. The numbers in each row represent a chi-square sampling distribution for a certain number of degrees of freedom. To use the table, the supervisor finds the intersection of the row for 3 df and the column for the 0.05 level of significance and determines that the smallest value needed to reject the null hypothesis is 7.82. Since her χ^2 value is 16.40, the supervisor rejects the null hypothesis and concludes that the results support her belief that there is systematic bias in the assignment of noncomplying patients to nurses. It should be noted that χ^2 in this case does not tell the supervisor which of the observed differences is statistically significant from the others, that is, she cannot conclude that Nurse B receives more noncomplying patients than Nurses A, C, or D. Rather, χ^2 is a test of the significance of the differences in the total set of data. Only in those instances in which χ^2 is used to compare two categories is it possible to speak to the nature of the differences on the basis of the χ^2 results. If a chi-square test is significant when more than two categories are compared, then further statistical analysis is required in order to single out specific differences.

Chi-square, when used in this manner, tests whether or not the frequencies in a two-or-more-category discreet variable differ by chance. In the example, there was one variable, nurses. This variable had four categories or levels, A, B, C, D.

Chi-square analysis can also be used to determine whether or not two groups are independent of each other. The hypothesis tested is that the two groups differ with respect to some characteristic and therefore with respect to the relative frequency with which group members fall in several categories. To test this hypothesis, the researcher counts the number of cases from each group that fall in various categories, and compares the proportion of cases from one group in the various categories with the proportion of cases from the other group.

(Formula 10-2)[23]

$$\chi^2 = \sum_{i=1}^{r} \sum_{j=1}^{K} \frac{(O_{ij} - E_{ij})^2}{E_{ij}}$$

where:

χ^2 = chi-square statistic for two independent samples

O_{ij} = observed number of cases categorized in the i-th row of the j-th column

E_{ij} = number of cases expected under the null hypothesis to be categorized in the i-th row of j-th column

$\sum_{i=1}^{r} \sum_{j=1}^{K}$ = sum over all rows (r) and all columns (K), i.e., sum over all cells

The values of χ^2 yielded by this formula are tested with df = $(r - 1)$, $(K - 1)$, where r = the number of rows and K = the number of columns. To determine the expected frequency for each cell (E_{ij}), multiply the two marginal totals common to a particular cell, and then divide this product by the total number of cases, N.

Example

A researcher is interested in determining whether BSN nursing graduates and AA nursing graduates differ with respect to leadership qualities. The researcher samples nurses from each of the two settings and categorizes them as leaders, followers, or unclassifiable. The resulting data are shown in Table 10-1.

TABLE 10-1. Type of Program and Leadership

	BSN	AA	
LEADER	30	10	40
FOLLOWER	10	30	40
UNCLASSIFIABLE	10	10	20
TOTAL	50	50	100

Table 10-1 is called a *contingency table.* Specifically, it is a 2 × 3 contingency table because there are two categories for the variable type of program and three categories for the variable leadership.

In each case, the researcher multiplies the two marginal totals common to a particular cell and then divides the product by N to obtain the expected frequency (Table 10-2).

TABLE 10-2. Type of Program and Leadership: Observed and Expected Frequencies

	BSN	AA	
LEADER	30 (20)	10 (20)	40
FOLLOWER	10 (20)	30 (20)	40
UNCLASSIFIABLE	10 (10)	10 (10)	20
TOTAL	50	50	100

For example, the expected frequency for the lower right-hand cell in the above table is

$$E_{32} = \frac{(50)\,(20)}{100}$$

$$= 10$$

As before, if the observed frequencies are in close agreement with the expected frequencies, the differences $(O_{ij} - E_{ij})$ will be small and thus the value of χ^2 will be small. A small χ^2 will not lead to the rejection of the null hypothesis that the two sets of characteristics are independent of each other. On the other hand, if some or many of the differences are large, χ^2 will be large, and the larger χ^2 the more likely it is that the two groups differ with respect to type of program and leadership.

The computation of χ^2 for the data in Table 10-2 is straightforward:

$$\chi^2 = \sum_{i=1}^{r} \sum_{j=1}^{K} \frac{(O_{ij} - E_{ij})^2}{E_{ij}}$$

$$= \frac{(30 - 20)^2}{20} + \frac{(10 - 20)^2}{20} + \frac{(10 - 10)^2}{10} +$$

$$\frac{(10 - 20)^2}{20} + \frac{(30 - 20)^2}{20} + \frac{(10 - 10)^2}{10} +$$

$$= 5 + 5 + 0 + 5 + 5 + 0$$

$$= 20$$

The df for testing this χ^2 statistic is $(r - 1)(K - 1)$ or $(3 - 1)(2 - 1) = 2$. To determine the significance of $\chi^2 = 20$ with df $= 2$, Table 2 in the Appendix is used. The table shows that this value of χ^2 is significant beyond the 0.05 level. Therefore, the researcher can reject the null hypothesis of no differences and accept the alternative hypothesis that there is a relationship between type of program and leadership. In order to talk about the nature of the relationship, however, the investigator would need to employ additional statistical procedures.

Two requirements must be met in order to use χ^2. First, the expected frequency in any cell must be greater than zero. Second, the expected frequencies in at least 80 percent of the cells must exceed five. Small expected frequencies may result in spuriously high values for the χ^2 statistic.

These requirements have led to the technique of collapsing or combining categories in order to increase the expected frequencies. Fisher's Exact Test[23] is another alternative that may be used when low expected cell frequencies occur.

When the researcher has three variables and a very large sample, an analysis of crossbreaks may be a useful procedure. For each category of the third variable, a contingency table is constructed using the other two variables. The resulting chi-square statistics are then compared to ascertain whether or not the presence of the third variable affects the relationship between the first two variables. In the example of the relationship between type of program and leadership, the researcher might have wished to consider whether this association differs according to experience.

The researcher would gather data from twice as many subjects, half with less than 10 years of nursing experience and half with 10 or more years of experience. The researcher would then construct two contingency tables. One table would include only subjects with less than 10 years of nursing experience and the other only subjects with 10 or more years of experience. If the chi-square statistic for the 10 years or more experience group was significant and the statistic for the less than 10 years experience group was not, the researcher would conclude that there is an association between type of program and leadership for nurses with more than 10 years of experience, but for those with less than 10 years of experience there is not.

χ^2-BASED MEASURES OF ASSOCIATION

The χ^2 statistic merely tells the researcher whether or not there is a relationship between the variables investigated, it does not speak to the nature or strength of the relationship. In order to ascertain the nature and extent of the relationship, the researcher must follow up the χ^2 analysis with one of the following statistical procedures: phi, Cramer's V, or contingency coefficient. The discussion in this section closely parallels that of Nie and associates[18] and therefore should facilitate the reader's utilization of the SPSS package for computer analysis.

Phi

Phi (ϕ) is a measure of the relationship between two nominal, dichotomous variables. It is especially appropriate for utilization when data are arranged in a 2 × 2 contingency table such as Table 10-3.

TABLE 10-3. Example of a 2 × 2 Contingency Table

	VARIABLE X 0	VARIABLE X 1	TOTALS
VARIABLE Y	0	1	TOTALS
1	a	b	a+b
0	c	d	c+d
TOTALS	a+c	b+d	n

$$\text{(Formula 10-3)} \qquad \phi = \frac{bc - ad}{\sqrt{(a + c)\ (b + d)\ (a + b)\ (c + d)}}$$

where:
  a = frequency in cell a
  b = frequency in cell b
  c = frequency in cell c
  d = frequency in cell d

Example

Sixty obese patients who fail to comply with their treatment regimens are observed on the two variables, diet and clinic attendance. Arbitrarily, one (1) indicates followed diet and zero (0) indicates did not. Similarly, one indicates attended clinic regularly and zero, did not. Data are arranged as shown in Table 10-4.

TABLE 10-4. Adherence to Diet and Clinic Attendance

CLINIC ATTENDANCE (Y)	DIET (X)		TOTALS
	DID NOT FOLLOW (0)	DID FOLLOW (1)	
ATTENDED (1)	10 _a_	20 _b_	30 _a+b_
DID NOT ATTEND (0)	25 _c_	5 _d_	30 _c+d_
TOTALS	35 _a+c_	25 _b+d_	60 _n_

Frequencies in the table show the four possible pairs of characteristics of the 60 patients. For example, 10 people did not follow their diet, but attended clinic regularly (cell a). The marginal totals for rows present the numbers of patients at both levels of clinic attendance irrespective of their diet. Similarly, the marginal totals for columns present the numbers of patients at both levels of diet irrespective of their clinic attendance. The phi coefficient is then computed to measure the relationship between diet and clinic attendance.

$$\phi = \frac{bc - ad}{\sqrt{(a + c)\,(b + d)\,(a + b)\,(c + d)}}$$

$$= \frac{(25)\,(20) - (10)\,(5)}{\sqrt{(35)\,(25)\,(30)\,(30)}}$$

$$= \frac{500 - 50}{\sqrt{787500}}$$

$$= \frac{450}{887.4}$$

$$= 0.507$$

Those readers who have forgotten how to determine the square root of a number will find the book *Mathematics Made Simple*[24] extremely useful. The value for phi is found to be 0.507, indicating a moderate relationship between clinic attendance and diet in the sample of 60 patients. Phi ranges between -1 and $+1$. It should be noted that phi can assume the value $+1$ only when $a + b$ and $b + d$ are equal in the 2×2 contingency table. When there is no relationship between the two variables, phi will assume a zero value; when there is a perfect relationship, it assumes the value 1. The sign of the statistic indicates whether the two variables vary together $(+)$ or inversely $(-)$.

When phi is used with larger than a 2×2 table there is no upper limit to the value the statistic may assume. Some regard this as a real disadvantage of phi. Cureton[4] and Carroll[3] have proposed solutions to this problem that may be of interest to some readers encountering such a situation. Another, perhaps more viable, alternative to this problem is to select another statistic instead of phi, for example, Cramer's V.

Cramer's V

Cramer's V is a modified version of phi that is used for tables larger than 2×2. The value of this statistic ranges from 0 to 1 when several nominal categories are involved. In order to compute Cramer's V, one first determines phi and then inserts the resulting value into the following formula to obtain V:

(Formula 10-4)[18]
$$V = \sqrt{\frac{\phi^2}{\min (r - 1) (c - 1)}}$$

where:

ϕ^2 = phi coefficient squared

$\min$ = minimum value for r and c, respectively

r = number of rows

c = number of columns

A large value obtained for Cramer's V indicates a high degree of association between the variables, but it does not give information regarding the manner in which the variables relate (that is, positively or negatively).

Contingency Coefficient

The contingency coefficient (C) is a measure of the extent of association between two sets of attributes. It is useful when variables are measured at the nominal level and may be employed with any size table. In order to compute C, one first must determine the value of chi-square using Formula 10-1 and then insert that value into the following formula to obtain C:

(Formula 10-5)[23]
$$C = \sqrt{\frac{\chi^2}{N + \chi^2}}$$

where:

$$\chi^2 = \sum_{i=1}^{r} \sum_{j=1}^{K} \frac{(O_{ij} - E_{ij})^2}{E_{ij}}$$

N = total number of subjects

The contingency coefficient will equal zero when there is a complete lack of association between the variables. However, even when the variables are perfectly correlated, C cannot attain unity, that is, will not equal 1. The upper limit for C is a function of the number of categories. When K = r, the upper limit for C, the C that would occur for two perfectly correlated variables, is

$$\sqrt{\frac{K - 1}{K}}$$

For example, the upper limit of C for a 2×2 table is $\sqrt{1/2} = 0.707$. Thus, two contingency coefficients are not comparable unless they result from contingency tables of the same size.

OTHER MEASURES OF ASSOCIATION

In addition to the χ^2-based measures of association, there exist a number of other nonparametric measures of association that have utility in nursing research: lambda, gamma, tau and Somer's D.

These measures of association are based on the concept of *proportional reduction in error*. Simply stated, this means that a measure of association is derived so that it selects the category with the most cases (model category) to minimize the number of errors in predicting one variable from another.

Lambda

Lambda (λ) is a measure of association between two variables both measured at the nominal level. *Asymmetric lambda* indicates the ability to predict the value of the dependent or criterion variable given the value of the independent or predictor variable. The formula for asymmetric lambda (lambda$_a$) is:

(*Formula 10-6*)[18] $\text{Lambda}_a = \dfrac{\Sigma \max f_{jk} - \max f_k}{N - \max f_k}$

where:
  $\Sigma \max f_{jk}$ = sum of the maximum values of the cell frequencies in each column of the contingency table
  $\max f_k$ = maximum value of the row totals
  N = total number in the sample

The maximum value lambda can assume is +1.0 and occurs when the criterion variable can be perfectly predicted by the predictor variable. When the predictor variable does not allow one to predict the criterion variable, lambda equals zero.

Symmetric lambda (lambda$_s$) makes no assumptions about which of the two variables is dependent and it measures the overlap between the two variables.

(Formula 10-7)[18] $$\text{Lambda}_s = \frac{\sum_k \max f_{jk} + \sum_j \max f_{jk} - \max f_k - \max f_j}{2N - \max f_k - \max f_j}$$

where:

$\sum_k \max f_{jk}$ = sum of the maximum values of the cell frequencies in each column of the contingency table

$\max f_k$ = maximum value of the row totals

$\max f_j$ = maximum value of the column totals

$\sum_j \max f_{jk}$ = sum of the maximum values of the cell frequencies in each row of the contingency table

Note: The formula for symmetric lambda amounts to an average of two asymmetric values. Symmetric lambda ranges from 0 to 1. The value obtained for either of the lambda statistics will be affected by the marginal distributions. That is, if the marginal distributions are skewed, a zero value for lambda may occur even though a relationship exists.

So, when the researcher uses asymmetric lambda it is necessary to specify an independent and dependent variable. The researcher may then talk about the ability to predict the dependent variable given information about the independent variable. The researcher cannot, however, speak to the ability to predict the independent variable on the basis of the dependent variable unless the researcher computes a second asymmetric lambda specifying the independent variable as the dependent variable in the new analyses. If the researcher makes no assumptions regarding which variable is dependent, symmetric lambda is selected as a measure of the overall association between the two variables. Using symmetric lambda, the researcher can then speak to the amount of variance in variable one that can be explained on the basis of what is known about variable two and vice versa.

Gamma, Tau, and Somer's D are measures of association between two ordinal level variables. When ordinal data is employed, tied ranks may occur. If the researcher has tied ranks in the data, it is necessary to select a measure of association that corrects for tied ranks.

Gamma

Gamma is not an appropriate statistic to use when tied ranks occur because it makes no adjustments for ties. When gamma is calculated, tied pairs are eliminated from the analyses, the number of categories is thus diminished, and an inflated gamma may overestimate the extent of the relationship between the two variables.

Gamma is based on the concept of *concordant* and *discordant* pairs. That is, when gamma is computed each pair of variables is assessed to determine if their relative ordering on the first variable is the same as their relative ordering on the second variable. If the order is the same, the pair is *concordant*. If the order is reversed, they are *discordant*. For example, suppose that three subjects, A, B, and C, received the scores shown in Table 10-5 on variables X and Y.

TABLE 10-5. Scores of Three Subjects on Variables X and Y

SUBJECT	VARIABLE	
	X	Y
A	1	7
B	5	8
C	6	2

To determine the gamma statistic, it is necessary to consider the relative ordering of the three pairs of subjects' scores, AB, AC, and BC, on variables X and Y. From the display, it can be seen that on variable X, B ranked higher than A (5,1) and on variable Y, B ranked higher than A (8,7). Hence the pair AB is concordant. On variable X, C scored higher than A but on the Y variable, C scored lower than A. Thus, the pair AC is discordant. Similarly, on variable X, C ranked higher than B but on variable Y, C ranked lower than B. Hence, the pair BC is discordant. Therefore, there are two discordant pairs and one concordant pair in the data. When the number of discordant pairs is greater than the number of concordant pairs, the gamma statistic will assume a negative value. When the number of concordant pairs dominates, the gamma statistic has a positive sign. If the number of concordant pairs is equal to the number of discordant pairs, gamma will equal zero. In addition to considering the sign of gamma, it is possible to determine numerically the probability of correctly guessing the order of a pair of cases on one variable once their ordering on the other variable is known. This numerical value is found by inserting the information regarding the number of concordant and discordant pairs into the following formula:

(Formula 10-8)[18] $$\text{Gamma} = \frac{P - Q}{P + Q}$$

where:
   P = number of concordant pairs in the data set
   Q = number of discordant pairs in the data set

The value of the resulting gamma statistic ranges from -1 to $+1$. The value 1 indicates a 100 percent probability of correctly guessing the order of a pair of cases on one variable given information about the relative ordering on the other variable, while 0 indicates zero probability of correctly guessing the order.

Example

Using the data from the display, in which the number of discordant pairs was two and the number of concordant pairs was one, gamma may be determined in the following manner:

$$\text{Gamma} = \frac{P - Q}{P + Q}$$

$$= \frac{1 - 2}{1 + 2}$$

$$= \frac{-1}{3}$$

$$= -0.33$$

The resulting gamma value of -0.33 indicates that discordant pairs dominate in the data set and that the probability of correctly guessing the order of a pair of cases on one variable once the ordering on the other variable is known is 33 times per 100 guesses or one time in every three.

Zero-order gamma (Formula 10-8) simply measures the relationship between two variables without controlling for other variables. When a contingency table has three or more dimensions, it is possible, in addition to a zero-order gamma, to compute a partial gamma. *Partial gamma* measures the relationship between two variables controlling for one or more other variables. The zero-order gamma for a contingency table having three or more dimensions is obtained by collapsing across all control variables and then computing gamma for the resulting 2×2 table. The gamma value resulting from a collapsed contingency table will not be exactly equal to the gamma for the original 2×2 table for the same two variables. The formula for partial gamma is:

(Formula 10-9) $$\text{Partial Gamma} = \frac{\Sigma_i \, (P_i - Q_i)}{\Sigma_i \, (P_i + Q_i)}$$

where:
    Σ_i = sum of all subtables in the contingency table
    P_i = number of concordant pairs in all subtables in the contingency table
    Q_i = number of discordant pairs in all subtables in the contingency table

By comparing the value of the zero-order gamma for two variables with the partial gamma, the researcher can assess the effect of the control variable on the relationship between the two variables.

Tau

Tau is a measure of association between two ordinal variables. Like gamma, tau is based on the concept of concordant/discordant pairs. There are three forms of tau: a, b, c. Tau a is not appropriate for data in which tied ranks occur in that it cannot attain 1 even with a perfect relationship. Tau b and c both correct for ties. Tau b is appropriate for nongrouped data presented in a square table, that is, a table in which the number of rows is equal to the number of columns. Tau c is for grouped data and rectangular tables. The formulas for Tau b and c are:

(Formula 10-10)

$$\text{Tau b} = \frac{P - Q}{[\frac{1}{2}[N(N - 1) - T(T_1 - 1)]\frac{1}{2}[N(N - 1) - T_2(T_2 - 1)]]^{1/2}}$$

where:
T_1 = the number of ties on the row variables
T_2 = the number of ties on the column variables

(Formula 10-11)[18]

$$\text{Tau c} = \frac{2m(P - Q)}{N^2(m - 1)}$$

where:
m = total number of pairs adjusted for the numbers of rows or columns, whichever is smaller

Tau ranges from −1 to +1 and is interpreted in the same manner as gamma.

Somer's D

Somer's D is for ordinal variables, takes ties into account, and has asymmetric and symmetric versions. *Asymmetric Somer's D* is computed as follows when the row variable is considered to be the dependent variable:

(Formula 10-12)[18]

$$\text{Somer's D}_a = \frac{P - Q}{P + Q + T_1}$$

When the dependent variable is columns the formula is:

(Formula 10-13)[18]

$$\text{Somer's D}_a = \frac{P - Q}{P + Q + T_2}$$

Symmetric Somer's D is calculated in the following manner:

(Formula 10-14)[18]

$$\text{Somer's D}_s = \frac{P - Q}{P + Q + \frac{1}{2}(T_1 + T_2)}$$

SUMMARY

The selection of a nonparametric measure of association will depend on (1) the level of measurement of the variables, (2) table size, and (3) assumptions regarding the presence of independent/dependent variables. Those measures of association for two variables measured at the nominal level are chi-square, Cramer's V, contingency coefficient, and lambda. The association between two ordinal variables may be assessed using tau a, b, or c, gamma, or Somer's D.

Parametric Measures of Relationship

Parametric measures of relationship are more powerful statistical procedures than their nonparametric counterparts. Similarly, multivariate parametric procedures have more power than bivariate parametric statistics. In this section, attention is given to bivariate and multiple correlation and regression procedures.

BIVARIATE CORRELATION

A bivariate correlation procedure is employed when the researcher is interested in the nature and extent of the relationship between two variables.

A *scatterplot* or *scattergram* is a two dimensional representation of a set of ordered pairs and is very useful for envisioning the nature of the relationship that exists between two variables. Suppose five subjects were measured using two forms of a 12-item summated rating scale and the results shown in Table 10-6 were obtained.

TABLE 10-6. Presentation of Subjects' Scores Using a Tabular Format

SUBJECT	SCORE	
	SCALE 1	SCALE 2
A	12	7
B	10	8
C	8	6
D	7	5
E	5	3

The scatterplot for these scores is shown in Figure 10-1. In addition to using the information in a scatterplot to assess the nature of the relationship between two variables, it is often useful to determine the extent of the relationship between the two variables by employing an appropriate correlational statistic

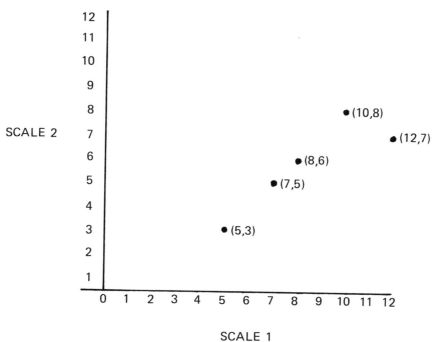

FIGURE 10-1. Scatterplot of scores of five subjects (see text for discussion).

as well. The product moment correlation coefficient (r_{xy}) is the statistic most frequently employed to quantitatively summarize the information in the scatterplot. It should be noted that the r_{xy} statistic requires data measured at the interval level. Variations of and approximations to r_{xy} are available for data measured at other than the interval level and are discussed later in this chapter.

The left scatterplot in Figure 10-2 presents an example of a scatterplot likely to result in an r_{xy} of +1.00. If the line slopes downward from left to right, as in the scatterplot on the right in Figure 10-2, r would equal −1.00.

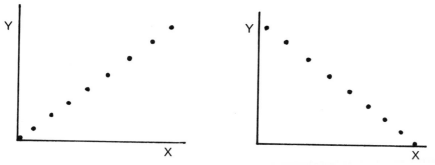

FIGURE 10-2. *Left,* Example of a perfect positive linear relationship, r_{xy} = +1.00. *Right,* Example of a perfect negative linear relationship, r_{xy} = −1.00.

If a change in score on one measure is not perfectly correlated with changes in score on the other measure, patterns similar to those shown in Figure 10-3 may occur.

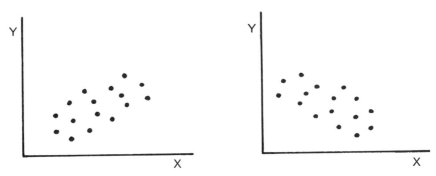

FIGURE 10-3. *Left*, Example of a positive linear relationship, r_{xy} is less than $+1.00$ but greater than 0. *Right*, Example of a negative linear relationship, r_{xy} is less than 0 but greater than -1.

In the scatterplot on the left in Figure 10-3, increases in the value of Y tend to be associated with increases in the value of X. In the scatterplot on the right, increases in the value of Y tend to be associated with decreases in the value of X. It should be noted that a lack of perfect correlation results in a scattering of the points away from the straight line best summarizing the trend. The more the scatter, the less well defined the trend and the closer r is to zero.

The correlation coefficient may assume a zero value when (a) the pattern in the scattergram looks like the left scatterplot in Figure 10-4 or (b) the pattern seems to follow a well defined curve as in the right scatterplot in Figure 10-4.

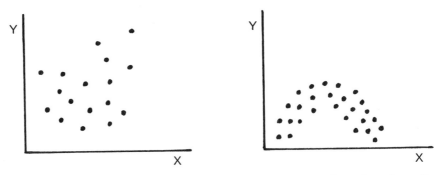

FIGURE 10-4. The correlation coefficient may assume a zero value when the pattern in the scattergram lacks a well defined shape *(left)* or seems to follow a well defined curve *(right)*.

There is no useful relationship between the variables in the left scatterplot Figure 10-4 and this is accurately reflected in the correlation coefficient value of zero. A useful relationship may exist between the variables in the right scatterplot and in this instance the value of the correlation coefficient may be quite misleading. A statistical index that is appropriate for measuring the degree of curvilinear association between variables is eta.[8]

The interpretation of correlation study results is usually in terms of the percent of the variance shared by the two variables. This is obtained by squaring the r value obtained for the correlation between two variables (Fig. 10-5).

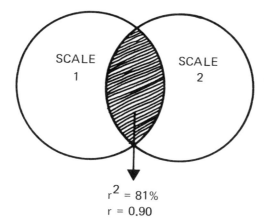

$r^2 = 81\%$

$r = 0.90$

FIGURE 10-5. Venn diagram of the percent of variance shared by Scales 1 and 2.

In Figure 10-5, each of the variables in the preceding example is represented by a circle. The area common to both, or r^2, represents the percent of the variance shared by the two variables, that is, the area common to both. Similarily, r^2 may be interpreted on the basis of predicting one variable given information about the second variable. For example, the researcher may conclude on the basis of the results in Figure 10-5 that 81 percent of the variance in Scale 1 can be predicted or explained on the basis of Scale 2 or equivalently that 81 percent of the variance in Scale 2 may be explained or predicted on the basis of Scale 1. It should be noted that correlation results are *reversible* and there is no independent or dependent variable per se.

As stated earlier, the correlation coefficient of choice is the Pearson product moment correlation coefficient (r_{xy}). In order to use this coefficient, the following assumptions must be met:

1. Both variables must be measured at the interval level or higher.
2. The variables must distribute normally and independently in the population.
3. Homoscedasticity must exist, that is, scores on both variables must have equal variances or be equally dispersed about the line.

The Pearson product moment correlation coefficient (r_{xy}) is computed in one of two ways, from raw scores or from Z scores.

Computing r_{xy} from *raw scores*:

(Formula 10-15)[7] $\quad r_{xy} = \dfrac{n\Sigma XY - (\Sigma X)(\Sigma Y)}{\sqrt{[n\Sigma X^2 - (\Sigma X)^2][n\Sigma Y^2 - (\Sigma Y)^2]}}$

where:

ΣXY = the sum of the products of each individual's X and Y scores

(ΣX) = the sum of all X scores

(ΣY) = the sum of all Y scores

n = the number of subjects

ΣX^2 = the sum of all squared X scores

$(\Sigma X)^2$ = the square of the sum of all X scores

ΣY^2 = the sum of all squared Y scores

$(\Sigma Y)^2$ = the square of the sum of all Y scores

Example: Determine the relationship between five subjects' (A, B, C, D, E) scores on variables X and Y.

Subject	X	Y	XY	X²	Y²
A	2	2	4	4	4
B	8	4	32	64	16
C	6	5	30	36	25
D	14	6	84	196	36
E	10	8	80	100	64
	$\Sigma X = 40$	$\Sigma Y = 25$	$\Sigma XY = 230$	$\Sigma X^2 = 400$	$\Sigma Y^2 = 145$

$$(\Sigma X)^2 = 1600 \qquad (\Sigma Y)^2 = 625$$

$$r_{xy} = \frac{n\Sigma XY - (\Sigma X)(\Sigma Y)}{\sqrt{[n\Sigma X^2 - (\Sigma X)^2][n\Sigma Y^2 - (\Sigma Y^2)]}}$$

$$= \frac{5(230) - (40)(25)}{\sqrt{[5(400) - (1600)][5(145) - (625)]}}$$

$$= \frac{1150 - 1000}{\sqrt{(2000 - 1600)(725 - 625)}}$$

$$= \frac{150}{\sqrt{40000}}$$

$$= \frac{150}{200}$$

$$= 0.75$$

The value of 0.75 for r_{xy} may be squared and then interpreted to mean that 56 percent of the variance in X maybe explained on the basis of Y and vice versa.

Calculating r_{xy} from Z scores:

(Formula 10-16) $$r_{xy} = \frac{\Sigma(Z_x Z_y)}{N}$$

where:

Z_x = Z score of a particular person on variable X

Z_y = Z score of the same person on variable Y

N = total number of products entering the sum

$\Sigma(Z_x Z_y)$ = sum of the Z score products

Example: Determine the relationship between five subjects' (A, B, C, D, E) scores on variables X and Y in the preceding example using the Z score formula for r_{xy}. First convert all raw scores on X and Y to Z scores using Formula 8-6 in Chapter 8. Then proceed in the following manner.

Subject	Z_x	Z_y	$Z_x Z_y$
A	−1.5	−1.5	2.25
B	0	−0.5	0.00
C	−0.5	0.0	0.00
D	1.5	0.5	0.75
E	0.5	1.5	0.75

$$\Sigma(Z_x Z_y) = \overline{3.75}$$

$$r_{xy} = \frac{3.75}{5}$$

$$= 0.75$$

The resulting r = 0.75, if squared, indicates 56 percent of the variance in X and Y is common or shared variance.

It should be noted that for the same data set, using either Formula 10-15 or 10-16 will result in the same numerical value for r_{xy}. Formula 10-15 is frequently referred to as the computational formula for determining r_{xy} because it lends itself to computation utilizing a hand calculator.

Several variations on r_{xy} are available for use with other than interval level data, some of which are discussed in the section on nonparametric techniques. For convenience, these coefficients are summarized in Table 10-7. Formulas and other specifics regarding the utilization of those statistics not discussed earlier can be found in Glass and Stanley,[7] Kirk,[13] Nunnally,[19] or Siegel.[23]

TABLE 10-7. Coefficients for Use with Various Types of Data

VARIABLE Y	VARIABLE X		
	NOMINAL	ORDINAL	INTERVAL OR RATIO
NOMINAL	PHI (ϕ) CONTINGENCY (C) TETRACHORIC (r_{tet})	CURETON'S RANK BISERIAL (r_{rb})	BISERIAL (r_b, r_{bis}) POINT BISERIAL (r_{pb})
ORDINAL	CURETON'S RANK BISERIAL (r_{rb})	SPEARMAN RHO (P, r_s) KENDALL'S TAU (τ)	TAU (τ)
INTERVAL OR RATIO	BISERIAL (r_b, r_{bis}) POINT BISERIAL (r_{pb})	TAU (τ)	PEARSON PRODUCT MOMENT (r_{xy})

Of those coefficients listed in Table 10-7, phi, r_s, and r_{pb} are equal to r_{xy}. That is, they are simply the product moment correlation coefficient formula applied to nominal and ordinal data. The remaining coefficients, r_{tet} and r_{bis}, are attempts to approximate r_{xy}.

When the researcher desires to control or remove the effect or variance due to a third variable from the relationship between two other variables, the researcher uses *partial correlation* (Fig. 10-6).

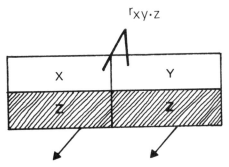

FIGURE 10-6. Venn diagram of a partial correlation.

In Figure 10-6, the researcher is interested in the correlation between variables X and Y, partialling out, removing the effect of, or holding Z constant ($r_{xy \cdot z}$). The Venn diagram illustrates that a partial correlation coefficient reflects the relationship between two variables after the overlap or factors each have in common with the third variable have been removed from the analysis.

The formula for determining a partial correlation coefficient is:

(Formula 10-17)[7]
$$r_{xy \cdot z} = \frac{r_{xy} - r_{xz}r_{yz}}{\sqrt{1 - r_{xz}^2}\,\sqrt{1 - r_{yz}^2}}$$

where:

r_{xy} = Pearson product moment correlation coefficient for X and Y
r_{xz} = Pearson product moment correlation coefficient for X and Z
r_{yz} = Pearson product moment correlation coefficient for Y and Z

Example:

$r_{xy} = 0.80$
$r_{xz} = 0.30$
$r_{yz} = 0.40$

$$r_{xy \cdot z} = \frac{(0.80) - (0.30)\,(0.40)}{\sqrt{(1 - 0.09)}\,\sqrt{(1 - 0.16)}}$$

$$= \frac{0.80 - 0.12}{\sqrt{0.91}\,\sqrt{0.84}}$$

$$= \frac{0.68}{(0.95)\,(0.92)}$$

$$= \frac{0.68}{0.87}$$

= 0.78, i.e., the nature and size of the relationship between X and Y after removing the effects of the third variable, Z.

Partial correlations are useful in essentially two ways:

1. They allow the researcher to assess the effect of a confounding variable that cannot be controlled by the research design or sampling procedure.
2. They are an integral part of the multiple correlation and regression procedures that are discussed later.

CROSS-LAGGED PANEL CORRELATION ANALYSIS

In a cross-lagged panel correlation analysis (CLPC), the same two variables are restudied on two or more occasions using the same subjects. The intent of this quasi-experimental approach is to produce an index of the direction and strength of causation between the two variables.[2, 11]

The strategies employed in a CLPC analysis are best illustrated by example. The intent of the following discussion is to introduce the reader to the logic and basic elements of the CLPC procedure. The purpose is not to present sufficient detail to enable the reader to carry out the procedure independently. A study was undertaken by one of the authors[27] to examine evidence for the convergence of students' preferences for nursing practice with the preferences of the faculty member who directed their clinical nursing experiences. A preference index was administered to all faculty (N = 14) teaching a clinical nursing course to junior students at three points in time: (1) before the students had any contact with the faculty in the course or clinical experiences, (2) six weeks later, after the students had received their first formal clinical evaluations from their clinical faculty member, and (3) at the completion of the clinical course. The same preference scale was administered to 170 junior nursing students at the same three points in time that it was administered to faculty. Faculty and students completed the scale separately but on the same day and at the same time during a regularly scheduled class period. Each member of the faculty included in this study directed the clinical nursing experiences of the same group of students during the entire 14 weeks of the course. Thus, each group of students had contact with the same faculty member for all clinical nursing experiences they had in the course. Furthermore, since students took only one clinical course per semester, each intact group of students had contact in the clinical area with only one faculty member during the semester of data collection.

A mean preference score was obtained for each group of students at the time of each data collection. The result was 14 student scores, each representative of the mean preference score for a group of students linked with the score of their respective faculty member on each of the three testing occasions. For example, at Time 1, 14 student scores were obtained, each representing the mean preference score for a group of students, and each group score was linked with the preference score of the respective clinical faculty member. The mean scores obtained for each group of students were then correlated with their respective faculty member's score. The product moment correlation coefficients obtained for Time 1, Time 2, and Time 3 were indicators of the correlation between faculty and student preferences as measured by the preference scale.

The elements of the CLPC included two constructs, faculty preferences and student preferences, measured at three different points in time. Figure 10-7 presents the CLPC paradigm.

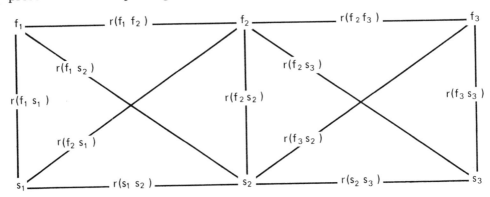

FIGURE 10-7. The cross-lagged panel correlation paradigm.

From Figure 10-7, it can be seen that the two constructs and three times generated six variables: f_1, f_2, f_3, s_1, s_2, s_3. These six variables then generated eleven correlations: four *autocorrelations*, $r(f_1f_2)$, $r(f_2f_3)$, $r(s_1s_2)$, $r(s_2s_3)$, three *synchronous* correlations, $r(f_1s_1)$, $r(f_2s_2)$, $r(f_3s_3)$, and four *cross-lagged* correlations, $r(f_1s_2)$, $r(f_2s_1)$, $r(f_2s_3)$, $r(f_3s_2)$.

The strategy employed by the CLPC involves the comparison of the cross-lagged correlations, which can be expressed as cross-lagged differentials:

$$r(f_1s_2) - r(f_2s_1) = \text{cross-lagged differential I}$$
$$r(f_2s_3) - r(f_3s_2) = \text{cross-lagged differential II}$$

In other words, the first cross-lagged differential is the value found when the correlation coefficient between faculty scores at the Time 2 measurement and student scores at the Time 1 measurement is subtracted from the correlation coefficient between faculty scores at the Time 1 measurement and student scores at the Time 2 measurement. Similarly, the second cross-lagged differential is the value found when the correlation coefficient between faculty scores at the Time 3 measurement and student scores at the Time 2 measurement is subtracted from the correlation coefficient between faculty scores at the Time 2 measurement and student scores at the Time 3 measurement. The logic underlying the interpretation of the cross-lagged differential is that in order for one variable to be argued as causing a second variable it must occur first in time, and the variation in the first variable should be mirrored by similar variation in the second. If faculty preferences influence student preferences, then the correlation coefficient between faculty preferences at Time 1 and student preferences at Time 2 would be greater in size than the correlation coefficient between faculty preferences at Time 2 and student preferences at Time 1, and the correlation between faculty preferences at Times 1 and 2 would be significant. In this case, the value of the cross-lagged differential would be positive in sign and its absolute size would be indicative of the amount of change that occurred in student preferences from the Time 1 to the Time 2 measurement that brought these more in line with faculty preferences. On the other hand, given that student preferences at Time 1 and Time 2 remain highly correlated and the correlation between faculty preferences at Time 2 and student preferences at Time 1 was greater than the correlation between faculty preferences at Time 1 and student preferences at Time 2, the cross-lagged differential would be negative in sign and would provide evidence that student preferences influenced the preferences of the faculty.

The null hypothesis tested by equality of the cross-lags is that the relationship between faculty and student preferences for nursing practice is due to an unmeasured third variable and not causation. Any unmeasured third variable that would affect the preferences of both students and faculty in a similar fashion is a plausible rival hypothesis for the relationship observed between faculty and student preferences. For example, if direct patient care involvement was the social norm, and this social norm had effects on both faculty and student preferences, any correlation observed between faculty and student preferences could be explained by this unmeasured third variable without assuming any effect of the faculty on student preferences per se. Before causal models are entertained, the third variable effect (that is, spuriousness) needs to be ruled out by the detection of a statistically significant difference between the cross-lagged correlations.

A second hypothesis investigated in the CLPC is the equality of the synchronous correlations to test for stationarity. The rationale underlying CLPC is based on two assumptions, synchronicity and stationarity. By *synchronicity* it is meant that the two constructs, faculty and student preferences, are measured at the same point in time. The two major threats to this assumption derive from retrospection (questions in panel studies that ask subjects directly or indirectly to recall behavior, attitudes, or experiences in the past) and aggregation (variables that are aggregated or averaged over time). The justification for the tenability of the synchronicity assumption rests for the most part on the design of the research. *Stationarity* means that the causal or structural equation for a variable is not different at the three points of measurement. Stationarity is different from stability. *Stability*, measured by the autocorrelations, refers to a lack of change over time of the empirical values of a variable, while *stationarity* refers to a lack of change over time of strength and direction of the causes of the variable. Stationarity presumes that the causal mechanisms did not change during the interval measured. A lack of synchronicity or stationarity is a potential explanation of a difference between the cross-lagged correlations. The tenability of both stationarity and synchronicity together would imply equal cross-lags. The null hypothesis that the cross-lagged differential is zero is then a test of spuriousness. Asymmetric cross-lags may indicate a causal effect or, more likely, that there is a factor that causes one of the measured variables and causes the other variable at a later point in time.[11]

A major difficulty with interpreting cross-lagged differentials arises from competing confounded pairs of hypotheses. There are two sources of an effect, f and s, and two directions of that effect, positive and negative, making a total of four possible hypotheses. Within the context of the CLPC design, finding $r(f_1 s_2)$ greater than $r(f_2 s_1)$ is consistent with both faculty causing an increase in student preferences and students causing a decrease in faculty preferences. Finding $r(f_1 s_2)$ less than $r(f_2 s_1)$ is consistent with both students causing an increase in faculty preferences and faculty causing a decrease in student preferences. To test the confounded hypotheses within the framework of this design, a no-cause baseline can be computed.[11, 21] The logic of the no-cause baseline is that the cross-lags should be less than the synchronous correlation by some factor. This factor (that is, no-cause baseline) is estimated from the autocorrelations. The value of the no-cause baseline represents the size of the difference that could exist between the synchronous correlations and the cross-lagged differential as a result of chance alone, that is, in the absence of influence on the part of either faculty or students.

The no-cause baseline requires estimates of the reliability of each variable and tenability of the assumption of *homogeneous stability* (that all the non-errorful causes of f and s change at the same rate over time). Evidence consistent with this assumption is that the unattenuated autocorrelations for the faculty and student variables are equal. The sign of the synchronous correlation is suggestive of the direction of the effect. If the synchronous correlations are positive, they support faculty causing increases in student preferences. Negative synchronous correlations suggest decreases. Given homogeneous stability, the cross-lags should always be smaller in absolute value than the synchronous correlations, given spuriousness, stationarity, and synchronicity. So a cross-lag larger than the synchronous correlation (that is, above the value of the no-cause baseline), given stationarity, is indicative of a causal effect. A cross-lag larger or smaller than the synchronous correlation, but within the range represented by the no-cause baseline values, is indicative of chance variation alone and not a causal effect.[11]

Given a nonsignificant difference between the cross-lagged correlations, the null hypothesis of spuriousness cannot be rejected, that is, the hypothesis that the variables do not cause each other but are a symptom of some set of common causes. Alternate explanations include: (1) f and s may cause each other in a positive feedback loop, (2) it may be that f causes s or vice versa, but the magnitude of the effect is too small to be detected, or (3) the measured lag may not correspond to the causal lag.

The patterns of correlations examined in this study are presented in Figure 10-8.

Evidence for convergence existed if the following relationships held during the first six weeks of the course: (1) $r(f_1 f_2) > 0$, the preference scores of faculty were reliable and stable over testing occasions; (2) $r(f_2 s_2) = r(f_1 s_1)$, the correlation between faculty preference scores Time 2 and student mean scores Time 2 was equal to the correlation between faculty scores Time 1 and student mean scores Time 1 (This finding was necessary to support the tenability of the assumption of stationarity underlying the utilization of the CLPC design.); (3)

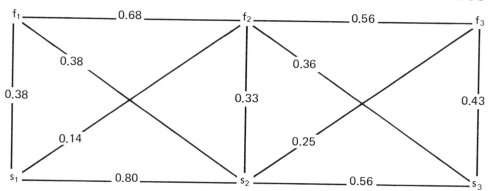

FIGURE 10-8. Cross-lagged panel correlations between faculty FSP scores and the mean FSP score of their respective student groups (N = 14).

$r(f_1s_2) > r(f_2s_1)$, the correlation between faculty scores Time 1 and student mean scores Time 2 was greater than the correlation between faculty scores Time 2 and student mean scores Time 1.

Additional support for convergence existed if: (1) $r(f_2f_3) > 0$, the faculty scores Time 2 and Time 3 were reliable and stable; (2) $r(f_3s_3) = r(f_2s_2)$, the correlation between faculty scores Time 3 and student mean scores Time 3 was equal to the correlation between faculty scores Time 2 and student mean scores Time 2; (3) $r(f_2s_3) > r(f_3s_2)$, the correlation between faculty scores Time 2 and student mean scores Time 3 was greater than the correlation between faculty scores Time 3 and student mean scores Time 2.

The specific hypotheses tested were: (1) $r(f_2s_2) = r(f_1s_1)$, $r(f_3s_3) = r(f_2s_2)$, to test the tenability of the assumption of stationarity, and (2) $r(f_1s_2) - r(f_2s_1) > 0$, $r(f_2s_3) - r(f_3s_2) > 0$, to reject the null hypothesis of spuriousness. Dependent Z tests[20] were used to test the significance of these synchronous and cross-lagged differentials.

Thus, to obtain evidence for convergence of students' preferences with those of their clinical faculty, it was first necessary to assess the tenability of the synchronicity assumption (that the two constructs, student preferences and faculty preferences, were measured at the same point in time). The threats to this assumption, aggregation and retrospection, were ruled out on the basis of the study design. Care was taken to avoid questions on the preference scale that required students or faculty to recall information; both students and faculty were administered the instrument at the same time on all three measurement occasions; and questions involving aggregate variables were avoided. It is possible that faculty with more experience in nursing practice might recall past experiences in similar situations in answering the preference questions while students who had less experience to draw upon might not. This possibility, although recognized, was not considered a serious threat to synchronicity in that items on the scale were designed to avoid situations requiring specific prior knowledge of content or experience in nursing practice.

Given the tenability of the synchronicity assumption, the reliability and stability of the empirical values for each of the variables were determined by the size of the autocorrelations. The uncorrected values for the autocorrelations were presented in Figure 10-8; corrected values are shown in Figure 10-9.

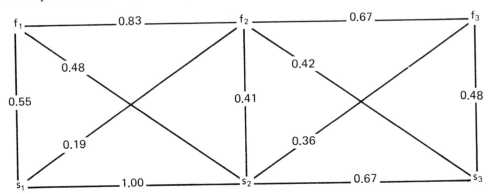

FIGURE 10-9. Corrected (using Nunnally's[21] formula) cross-lagged panel correlations between faculty FSP scores and the mean FSP score of their respective student groups (N = 14).

The size of the values obtained for both students and faculty were reasonable. All four autocorrelations were significantly different from zero at the 0.05 level. Thus, the predictions that $r(f_1f_2) > 0$ and $r(f_2s_3) > 0$ were confirmed.

From Figure 10-8 it should be noted that while the autocorrelations for the faculty Times 1 and 2 and for faculty Times 2 and 3 were consistent, the autocorrelation for students Times 2 and 3 was lower than the autocorrelation for students Times 1 and 2. This finding may represent unreliability in the student measure or, more likely, may be indicative of a change in student preferences for nursing practice from the Time 2 to Time 3 measurement. When change is an issue, the reliability of measures is better estimated utilizing an internal consistency measure such as the alpha coefficient.[19, 22] The alpha coefficients obtained for faculty on each of the three measurement occasions were 0.81, 0.82, and 0.88, respectively. The alpha coefficients for students were 0.60, 0.78, and 0.91, respectively. These findings suggest an increase in the reliability of the student measures over the three occasions, while the faculty reliability estimates remained consistent. Given the variability of the values obtained for the measures of stability and reliability of student responses to the scale, it should be noted that this may represent a potential alternative explanation for any cross-lagged differential obtained in this study.

Given sufficient reliability and stability of the empirical values of the variables, next the tenability of the assumption of stationarity was assessed by examining the equality of the synchronous correlations. Some degree of stationarity was expected in this study because it was believed that the same variable was repeatedly measured in the panel. In addition, it was believed that the causes of this variable would not have changed during the study for the following reasons: students had the same faculty member for clinical experiences for the en-

tire semester, and faculty teaching the course had responsibility for both direct-
ing the clinical experiences of a group of students and teaching theory portions
of the course. Therefore, the general course experiences and contacts between
faculty and students as a whole were invariant for all students and faculty, and
variation was limited to student-faculty contact in the clinical portion of the
course. No major changes within the College of Nursing or within the profession of nursing were noted during the course of the study that might influence
changes in the preferences of either students or faculty. Neither of the synchronous differentials was statistically significant. Thus, the predictions that
$r(f_1s_1) = r(f_2s_2)$ and $r(_2s_2) = r(f_3s_3)$ were supported. This evidence suggests a lack
of change over time of the strength and direction of causes of the variables and
supports the tenability of the assumption of stationarity.

Given the tenability of synchronicity and stationarity, the equality of the
cross-lagged correlations was examined to test the null hypothesis of spuriousness. The relationship between the corrected and uncorrected cross-lagged correlations can be seen in Figures 10-8 and 10-9. As predicted, $r(f_1s_2)$ was greater in size than $r(f_2s_1)$. Similarly, as predicted, $r(f_2s_3)$ was greater than $r(f_3s_2)$.
These findings suggest that student preferences were influenced by faculty
preferences. If homogeneous stability is the case, that is, that the corrected
autocorrelations are not statistically significantly different, the cross-lagged
correlations should always be smaller in absolute value than the synchronous
correlations given spuriousness, stationarity, and synchronicity. Therefore, a
cross-lagged correlation greater than the synchronous correlation as in the
Times 1 and 2 measurement is indicative of faculty preferences influencing student preferences. If, on the other hand, faculty "cause" a decrease in student
preferences and homogeneous stability holds, then the cross-lagged correlations
would be smaller than the synchronous correlations. This is the finding at the
Times 2 and 3 measurement. Neither of the cross-lagged differentials was statistically significant. A no-cause baseline[11, 21] was obtained by averaging the
test-retest correlations of both variables corrected for attenuation and then multiplying the resulting value by the average of the two synchronous correlations.
The no-cause baseline was 0.47 for the first cross-lagged differential and 0.25
for the second cross-lagged differential. Both cross-lagged differentials were
below the no-cause baseline. Therefore, the null hypothesis of spuriousness
could not be rejected, and no support was found for the prediction that $r(f_1s_2) -
r(f_2s_1) > 0$ and $r(f_2s_3) - r(f_3s_2) > 0$. It should be noted that the detection of a sig-
nificant difference between cross-lagged panel correlations given the low power of CLPC procedures is largely dependent on the size of the study sample.
Increased power to reject the null hypothesis of spuriousness is directly related
to increased sample size. Kenny[11] emphasizes that it is difficult to obtain statistically significant differences between cross-lagged correlations even when
the sample size is moderate (50 to 300). The failure to reject the null hypothesis
in this study, given the evidence provided by the relative sizes of the cross-
lagged correlations and the small number of subjects (14) suggests that the
findings of this study were limited to some extent by the size of the study
sample.

The potential of the CLPC procedure for investigating nursing research questions of a longitudinal nature has not been fully realized. For this reason, readers are encouraged to further consider the viability of this approach in their own work using the references listed at the end of the chapter.

BIVARIATE REGRESSION

The researcher who has reason to believe that one of the two variables will be a function of or change due to the influence of the other variable, will employ a bivariate regression procedure. Thus, regression procedures are appropriately used when one wishes to predict scores on one variable (the criterion or dependent variable) from the scores on a second variable (the predictor or independent variable). To state it yet another way, in regression studies, the interest is in how much variance in a dependent or criterion variable is explained or predicted by the independent or predictor variable.

The logic of prediction is best illustrated by example. A researcher desires to predict nurses' preferences for patient care, as measured by their scores on a preference index, on the basis of their personality characteristics, measured by a personality inventory. In this instance, then, the *criterion variable* (that is, the variable on which performance is to be *predicted*) is preference index scores. The *predictor variable* (that is, the variable being used as a basis for predicting preferences) is personality inventory scores. What strategies can the researcher employ to make an accurate prediction?

First, the researcher determines the preference scores of all individuals having the same personality score. This is called a *conditional* or *contingent* score distribution. For example, if 10 individuals obtained the following preference scores, there would be three conditional distributions.

Subject	Personality score
A	10
B	15
C	20
D	10
E	20
F	20
G	20
H	10
I	15
J	15

That is, subjects A, D, and H would be members of one conditional distribution, the distribution contingent on their having a personality score of 10. Subjects B, I, and J would be members of the distribution contingent on their having a score of 15, and subjects C, E, F, and G would be members of the distribution contingent on having a personality score of 20. Thus, inclusion of an individual in one of these three distributions is contingent upon that individual having the same personality score as other individuals in the group. It should be noted that a contingent distribution of criterion scores exists for each distinct predictor score as well.

Next, the researcher finds the mean of the preference scores in each conditional distribution. The mean of the respective contingent distribution to which an individual belongs is then used as the estimate of that individual's criterion performance. The result is referred to as a least squares estimate of that individual's performance. Suppose the 10 individuals in the preceding example had the following preference scores:

Subject	Personality Score	Preference Score
A	10	50
D	10	60
H	10	40
		$\overline{X} = 50$
B	15	70
I	15	75
J	15	80
		$\overline{X} = 75$
C	20	85
E	20	90
F	20	90
G	20	100
		$\overline{X} = 91$

The prediction policy would lead the researcher to estimate subject A's criterion performance to be 50, subject J's 75, and so forth.

It should be evident that this procedure is cumbersome and inefficient, especially when large numbers are involved. If two variables are linearly related, the means of the contingent distributions will fall in a straight line as shown below:

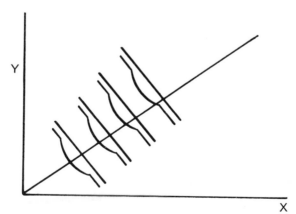

Therefore, finding this line or the equation that describes this line allows one to predict an individual's performance without going through calculations involved in finding the mean of each contingent distribution.

Linear Prediction Equation for Raw Score Data

The simplest case of linear prediction involves one predictor (X) and one criterion (Y) variable. The raw score prediction equation is:

(Formula 10-18) $Y' = \overline{Y} + B_{yx}(X - \overline{X})$

In words, an individual's predicted criterion score Y' is equal to the mean of the criterion score distribution, $\overline{Y}$, plus some multiplier, B_{yx}, of the person's distance from the mean (that is, the person's deviation score) in the predictor distribution $(X - \overline{X})$.

Note: If the researcher did not know an individual's score on the predictor variable, and thus took the mean of the predictor distribution as the best estimate of the person's performance on the predictor measure, the prediction equation would look like this:

$$Y' = \overline{Y} + B_{yx}(\overline{X} - \overline{X})$$
$$= \overline{Y} + B_{yx}(0)$$
$$= \overline{Y}$$

In other words, one would estimate criterion performance to be $\overline{Y}$, the mean of the criterion distribution.

On the other hand, if the researcher knew an individual's predictor performance (X), the prediction procedure would give a refined estimate of criterion performance, which depends on:

1. The individual's distance from the mean of the predictor distribution $(X - \overline{X})$.
2. The value of the constant multiplier B_{yx}.

Pictorally, a linear prediction or regression line for a given population would appear as shown below:

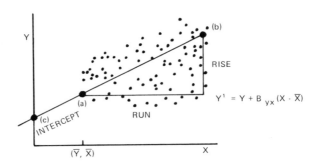

Note: 1. The prediction line passes through the point $(\overline{Y},\overline{X})$, that is, the point whose coordinates are the means of the criterion and predictor variables in this data set.

2. B_{yx} is the slope of the line, that is, the vertical distance between points b and a called the *rise* divided by the horizontal distance between the same two points, called the *run*.

3. The slope of a *straight line* can be determined using any two arbitrarily selected points on the line.

4. The rise and run are measured in whatever units are used in calibrating the vertical and horizontal axes, respectively.

5. The intercept (c) is determined by subtracting the product of the slope and the mean of the predictor distribution from the mean of the criterion score distribution, that is, $\overline{Y} - B_{yx}\overline{X}$.

Determining the Slope of the Regression Line

In the figure below, the line passes through the points (1,2), (2,4), and (3,6).

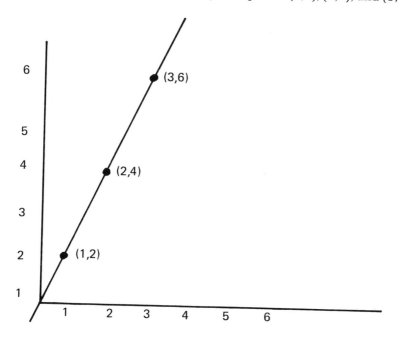

If the points (1,2) and (2,4) are used, the rise is 2 and the run 1; therefore, the slope is $\frac{2}{1}$ or 2. If one chooses any two other points and repeats the process, although the values of the rise and run may differ, their ratio will remain $\frac{2}{1}$ or 2.

To determine the slope of the regression line, B_{yx}, using raw scores, the following formula is employed:

(Formula 10-19)
$$B_{yx} = r_{xy}\left(\frac{SD_y}{SD_x}\right)$$

where:

r_{xy} = correlation between the predictor and criterion variables
SD_y = standard deviation of the criterion score distribution
SD_x = standard deviation of the predictor score distribution

Example: If r_{xy} is 0.50, the standard deviation of the predictor score distribution is 15, and the standard deviation of the criterion score distribution is 5, then the slope of the regression line is equal to:

$$B_{yx} = r_{xy}\left(\frac{SD_y}{SD_x}\right)$$
$$= 0.50\left(\frac{5}{15}\right)$$
$$= 0.50(0.33)$$
$$= 0.165$$

Once an individual's score has been predicted, the discrepancy between the person's actual criterion score, Y, and predicted criterion score, Y', is called an *error of estimate*, E. In other words, this prediction procedure effectively divides each criterion score, Y, into two parts: (1) an estimated criterion score (Y') and (2) an error of estimate, E = Y − Y' or, in other words, Y = Y' + E.

If the criterion score were estimated for each person in the population, three distributions of scores would be generated:

1. The distribution of *observed criterion* scores, Y.
2. The distribution of *predicted criterion* scores, Y'.
3. The distribution of *error* scores, E.

If it is *assumed* that:

1. The prediction line passes through the mean value of Y in each contingent X distribution.
2. The contingent distributions are all normal and display the same amount of variation:

$$VAR_y = VAR_{y'} + VAR_E$$

If this equation is divided by VAR_y (the variance of the observed criterion score distribution):

$$\frac{VAR_y}{VAR_y} = \frac{VAR_{y'}}{VAR_y} + \frac{VAR_E}{VAR_y}$$

$$1 = \sqrt{\left\{\frac{VAR_{y'}}{VAR_y} + \frac{VAR_E}{VAR_y}\right\}}$$

is the proportion of criterion variation
explainable using our prediction policy
is r^2

Linear Prediction Equation for Z Score Data

If an individual's X and Y scores, and the value of r_{xy} are known, the prediction equation for determining the regression line is:

(Formula 10-20) $Z_{y'} = r_{xy} \cdot Z_x$

That is, an individual's predicted criterion Z score ($Z_{y'}$) is equal to the person's Z score on the predictor variable (Z_x) times the linear correlation between the criterion and predictor variables.

Note: If raw scores are changed to Z scores, the resulting distribution will have a mean = 0 and standard deviation = 1.

Thus, the slope of the Z score prediction line will be:

$$B_{Z_y} \cdot Z_y = r_{yx}$$

Regardless of whether raw or Z score data are used in determining the regression equation, the quality of a particular predictor for estimating performance on a specific criterion variable depends only on the value of the correlation between the predictor and criterion (r_{cp}).

The higher the correlation, the closer the data points in the scatterplot cluster about the line of best fit (that is, the straight line running through the arithmetic means of the various contingent distributions). The closer the data points within these contingent distributions are to the straight line (and thus to the means of their respective contingent distributions), the smaller the value of the standard deviation of each of these distributions. Since each contingent distribution is a distribution of prediction errors, the standard deviation of each contingent distribution is called the *standard error of estimate* for that particular distribution. The larger the value of r_{xy}, the smaller the standard errors of estimate.

In practice, if it is assumed that (1) all the contingent distributions have the same shape, that is, are all normal in shape, and (2) all the contingent distributions display an equal amount of variability, then the average standard deviation of the various contingent distributions (the standard error of estimate) may be computed by the formula:

(Formula 10-21) $\sigma_{cp} = \sigma_c \sqrt{1 - r_{cp}^2}$

where:

σ_{cp} = average standard deviation of the various contingent distributions (the standard error of estimate)

σ_c = standard deviation of the criterion score distribution

r^2_{cp} = square of the predictor-criterion correlation coefficient

This average standard error of estimate can then be used as an indicator of the quality of the prediction.

The results of bivariate regression studies are usually interpreted in terms of the percent of variance in the criterion variable explained or predicted by scores on the predictor variable (r^2). Unlike the results from correlation studies, regression findings are not reversible. That is, the predictor and criterion variables are identified prior to data collection and statements are then restricted to the percents of variance explained and unexplained in the criterion variable on the basis of the predictor variable (Fig. 10-10).

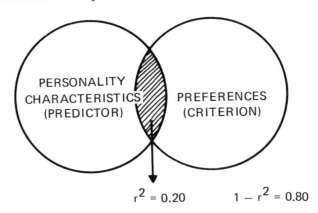

FIGURE 10-10. Venn diagram of prediction results.

The following interpretation may be made on the basis of the regression findings presented in Figure 10-10.

1. The nature of the relationship between personality characteristics and nurses' preferences is positive.
2. Twenty percent of the variance in nurses' preferences can be explained or predicted on the basis of personality characteristics.
3. Eighty percent of the variance in nurses' preferences is unexplained on the basis of personality characteristics.

MULTIPLE REGRESSION

Multiple regression procedures are extensions of the bivariate procedure that enable the researcher to consider the relationship between two or more predictor variables and one criterion variable.

Table 10-8 illustrates how bivariate regression is extended to account for

TABLE 10-8. Bivariate Regression Extended to Multiple Regression

	Bivariate	*Multiple*
No. of variables	one predictor one criterion	two or more predictors one criterion
Algebraic model	$Z_{y'} = r_{xy}Z_y$ $Z_{y'}$ = predicted criterion Z score r_{xy} = slope of line of best fit Z_x = Z score on the predictor variable	$Z_{y'} = B_1Z_1 + B_2Z_2 +$ intercept $Z_{y'}$ = predicted criterion Z score B = beta weight for each predictor Z = Z score on each predictor. intercept = the point on the Y axis where the line of best fit crosses; when Z scores are employed this value is always 0.
Assumptions	1. Variables are linearly related. 2. Variables measured at the interval level. 3. Distributions of both variables are normal. 4. Variables are independent of each other. 5. Scores on both variables have equal variances, that is, scores for both variables are equally dispersed or scattered about the line of best fit.	1. Variables are linearly related, that is, an additive composite of predictor variables will equal the criterion. 2. Variables measured at the interval level. 3. Distributions of variables are multivariate normal. 4. Variables are independent of each other. 5. Scores for variables are equally dispersed or scattered about the line of best fit, that is, scores are homoscedastic.

multiple predictor variables. In multiple regression, the task is to determine the values for the beta weights that will minimize the sum of squared errors or residuals. The beta weight for each predictor indicates the relative contribution the variable makes to the prediction of the criterion. That is, the larger the value of the beta weight for a given variable, the greater the contribution of that variable to the prediction of the criterion. The multiple regression coefficient (R), which ranges from 0 to 1, indicates the strength of the relationship between the criterion and all the predictors taken together. R^2 represents the proportion of variance in the criterion variable scores that is predictable or explained by all predictor variables. The R, then, in multiple regression is an average measure of prediction given all predictor variables.

Table 10-9 presents the results of a regression where the researcher's interest was in predicting students' preferences for a particular type of patient care

TABLE 10-9. FSP_3 as a Function of FSP_1

		df		F
Multiple R $= 0.46011$		Regression	1	44.57892^*
$R^2 = 0.21170$		Residual	166	
Variable	B	Beta	Standard Error Beta	F
FSP_1	0.48025	0.46011	0.07193	44.579^*
Constant	22.93087			
				$^*p < 0.05$

involvement after a clinical nursing course (FSP_3) on the basis of the students' preferences before the course (FSP_1).

Since the information in the table resulted from a regression analysis employing only two variables (FSP_1 and FSP_3), the resulting multiple R is simply r_{xy}, that is, it is a bivariate regression. The F is a test of the significance of the overall prediction and in this instance is significant at the 0.05 level. The B weight is the weight assigned to a given predictor when raw scores are used in the analysis instead of Z scores. Beta weights, which result when Z scores are employed, are preferred over B weights because they are more stable and less likely to vary over repeated regression analysis.

It should be noted that in this instance the beta weight is equal in value to the multiple R. This makes sense because the slope of the line in a bivariate regression is r_{xy} (that is, $Z_{y'} = r_{xy}Z_x$). On the basis of the findings in Table 10-9, the researcher would conclude that 21 percent of the variance in FSP_3 can be predicted on the basis of FSP_1 and this amount is significant at the 0.05 level. Alternatively, 79 percent of the variance in FSP_3 is not explainable on the basis of FSP_1.

Suppose this researcher has reason to believe that FSP_3 is a function not only of FSP_1, but is affected as well by:

1. Student preferences after six weeks of the course (FSP_2).
2. Student perceptions of the link between the content taught and faculty activities (Scale 1).
3. Student perceptions of the faculty who set standards for the course (Scale 2).
4. Preferences and reputation attributed to faculty by students (Scale 3).
5. Student perceptions of their clinical experience's relevance to nursing issues, roles, and their own goals (Scale 4).

Thus, the researcher decides to do a multiple regression analysis to ascertain the amount of variation in FSP_3 that can be explained on the basis of these six variables taken together. The results are presented in Table 10-10.

By including the additional predictors in the analysis, the researcher is able to explain 28 percent of the variance in FSP_3. The F (10.63910) test of the overall regression is significant at the 0.05 level. By considering the beta weights for each of the predictor variables, the researcher is able to ascertain (1) the relative contribution of each predictor to the overall prediction and (2) the nature of the

TABLE 10-10. Regression of FSP_1, FSP_2, and Scales 1, 2, 3, and 4 Scores on FSP_3

			df		F
Multiple R	= 0.53284		Regression	6	10.63910*
R^2	= 0.28392		Residual	161	

Variable	B	Beta	Standard Error Beta	F
FSP_1	0.33123	0.31734	0.08069	16.851*
FSP_2	0.28945	0.27697	0.08056	12.910*
Scale 1	−0.00770	−0.02226	0.03123	0.061
Scale 2	0.08669	0.09727	0.07681	1.274
Scale 3	−0.04395	−0.13189	0.02570	2.924*
Scale 4	−0.02597	−0.02386	0.08650	0.090
Constant	17.75534			

*$p < 0.05$

relationship between each predictor variable and the criterion variable. The F tests opposite the values for each variable allow the researcher to test the significance of the contribution of each variable, and are referred to as F tests of the beta weights. The researcher determines that the F tests of the beta weights for FSP_1, FSP_2, and Scale 3 are significant at the 0.05 level. Thus, these three variables are contributing significantly to the prediction of FSP_3 and Scales 1, 2, and 4 scores are not. Furthermore, by comparing the relative sizes of the beta weights for FSP_1, FSP_2 and Scale 3, the researcher sees that FSP_1 is the most important contributor and then FSP_2 and Scale 3, respectively. In addition, by considering the sign of the beta weight for each of the three variables the researcher concludes that FSP_1 and FSP_2 are positively related to FSP_3, while Scale 3 scores are inversely (−) related to FSP_3. In order to estimate the accuracy or quality of the prediction, the researcher considers the size of each beta weight relative to the size of the standard error of the beta. The smaller the size of the error and the higher the size of the beta, the more accurate the prediction. As the difference between the size of the beta and the size of the error diminishes, the researcher becomes less willing to put a great deal of emphasis on the results. Similarly, when the size of the beta is less than the size of the error, the probability of misinterpretation is highest.

From this example, it is apparent that multiple regression provides the researcher with additional information regarding the nature and strength of the contributions of each variable to the prediction as well as increases the amount of variance in the criterion that may be explained by the predictors. On the other hand, multiple regression increases the cost to the researcher in that the researcher must employ more instruments, collect more data, and request more time and effort from the subjects. Thus, a very pragmatic concern is: when does multiple regression buy the researcher enough information to warrant its increased cost? One approach to answering this question is to determine the significance of the increment in R^2 when multiple regression is employed rather than bivariate regression. That is, if a multiple regression procedure significantly increases the ability to predict the criterion, than it is preferable to a bivariate procedure.

A convenient formula that allows the researcher to test the significance of the difference between two regressions is:

(Formula 10-22)[12]

$$F = \frac{(R^2_{K1} - R^2_{K2})/(K_1 - K_2)}{(1 - R^2_{K1})/N - K_1 - 1}$$

$$df = (K_1 - K_2), (N - K_1 - 1)$$

where:

R^2_{K1} = the R^2 obtained from the first regression analysis
R^2_{K2} = the R^2 resulting from the second regression analysis
K_1 = the number of variables used in the first regression analysis
K_2 = the number of variables used in the second regression analysis
N = the total number of subjects

Example

The researcher conducts two separate regression analyses using the same 168 subjects. The first analysis results are presented in Table 10-9 and the second set of results in Table 10-10. To determine the statistical significance of the increment in R^2 when seven variables are employed rather than two, the researcher uses Formula 10-22.

$$F = \frac{(0.28392 - 0.21170)/(7 - 1)}{(1 - 0.28392)/(168 - 7 - 1)}$$

$$= \frac{0.07222/6}{0.71608/160}$$

$$= \frac{0.014444}{0.004448}$$

$$= 3.247$$

This F with df 6 and 161 is significant at the 0.05 level. Thus, by using the additional predictor variables, the researcher in this example was able to significantly increase the ability to predict the criterion variable.

There are essentially two approaches to multiple regression analysis when a predictive framework is employed: (1) the general or overall approach, and (2) step in procedures including forward, backward, and true stepwise.

General Multiple Regression

In nursing, the researcher is often concerned with multiple forces operating within a situation. Furthermore, it is often difficult if not impossible to isolate any one of these forces or variables in reality. Rather, given a certain set of conditions, one can expect certain things to happen. For example, in treating the diabetic patient, one might say given that the patient understands and follows the diet regimen, the right type and amount of medication is prescribed and taken by the patient, and physical activity is regulated, one expects the patient's disease condition to be controlled or managed. In this instance, it does not make sense to talk about diet or drug therapy in isolation, but rather to consider all these variables together and their impact on the diabetic patient's condition. The multiple regression analysis presented in Table 10-10 is an example of a *general multiple regression*. That is, the researcher's interest was in the ability to predict FSP_3 given FSP_1, FSP_2, and Scales 1, 2, 3, and 4 scores taken together.

When the general approach is used, all predictors are entered together and the average correlation between the criterion variable and all predictor variables is obtained. This is R. This R is then squared and subtracted from 1 to determine how much variance is left unexplained by the set of predictors. To ascertain the extent to which the variables are independent of each other, the matrix of intercorrelations is considered. If predictor variables are highly correlated with each other, there will be less clarity in the interpretation of results and the possibility of less stability over replication is increased. Similarly, when high intercorrelations exist, the researcher may expect to find variables that do not contribute significantly to the prediction per se aside from their relationship to other predictors. Such variables can usually be eliminated from subsequent analyses. On the basis of the size and direction of the bivariate correlations between each predictor variable and the criterion variable, the researcher can get a feel for the variables that may be potentially important predictors. The matrix of intercorrelations for the six variables is presented in Table 10-11.

The range of intercorrelations among predictors in Table 10-11 is from 0.01 between Scale 2 and FSP_2 to 0.57 between Scales 1 and 2. The size of the intercorrelations between FSP_3 and the predictor variables suggest that the important variables may be FSP_1 and FSP_2. The fact that Scale 3 does not have a high bivariate correlation with FSP_3 and yet contributes significantly to the multiple regression illustrates the fact that a variable that does not correlate highly with the criterion may be important when considered with and enhanced by other predictors, that is, Scale 3.

It should be noted that beta weights tend to fluctuate from sample to sample and the likelihood of this phenomenon increases when predictor variables have high intercorrelations or sample size is small, or both. In regression analyses, it is desirable to have approximately 30 subjects per variable. The variable to subject ratio in this instance is 0.03. In a study with 10 variables and 30 subjects the ratio is 0.33. Thus, the lower the variable to subject ratio, the less the betas are likely to fluctuate from sample to sample and the less likely the researcher is to make erroneous interpretations on the basis of the results.

In summary, the researcher interprets the results of a general regression analysis by:

1. Looking at the standard deviation for each variable; low variances may explain a low multiple R.

TABLE 10-11. Matrix of Intercorrelations

	FSP_1	FSP_2	SCALE 1	SCALE 2	SCALE 3	SCALE 4	FSP_3
FSP_1	1.00000	0.49105	-0.06823	-0.02851	-0.06468	0.02153	0.46011
FSP_2	0.49105	1.00000	-0.01358	-0.01211	0.02087	-0.05615	0.43051
SCALE 1	-0.06823	-0.01358	1.00000	0.57537	0.45828	0.48787	-0.06379
SCALE 2	-0.02851	-0.01211	0.57537	1.00000	0.41585	0.45346	0.00639
SCALE 3	-0.06468	0.02087	0.45828	0.41585	1.00000	0.20573	-0.12130
SCALE 4	0.02153	-0.05615	0.48787	0.45346	0.20573	1.00000	-0.02647
FSP_3	0.46011	0.43051	-0.06379	0.00639	-0.12130	-0.02647	1.00000

2. Considering the matrix of intercorrelations to determine:
   a. The lowest and highest bivariate correlations between predictors.
   b. The size of the majority of the intercorrelations to determine the likelihood of making erroneous interpretations.
   c. The bivariate correlation between each predictor and the criterion to identify potentially important predictors.
3. Ascertaining the size of the standard error of the beta weights relative to the size of each beta weight. A high beta weight and a low standard error are desirable.
4. Considering the size of the beta weight to speak to the strength of the relationship with the criterion, and the sign of the beta to speak to the direction of the relationship.
5. Determining the significance of the F tests of the beta weight to identify those predictors contributing to the prediction and those that may be eliminated in subsequent analyzes.
6. Considering R and R^2 and $1 - R^2$; R^2 allows the researcher to speak to the amount of variance in the criterion explained or predicted by all predictor variables together and $1 - R^2$ the proportion of unexplained variance.
7. Determining the significance of the F test of the overall regression to determine if the variance explained by all predictors is a more than chance occurrence.

Step in Regression Procedures

Step in regression procedures are employed when the researcher aims to select the minimum number of variables necessary to account for approximately as much variance as is accounted for by the total set. These procedures are particularly useful when constraints exist in terms of cost, time, availability of subjects, and the like.

In the *forward* procedure, first, the bivariate correlation between the criterion variable and each of the predictor variables is determined. Then, the variable that has the highest correlation with the criterion is entered first into the regression analyses. The R is squared and subtracted from one to determine how much variance is left unexplained by the first or best predictor. Each of the remaining predictors is then correlated with this residual $(1 - R^2)$. The resulting correlations are similar to partial correlations in that the effects or variances due to the first predictor are removed from the correlation now computed between the residual and other predictors. The predictor with the highest value is chosen and becomes the second best predictor. The same process continues, each time removing from the residual the effects or variance due to all the predictors that have already been estimated.

A weakness in the forward approach is that the variables entered into the equation are retained despite the fact that they may have lost their usefulness in the light of the contributions made by variables entered at later stages.

An example may help to clarify the forward procedure. The intercorrelation matrix for the variables FSP_1, FSP_2, FSP_3, and Scales 1, 2, 3, and 4 was presented in Table 10-11. On the basis of the information in the table, FSP has the highest bivariate correlation with FSP_3 and thus is entered first into the regression analysis. Table 10-12 presents the results of the first step of a forward step in regression of FSP_1, FSP_2, and Scales 1, 2, 3, and 4 on FSP_3.

TABLE 10-12. Results of First Step in Forward Regression

Dependent variable ... FSP_3
Variable(s) entered on Step Number 1 ... FSP_1

		df		F
Multiple R = 0.46011		Regression	1	44.57892*
R^2 = 0.21170		Residual	166	

Variables in the Equation

Variable	Beta	Standard Error Beta	F
FSP_1	0.46011	0.07193	44.579*
Constant	22.93087		

Variables not in the Equation

Variable	Partial	F
FSP_2	0.26450	12.412
Scale 1	−0.03657	0.221
Scale 2	0.02198	0.080
Scale 3	−0.10331	1.780
Scale 4	−0.04098	0.277

*$p < 0.05$

From the table, it can be seen that 21 percent of the variance in FSP_3 is explained by FSP_1 and this is significant at the 0.05 level. Similarly, 79 percent of the variance in FSP_3 is still unexplained. The values in the column *Partial* under the subheading *Variables Not in the Equation* reflect the correlations of each variable with the residual $(1 - R^2)$. For example, 0.26450 is the correlation between FSP_2 and FSP_3 holding FSP_1 constant. Bivariate correlations are sometimes referred to as *zero order* correlations because nothing has been partialled out. The correlation 0.2450 is a *first order* correlation because one variable, FSP_1, has been removed. A *second order* correlation would be a partial correlation in which two variables have been removed, and so forth.

Since FSP_2 has the highest partial correlation with the criterion, it would be entered next into the regression. Table 10-13 presents step two of this regression.

From Table 10-13 it can be seen that, in fact, FSP_2 is entered next. The multiple R^2 of 0.26685 indicates that 27 percent of the variance in FSP_3 can be predicted by FSP_1 and FSP_2 and this is significant at 0.05. The F test of multiple R^2 in this instance is a test of the significance of R^2 when FSP_2 is added to FSP_1. The F test of the beta weights for both FSP_1 and FSP_2 are significant, indicating they are both contributing to the prediction of FSP_3. Looking at the second order partial correlations for the variables not in the equation, Scale 3 has the highest correlation with FSP_3 when FSP_1 and FSP_2 are removed, and hence will be entered next into the regression equation.

TABLE 10-13 Results of Second Step in Forward Regression

Dependent Variable ... FSP_3
Variable(s) entered on Step Number 2 ... FSP_2

		df		F
Multiple R = 0.51657		Regression	2	
R^2 = 0.26685		Residual	165	30.02752*

Variables in the Equation

Variable	Beta	Standard Error Beta	F
FSP_1	0.32773	0.07987	18.344*
FSP_2	0.26958	0.07997	12.412*
Constant	16.71126		

Variables not in the Equation

Variable	Partial	F
Scale 1	−0.04422	0.321
Scale 2	0.02220	0.081
Scale 3	−0.12396	2.559
Scale 4	−0.02154	0.076

*$p < 0.05$

The analysis continues in this manner. There are basically two types of criteria for terminating a regression analysis—statistical significance and meaningfulness. At each step of the analysis, the researcher can test whether an increase in R^2 attributed to a variable is statistically significant. When increases cease to be significant, the analysis is terminated. Meaningfulness involves a decision by the researcher as to whether or not an increment is substantively meaningful. Meaningfulness is specific to the research situation, that is, what has value in one situation may not in another. For example, if the researcher is doing an exploratory study in an area in which little previous investigation has occurred, the ability to predict a small amount of variance, even though it is not statistically significant, may be meaningful enough to warrant further studies in the area. Since statistical significance has little value unless the results are meaningful, the authors' recommend that both criteria be given equal importance.

In a *true stepwise* regression, at each step of the analysis, F tests are performed to determine the contribution of each variable in the equation as if it were the last to enter. Thus, it is possible to discard a variable that was initially a good predictor if its predictive power diminishes as other variables are entered. A true stepwise procedure is then just a more precise variation of the forward procedure.

The *backward* step in procedure starts by entering all predictors and then deleting variables one at a time, assessing the statistical significance of the decrement in R^2 at each step.

An important consideration to be made in interpreting the results of multiple regression is the notion of the *shrinkage of R*. The choice of a set of beta weights is designed to yield the highest possible correlation between the predictors and criterion variable. The value of R can be expressed as the correlation between the predicted scores based on the regression equation (Y′) and the observed criterion scores (Y). If the researcher applies the set of weights derived from the study to the predictor scores of another sample in another study and then correlates these predicted criterion scores (Y′) with the observed criterion scores (Y), the resulting R will almost always be smaller than the R obtained in the sample for which the weights were originally calculated. This phenomenon is referred to as the shrinkage of R.

The reason for this shrinkage is that in calculating the weights to obtain a maximum value for R, the zero order correlations are treated as if they were error free, and this of course is never the case in reality. Consequently, there is a certain amount of capitalization on chance and the resulting R is biased upward. The degree to which R is overestimated will depend in part on the ratio of the number of predictor variables to the size of the sample. The higher the variable to subject ratio, the greater the overestimation of R. As a rule of thumb, a ratio of one variable per 30 subjects is recommended. Similarly, the larger the sample size, the more stable regression results and hence large numbers of subjects are recommended. When all predictor variables are used in the analysis as in the general approach, the capitalization on chance is less than when a step in regression procedure is used because the best set of predictors is selected from a larger pool and is bound to have errors due to the correlation of these variables with the criterion as well as errors due to the intercorrelations among the predictors. Therefore, in an attempt to reduce these errors when a step in procedure is employed, very large samples are recommended.

Although it is not possible to determine the exact degree of the overestimation of R, there are formulas available that allow one to estimate the amount of shrinkage and several procedures exist that facilitate the utilization of these formulas. Such procedures are called *cross-validation* procedures and all involve using two samples or subsamples in the following manner:

1. A regression analysis is performed and R^2 and the regression equation obtained. This is called the *screening* sample.
2. A second sample is obtained and the regression weights from the first analysis are applied to the predictor variable scores for this second, *calibration*, sample. That is, Y′ is determined for each subject using the equation $Y' = Beta_1 X_1 + Beta_2 X_2 + \ldots$. The result is a set of Y′ scores, one for each subject.
3. A Pearson r is then calculated between these predicted criterion scores (Y′) and the observed criterion scores (Y) for members of this calibration sample. The resulting $r_{y'y}$ is analogous to a multiple regression coefficient such as the R obtained in the screening sample.
4. The size of the R from the screening sample is then compared with the new R (that is, R = y′y) to estimate the expected amount of shrinkage.

In multiple regression studies in which explanation is the aim, the researcher will generally employ one of two procedures, commonality analysis or path analysis.

Commonality Analysis

Commonality analysis, sometimes referred to as elements analysis, is a method of analyzing the variance of a criterion variable into common and unique variances to help identify the relative influences of independent variables.[12] The unique contribution of a predictor variable is defined as the variance attributed to it when it is entered last in the regression equation. In other words, the unique contribution is a squared partial correlation between the criterion variable and the predictor variable of interest after partialling out all other predictor variables. For example, for the following two predictor variables, the unique contribution of variable 1 is:

(Formula 10-23)[12]
$$U(1) = R^2_{y \cdot 12} - R^2_{y \cdot 2}$$

where:
  $U(1)$ = unique contribution of variable 1
  $R^2_{y \cdot 12}$ = squared multiple correlation of Y with variables 1 and 2
  $R^2_{y \cdot 2}$ = squared multiple correlation of Y with variable 2

Similarly, the unique contribution of variable 2 is:

$$U(2) = R^2_{y \cdot 12} - R^2_{y \cdot 1}$$

where:
  $U(2)$ = unique contribution of variable 2
  $R^2_{y \cdot 12}$ = squared multiple correlation of Y with variables 1 and 2
  $R^2_{y \cdot 1}$ = squared multiple correlation Y with variable 1

The commonality of variables 1 and 2 is:

$$C(1,2) = R^2_{y \cdot 12} - U(1) - U(2)$$

where:
  $C(1,2)$ = commonality of variables 1 and 2
  $U(1)$ = unique contribution of variable 1
  $U(2)$ = unique contribution of variable 2

As a result of determining the unique and common contributions of variables, it is possible to express the correlation between any predictor variable and the criterion variable as a composite of the unique contribution of the variable of interest plus its commonalities with other predictor variables. $R^2_{y \cdot 1}$ in the example can be expressed as:

$$R^2_{y \cdot 1} = U(1) + C(1,2)$$

In theory, this type of analysis should enable the researcher to assign relative importance to variables on the basis of their unique contribution. That is, those variables that make the greatest unique contribution are deemed the most important. In practice, however, problems arise in the interpretation of commonality analysis because unique and common contributions are affected by the intercorrelations among the predictor variables. That is, uniqueness by definition is the increment in R^2 accounted for when a given predictor variable is entered last in the regression equation. Thus, the uniqueness of variables depends on the relations among the specific set of predictors under study. The higher the intercorrelations among predictors, the larger the commonalities and the smaller the unique components. Similarly, the addition or deletion of variables may drastically change the uniqueness attributed to some or all of the remaining variables. For these reasons, some authors argue that commonality analysis can make a greater contribution in a predictive rather than explanatory framework.

Path Analysis

Path analysis is a method designed to determine the tenability of a theoretical model formulated by the researcher. The researcher designs the study on the basis of a theoretical formulation, explanatory scheme, or causal model and then determines whether the resulting data are consistent or inconsistent with the model. If the data are inconsistent with the model, doubt is cast on the model that generated it. Consistency of the data with the model is not proof of the model, but lends support to it. The following discussion focuses on some of the basic principles of path analysis. More detailed information may be obtained from Wright,[28] Tukey,[25] Li,[15] Turner and Stevens,[26] Land,[14] and Heise.[9]

The *path diagram* is a useful device for displaying graphically the pattern of causal relations among a set of variables. An *exogenous variable* is a variable whose variability is assumed to be determined by causes outside the theoretical model.[12] Consequently, no attempt is made to explain the variability of an exogenous variable or its relations with other exogenous variables. An *endogenous variable* is one whose variation is explained by exogenous or endogenous variables in the model.[12] The distinction between the two types of variables is illustrated below:

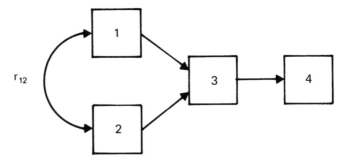

Variables 1 and 2 are exogenous. The correlation between exogenous variables is depicted by a curved line with arrowheads at both ends, indicating that the researcher does not conceive of one variable being the cause of the other. Thus, in the analysis, a relation between exogenous variables (for example, r_{12}) is not considered.

Variables 3 and 4 in the diagram are endogenous. Paths, in the form of unidirectional arrows, are drawn from the variables taken as causes (independent) to the variables taken as effects (dependent). The two paths leading from variables 1 and 2 to variable 3 indicate that variable 3 is dependent on variables 1 and 2.

The path model depicted above is a *recursive* model. That is, the causal flow in the model is unidirectional. This means that at a given point in time a variable cannot be both a cause and an effect of another variable. For example, if variable 1 were taken as a cause of variable 3, then the possibility of variable 3 being a cause of variable 2 is ruled out.

An endogenous variable treated as dependent in one set of variables may also be conceived as an independent variable in relation to other variables. For example, variable 3 in the diagram above is dependent on variables 1 and 2, and an independent variable in relation to 4.

Since it is not possible to account for the total variance of a variable, *residual* variables are introduced to indicate the effect of variables not included in the model. In the diagram below, a and b are residual variables:

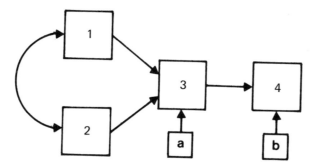

It is assumed in path analysis that residual variables are neither correlated with other residuals nor with other variables in the system. Thus, variable a is assumed to be not correlated with variable b or with variables 1, 2, and 4. To simplify the presentation of path diagrams, residuals are usually *not* represented in the diagram.

The major assumptions that underlie the application of path analysis are:

1. The relations among the variables in the model are linear, additive, and causal.
2. The residual variables are not intercorrelated nor are they correlated with other variables in the system.
3. There is a one-way causal flow in the system (that is, reciprocal causation between variables is ruled out).
4. The variables are measured on an interval scale.[12]

A *path coefficient* indicates the direct effect of an independent variable on a dependent variable. The symbol for a path coefficient is P with two subscripts, the first indicating the dependent variable and the second the independent variable. For example, the direct effect of variable 2 on variable 3 in the diagrams above would be symbolized P_{32}.

If the assumptions outlined earlier are tenable, path coefficients take the form of beta weights discussed in the section on multiple regression. It is therefore possible to determine path coefficients in the same manner used to solve for the betas. For example, for the variables in the first path diagram above, the researcher would regress variable 3 on variables 1 and 2. Each path coefficient is equal to the beta weight associated with the same variable. Thus, $P_{31} = B_{31.2}$ and $P_{32} = B_{32.1}$. It should be noted that $P_{31} \neq P_{13}$. P_{31} indicates the effect of variable 1 on variable 3, while P_{13} indicates the effect of variable 3 on variable 1. In unidirectional models it is not possible to have both P_{31} and P_{13}. The path coefficients that are calculated are those that reflect the causal model formulated by the researcher. If, as in the example, the model indicates that variable 1 effects variable 3, then P_{31} is determined.

There is an important difference between regular regression analysis and path analysis. In regular regression analysis, a dependent variable is regressed in a single analysis on all the independent variables under consideration. In path analysis, more than one regression analysis may be needed. At each stage, a dependent variable is regressed on the variables upon which it is assumed to depend. The resulting betas are the path coefficients for the paths leading from the particular set of independent variables to the dependent variable under consideration. For example, the model below requires three regression analyses for the calculation of all the path coefficients.

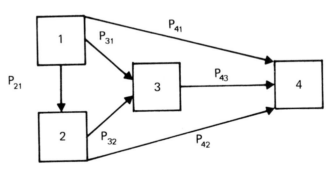

The path from 1 to 2 (P_{21}) is determined by regressing variable 2 on variable 1. P_{31} and P_{32} are obtained by regressing variable 3 on variables 1 and 2. P_{41}, P_{42}, and P_{43} are obtained by regressing variable 4 on variables 1, 2, and 3.

Through the application of path analysis, the researcher can determine whether or not a pattern of coefficients for a set of observations is consistent with a specific theoretical formulation. The researcher may believe the correlation between two variables is due to indirect effects only. By detecting such paths, the researcher may offer a more parsimonious causal model. Heise[9] suggests a pragmatic approach to the deletion of paths that he refers to as "theory trimming." Using this approach, first the researcher calculates all the path coefficients in the model and then employs one of two criteria for the deletion of paths: statistical significance or meaningfulness. Adopting the significance criterion, one may decide to delete paths whose coefficients are not significant at a prespecified α level. The problem with this approach is that minute path coefficients may be found significant when the analysis is based on fairly large samples. In view of this shortcoming of the significance criterion, some researchers prefer to use the criterion of meaningfulness and delete all paths whose coefficients they consider not meaningful. What may be meaningful for one researcher in one setting may be considered not meaningful by another researcher in another setting. Thus, a set of rules for determining meaningfulness is not available. In the absence of other guidelines some researchers recommend that path coefficients less than 0.05 be considered not meaningful.[16]

Summary

The researcher conducting a correlational study has a variety of both nonparametric and parametric statistical procedures available for analyzing the data. In addition to the research question or hypothesis, the selection of a statistical procedure will depend upon factors such as:

1. Level of measurement of the resulting data.
2. Assumptions regarding the population distribution from which subjects were drawn.
3. Sample size.
4. Power of the statistical test.
5. Number of variables to be investigated.
6. Resources available to the researcher (for example, time, money, computer access, and so forth).

In general, the researcher should strive to use the most powerful statistical procedure available. Thus, the researcher should aim for the highest possible level of measurement and large sample sizes.

USING THE COMPUTER TO ANALYZE DATA FROM CORRELATIONAL STUDIES

Historically, correlational studies preceded ANOVA and its related techniques, which were designed as shortcuts or abbreviations to avoid the arduous computations required in correlational studies when computers were not readily available for analysis of data. With the increased availability of a wide variety of computer programs, the advantages of correlational studies are once again being realized and their utilization is increasing rapidly.

The SPSS package includes five programs for analyzing data from correlational studies: CROSSTABS, NONPAR CORREL, SCATTERGRAM, PEARSON CORR, and REGRESSION. As with all the SPSS programs discussed to this point, once the basic deck setup is prepared, the researcher need only substitute one or two cards to run another program. The reader who wishes to utilize the SPSS package for correlational programs should consult the SPSS manual[18] Chapters 16, 18, 20 for step-by-step instructions.

CROSSTABS computes and displays two- to n-way crosstabulation tables for any discrete variables. Table 10-2 exemplifies a two dimensional table similar to that produced by CROSSTABS. Nominal and ordinal measures of relationship and tests of significance are also provided for most of the nonparametric statistical procedures discussed in the preceding section of this chapter, including chi-square, Cramer's V, contingency coefficient, asymmetric and symmetric lambda, Kendall's tau b and c, gamma. Somer's D, and so forth. Spearman and Kendall rank order correlations for ordinal data can be obtained using NONPAR CORREL. Those readers who wish to see a sample printout from the CROSSTABS, and NONPAR CORREL programs can find them in the SPSS manual[18] on pp. 220 and 292, respectively.

Two SPSS programs are available for obtaining parametric bivariate correlations: PEARSON CORR and SCATTERGRAM. PEARSON CORR provides Pearson product moment correlation coefficients for pairs of interval level variables. SCATTERGRAM prints two-variable scattergrams of data points similar to the ones presented in this chapter and calculates simple linear regression equations. Sample printouts of the PEARSON CORR and SCATTERGRAM programs can be found in the SPSS manual[18] on pages 287 and 299, respectively.

The multiple regression procedures discussed earlier are available via the REGRESSION program, which combines general and multiple regression and stepwise procedures in a manner that affords the researcher considerable control over the inclusion of predictor variables into the regression equation. It is also possible to obtain the components necessary for commonality and path analysis utilizing this program. Table 10-10 illustrates the type of table that results from the REGRESSION program when a general multiple regression procedure is employed. When a step in multiple regression procedure is employed, the REGRESSION printout resembles Tables 10-12 and 10-13. Additional examples of output from the REGRESSION program can be found in the SPSS manual[18] on page 364.

REFERENCES

1. Amborn, S. A.: *Clinical signs associated with the amount of tracheobronchial secretions.* Nurs. Res. 25(2):121, March–April, 1976.
2. Campbell, D. T. and Stanley, J. C.: *Experimental and Quasi-Experimental Designs for Research.* Rand McNally, Chicago, 1963.
3. Carroll, J. B.: *The nature of the data, or how to choose a correlation coefficient.* Psychometrika 26:347, 1961.
4. Cureton, E. E.: *Note on ϕ/ϕ max.* Psychometrika 24:89, 1959.
5. Deardorff, M., Denner, P., and Miller, C.: *Selected National League for Nursing Achievement Test scores as predictors of State Board Examination scores.* Nurs. Res. 25(1):35, January–February, 1976.
6. Elder, R. G.: *Orientation of senior nursing students toward access to contraceptives.* Nurs. Res. 25(5):338, September–October, 1976.

7. Glass, G. V. and Stanley, J. C.: *Statistical Methods in Education and Psychology.* Prentice-Hall, Englewood Cliffs, New Jersey, 1970.
8. Guilford, J. P.: *Fundamental Statistics in Psychology and Education,* ed. 4. McGraw-Hill, New York, 1965.
9. Heise, D. R.: *Problems in path analysis and causal inference.* In Borgatta, E. F. (ed.): *Sociological Methodology 1969.* Jossey-Bass, San Francisco, 1969.
10. Isaac, S. and Michael, W. B.: *Handbook in Research and Evaluation.* Edits Publishers, California, 1975.
11. Kenny, D. A.: *Cross-lagged panel correlation: A test for spuriousness.* Psychol. Bull. 82:887, 1975.
12. Kerlinger, F. N. and Pedhazur, E. J.: *Multiple Regression in Behavioral Research.* Holt, Rinehart, and Winston, New York, 1973.
13. Kirk, R. E.: *Experimental Design: Procedures for the Behavioral Sciences.* Brooks Cole, Monterey, Calif., 1968.
14. Land, K. C.: *Principles of path analysis.* In Borgatta, E. F. (ed.): *Sociological Methodology 1969.* Jossey-Bass, San Francisco, 1969.
15. Li, C. C.: *Population Genetics.* University of Chicago Press, Chicago, 1955.
16. Mayeske, G. W., et al.: *A Study of Our Nation's Schools.* U.S. Department of Health, Education and Welfare, Office of Education, Washington, D.C., 1969.
17. Mood, A. M.: *Partitioning variance in multiple regression analyses as a tool for developing learning models.* Am. Ed. Res. J. 8:191, 1971.
18. Nie, N. H., et al.: *Statistical Package for the Social Sciences,* ed. 2. McGraw-Hill, New York, 1975.
19. Nunnally, J. C.: *Psychometric Theory.* McGraw-Hill, New York, 1967.
20. Peters, C. C. and Van Voorhis, W. R.: *Statistical Procedures and Their Mathematical Basis.* McGraw-Hill, New York, 1940.
21. Rozelle, R. M. and Campbell, D. T.: *More plausible rival hypotheses in the cross-lagged panel correlation technique.* Psychol. Bull. 71:74, 1969.
22. Staropoli, C. and Waltz, C.: *Developing and Evaluating Educational Programs for Health Care Providers.* F. A. Davis, Philadelphia, 1978.
23. Siegel, S.: *Nonparametric Statistics for the Behavioral Sciences.* McGraw-Hill, New York, 1956.
24. Sperling, A. and Stuart, M.: *Mathematics Made Simple.* Doubleday, New York, 1962.
25. Tukey, J. W.: *Causation, regression and path analysis.* In Kempthorne et al. (eds.): *Statistics and Mathematics in Biology.* Iowa State College Press, Ames, 1954.
26. Turner, M. E. and Stevens, C. D.: *The regression analysis of causal paths.* Biometrics 14:236, 1959.
27. Waltz, C.: *Faculty influences on nursing students' preferences for practice.* Nurs. Res. 27(2):89, March–April, 1978.
28. Wright, S.: *Path coefficients and path regressions: Alternative or complementary Concepts.* Biometrics 16:189, 1960.
29. Popham, W. J.: *Educational Statistics.* Harper and Row, New York, 1967.

CHAPTER 11

SPECIAL TOPICS IN DESIGN AND STATISTICS

This chapter presents the rudiments of a number of designs and statistical procedures that are currently underutilized in nursing research but that have the potential for answering nursing research questions and testing hypotheses with more precision than many of the currently employed techniques. The discussion is divided into three sections: (1) selected multivariate procedures, (2) Bayesian analysis, and (3) primary, secondary, and meta-analysis of nursing research data. The references at the end of the chapter will facilitate the efforts of the reader who desires more detailed information.

SELECTED MULTIVARIATE PROCEDURES

The statistical procedures discussed in the preceding chapters can be grouped and classified in several ways, all of which possess a certain degree of arbitrariness. Keeping in mind the fact that the same data can often be appropriately analyzed using several different tests, let us dichotomize parametric statistical tests into two strains: one that measures differences (for example, ANOVA) and one that measures relationships from a correlational perspective (for example, regression).

Once so visualized, the specific ANOVA or regression procedure appropriate for a given purpose is primarily dictated by the number of variables involved. For example, if the study contains one independent variable and the researcher is interested in *differences* between levels or groups making up that variable, then a one-way analysis of variance is called for (or a t-test if only two groups are present). If two or more independent variables exist, then factorial ANOVA or ANCOVA is probably appropriate.

A similar situation exists with correlational data. Given two variables, neither of which takes precedence over the other (i.e., neither of which is designated an independent variable), then the Pearson r is the statistic of choice. Given three or more variables, one of which can be identified as the criterion, multiple regression is called for.

Within this framework, therefore, statistical tests exist for all possible contingencies involving one dependent variable as illustrated in Table 11-1.

TABLE 11-1. Statistical Tests for Studies Involving One Dependent Variable

	Differences	*Correlation*
two variables (1 IV + 1 DV or no designation)	t-test ANOVA	Pearson r Bivariate regression
three or more variables (2 or more IV + 1 DV)	Factorial ANOVA ANCOVA Nested, randomized block, and repeated measures ANOVA	Multiple regression

Hopefully, the alert reader will have noted a salient and artificial constraint inherent in this scheme. What about situations involving more than one dependent variable? Surely such problems can be conceptualized, such as cases in which a researcher wishes (1) to determine the effect of an experimental manipulation upon two or more *dependent* variables or (2) to predict variations in two or more *criteria*.

Not only can situations such as these be visualized, they are becoming increasingly more prevalent in nursing research. Statistical tests exist for this type of research, and as a group are called multivariate statistics. They are especially appropriate for nursing, which by its nature is essentially multivariate (as a profession, for example, nursing is usually interested in more than one aspect of the patient, more than one professional educational outcome, the assessment of more than one skill, affective dimension, and so forth).

Multivariate statistical procedures, although both conceptually and computationally more involved than univariate ones, can be visualized as direct extensions of the chart in Table 11-1, as shown in Table 11-2. If the researcher were dealing with the assessment of differences between groups and had more than one measure (that is, dependent variable) on each S, then a procedure called *discriminant analysis* could be employed. If the researcher wished to

TABLE 11-2. Statistical Tests for Studies Involving More Than One Dependent Variable

Differences		*Correlation*	
		three or more variables (no IV/DV designation) } factor analysis	
three or more variables (1 or more IV, 2 or more DV) }	discriminant analysis	three or more variables (2 or more IV, 2 or more DV) }	canonical correlation

describe the relationship between three or more variables without making independent/dependent distinctions, then *factor analysis* would be appropriate. If the researcher chose to designate two or more dependent variables and wished to employ a correlational procedure, then *canonical correlation* would be the analysis of choice. Despite their differences, all these analyses have one characteristic in common. They require a far larger number of subjects than their univariate counterparts, needing from 10 to 25 Ss *per variable* for any degree of confidence in their interpretability.

Although space constraints preclude a detailed discussion of these and other multivariate statistical procedures, a brief discussion of their power and utility should be helpful. Those readers desiring a more detailed description of these and other multivariate procedures should refer to either Cooley and Lohnes[7] or Tatsuoka.[24]

Factor Analysis

The statistics discussed in previous chapters assume either a very limited number of measures on each S in a study or some means by which a larger number of measurements can be reduced to a manageable size. In the simple contrast of an experimental treatment to the absence thereof, for example, a t-test or similar procedure was recommended based on the assumption that the experimental group would be compared with the control group according to *one* criterion.

It was possible of course that this one criterion might be comprised of a 50-item test, but the assumption still remained that those 50 items could be reduced to one composite score. Fifty separate t-tests would be extremely tedious to report as well as to consume. Furthermore, their interpretation would require some provision for the fact that (1) several would be expected to be statistically significant by chance alone, (2) a great deal of redundancy would accrue given the fact that some items might be highly correlated with one another, and (3) single items are often not reliable enough to yield statistically significant results.

Reduction of data to one total score is usually quite appropriate for a cognitive test whose items can be assumed to comprise a sample of a single domain of items. For other types of tests, however, the appropriateness of a single score is often suspect. It is very rare, for example, for a large number of attitudinal items to measure one and only one affective domain, especially if the instrument in question has not undergone extensive validation. The researcher could, of course, guess what the underlying dimensions of the instrument were and combine items to yield subscores accordingly. The researcher could even use whatever relevant theoretical framework happened to be available to enhance the guesses. With either of these options, however, guesswork would still be included and empirical justification would be necessary.

Factor analysis is that sort of device. It is an *empirical data reduction* tool of great utility and power that clusters individual items into linear combinations called factors, thereby greatly reducing an instrument's complexity. It is able, at the same time, to take the guesswork out of determining the different constructs underlying a set of items or variables.

Factor analysis has many potential uses. It can be used as an item selection device in the construction of a measuring instrument. (Items, for example, which are found to measure constructs different from the one(s) being sought can be deleted or altered.) It can also be used in an exploratory sense to determine exactly what an existing data collection instrument measures. In addition, it can be used in the testing of theory or in a confirmatory sense. (Given that Attribute A, for example, is hypothesized composed of three easily identified and distinct dimensions, can these three constituents be empirically documented?) Finally, factor analytic techniques can be used as an empirical method for determining subscores on an instrument that can constitute new dependent variables in future research.

EXAMPLE 11-1. Published Example of a Study Employing Factor Analysis

Title:	*Antecedents of nursing school attrition: Attitudinal dimensions.*
Source:	Hutcheson, LaRetta, and Lowe, Nursing Research, vol. 28, January–February, 1979, pp. 57–62.
Purpose:	1. To "identify attitudinal factors that influence attrition in a highly structured nursing program."
	2. To "determine how much attitudinal factors may operate despite variations in demographic characteristics and academic performance" (p. 57).
Procedure:	As a first step in accomplishing the above purposes, data were collected on 261 students in the graduating classes of a school of nursing between the years 1968–72. Specifically, three types of information were collected: Scholastic Aptitude Variables, Socioeconomic Status Variables, and Attitudinal Variables.
Analysis:	Each set of variables was subjected to a separate factor analysis followed by a varimax rotation.
Results:	1. The Scholastic Aptitude Variables yielded three independent factors: one dealing with reading and comprehension, one dealing with verbal usage, one involving mathematics.
	2. The Socioeconomic Status Variables yielded two classes of measures: one dealing with the father's status, one with the mother's.
	3. The Attitudinal Variables yielded three independent dimensions: attitudes toward professional and authority figures, social alienation, and attitudes toward individuals with health problems.
Interpretation:	These factors formed the basis for additional correlational procedures including path analyses designed to accomplish the above mentioned purposes and to test a hypothesized model of nursing school attrition.

Normal use of the procedure begins with multiple measures on the same group of subjects. These multiple measures (usually 10 or more) are often individual items, although, as illustrated in the example, complete tests can be used. The first statistical step consists of the construction of a matrix comprised of intercorrelations between every item and every other item.

This correlation matrix is then "examined" by the computer and manipulated in such a way that clusters of items that tend to measure the same dimensions (that is, are highly correlated with one another) are identified. This process is called factoring and can be accomplished in many ways, depending upon the researcher's objectives. For present purposes a procedure known as principal components, in which the diagonal of the correlation matrix is replaced by an estimate of the amount of variance shared by each item and the other items in the test, will be assumed.

The end result of this factoring process is a group of linear combinations of items called factors, each of which is independent of all other identified factors. Once constructed, each factor is then correlated with each item to produce *factor loadings*. (It might be helpful to conceptualize these factors as "lumps" of variance taken from items that tended to measure something in common, and the loadings as correlations between these lumps and the items comprising them.)

However they are conceptualized, the resulting factors will be relatively independent of each other. This is assured by the way in which the factors are constructed, in which the second factor is only defined *after* the variance of the first has been partialled out of each item; the third only after the variance of the first *and* second has been partialled out, and so forth.

Despite this basic independence between factors, several characteristics of this initial factor pattern conspire to limit its utility. In the first place, there are as many factors as there are items, which means that some will be *very* small, possessing less variance than contained in a single item. In addition, the first factor will often contain heavy loadings from most of the items, making it relatively uninterpretable. Finally, the same items may correlate with several factors, again limiting factor interpretability since the researcher must eventually be able to describe the factors in some meaningful, exclusive way. It will avail the researcher nothing to know that the instrument measures three different constructs, for example, if the researcher cannot "name" or describe those constructs.

Under normal circumstances a further step is therefore entailed. It involves a process called *rotation* in which the factors are repositioned in such a way as to give them more interpretability. Just as there are many techniques for arriving at an initial factor pattern, so are there many ways to rotate this initial solution. Again, the particular method chosen depends upon the researcher and the purposes of the study. For present purposes, the most common solution, the *varimax* rotation, will be assumed, in which:

1. Only the larger, hence more important, factors are considered.
2. Factors are rotated in such a way that items usually load substantially (that is, correlate with) only one factor.
3. The factors, once rotated, remain independent of one another.

Consider the following factor analysis of a course evaluation instrument administered to baccalaureate nursing students (data from only six items are included; actually, many more items were present). Most factor analytic programs (including SPSS) would yield the information shown in Table 11-3.

TABLE 11-3. Factor Analysis Output

(a)

Factor matrix using principal factors with iterations

Items	Factors I	II	III	IV .....
1. Overall instructor evaluation	0.67	0.04	0.42	0.21
2. Overall course evaluation	0.57	−0.03	0.23	0.16
3. Instructor's organization	0.42	−0.12	0.44	−0.17
4. Course workload	0.31	0.63	−0.00	0.17
5. Amount of outside reading	0.58	0.74	0.02	0.04
6. Course difficulty	0.59	0.42	0.18	0.22
.	.	.	.	.
.	.	.	.	.
.	.	.	.	.

(b)

Factor	Eigenvalue	Percent Variance
I	3.6	0.58
II	1.8	0.29
III	1.0	0.16
IV	0.5	0.08
.	.	.
.	.	.
.	.	.

(c)

Varimax rotated factor matrix

Items	Factors I	II	III
1. Overall instructor evaluation	0.86	0.06	−0.12
2. Overall course evaluation	0.69	0.00	−0.01
3. Instructor's organization	0.74	0.12	0.00
4. Course workload	0.09	0.67	0.20
5. Amount of outside reading	0.10	0.69	0.18
6. Course difficulty	−0.06	0.12	0.78
.	.	.	.
.	.	.	.
.	.	.	.

Factors are interpreted by examining the items loading upon each over and above a certain a priori set criterion (usually 0.30 is the minimum that will be considered). Note that the rotated factor pattern is more easily interpreted than the original one. Examination of the first set of factors yields very little of significance. Factor I contains loadings of 0.30 or better for all six items, hence is very general. Factor IV on the other hand is so small (accounting for only 4 percent of the total variance) that it is practically meaningless, especially given the fact that it contains no substantial item loadings at all. Furthermore, note that practically all of the items correlate substantially with more than one factor, further compounding the problem.

In contrast, the rotated factors are relatively clear-cut. To begin with, only the three largest factors have been rotated (usually the criterion for rotation is an eigenvalue of 1.0 or better, which indicates that a factor possesses at least as much total variance as contained in a single item). Furthermore, the clusters of items identified for each item conceptually "go together," hence making the naming of each factor feasible. Factor I, the largest, contains items dealing with overall satisfaction with the instructor, the course, and the instructor's degree of organization; hence, it might be classified as dealing with students' generalized satisfaction with the instructor and the course. Factor II contains only items dealing with workload as correlates (that is, amount of outside reading and the overall course workload); hence, it obviously involves a dimension concerned with students' perceptions of the amount of work required by the course *independent* of their overall satisfaction with the course and the instructor (Factor I). The final factor contains only one item loading substantially on it and that item deals with course difficulty, which, interestingly, appears to be independent of both overall satisfaction and perceptions of course workload.

These results are capable of being used in several ways. In the first place, following this analysis the researcher would know that student evaluations of a course and its instructor is not a unidimensional construct; it contains at least three different and independent aspects. Secondly, the researcher could, if desired, reduce the complexity of the data by reporting factor scores rather than item responses, both in terms of summary statistics *and* as dependent variables in future research. The computation of these factor scores is relatively straightforward. Each S's response on each of the six items in the scale is converted to a Z score ($\overline{X} = 0$, $\sigma = 1$), multiplied by its appropriate factor score coefficient (which is output after the rotated factor pattern), and summed.

When using factor scores, the researcher invariable requests that they be generated automatically by the computer. Some researchers, however, prefer a simpler strategy and that is to ignore the individual factor score coefficients and simply replace them with 1 if a particular item loading is above the a priori criterion (for example, 0.30), 0 if they are not. In this case, it is not necessary to convert each S's response to each item to a Z score. Instead, the actual raw responses are added on those items loading 0.30 or better (or whatever the criterion happens to be); those not doing so are ignored.

In other words, suppose that S_1's responses on the six item Likert scale were 5, 5, 4, 3, 3, and 2 respectively. Since Table 11-3 indicates that only Items 1 to 3 loaded substantially on the first factor, only the responses for those items would be added to achieve a composite score for Factor 1. S_1's score would therefore be $5 + 5 + 4 = 14$, or $(1 \times 5) + (1 \times 5) + (1 \times 4) + (0 \times 3) + (0 \times 3) + (0 \times 2) = 14$.

This latter strategy has the advantages of being computationally simple and takes into account the fact that the smaller loadings are probably chance correlations and treats them as 0. It loses a good deal with respect to precision, however, so researchers must simply make their own decisions. If a fairly large sample were used in arriving at the original factor score coefficients, their actual use in the computation of factor scores is probably preferable.

All factor analyses do not result in such easily interpretable factors as presented in Table 11-3, of course. (Although other studies involving student ratings have typically yielded similar results.) In general, the most difficult aspect of this statistical procedure, as well as the two that follow, is to objectively "name" or interpret the rotated factors. The researcher must be especially careful not to allow original predisposition or hunches color the interpretation because the interpretation of factor analyses (as well as most other multivariate statistical results) involves a certain amount of subjectivity. Perhaps the best rules of thumb to follow are: (1) choose a minimum loading to interpret, probably no less than 0.30, perhaps as high as 0.50, *before* the analysis is attempted, (2) in naming a factor, consider the relevant items in descending order with respect to the magnitude of their loadings, and (3) never ignore an item meeting a predetermined loading criterion simply because it does not "conceptually" fit with the rest of the items loading on a factor.

Discriminant Analysis

Discriminant analysis is an extension of factor analytic procedures to a situation in which the researcher wishes to reduce a set of variables to a more manageable number of independent dimensions and *then to use those dimensions to differentiate between two or more groups*. Discriminant analysis can therefore also be seen as a direct extension of analysis of variance procedures in the sense that it is a technique used to describe how groups differ with respect to two or more variables. (Discriminant analysis, like ANOVA, can be used with more than one independent variable although this particular application is relatively rare in nursing research.) Although most often used in correlational studies, the procedure is particularly well adapted to experimental research in which the objective is to describe *multiple* outcomes of a particular treatment.

As stated above, the procedure is quite similar to factor analysis in the sense that groups or clusters of items are identified that measure similar things. It is the criteria for selecting these factors (or functions, as they are called in discriminant analysis) that primarily differentiate the two procedures. In discriminant analysis, a "lump" of variance is identified upon which the various groups of Ss *most differ*. This variance is then partialled out of the total variance contained by the set of items and the process is repeated until $K - 1$ (where K = number of groups) discriminant functions have been identified.

Although several options exist, these functions are normally tested for significance with only those meeting a predetermined criterion being interpreted. Each discriminant function is a linear combination of the items in the dependent variable set, and like factors, each possesses item loadings. Those items loading on the same function are considered to operate in concert in the differentiation of the groups involved, with the exact configuration of the group differences being determined by the resulting group centroids.

Each discriminant function therefore contains its own set of item coefficients* that describe the parameters upon which the groups differ (which can be named like factors) and its own set of centroids (each of which describes a sort of average score for a particular group or a function) that can be used to geometrically plot the relative distance between each group with respect to that function. Besides having a significance level computed for each function, most computer programs provide canonical correlations that are interpreted as a sort of multivariate eta (R_{canon} = percent of a function's variance that can be explained by Ss' group membership).

Once computed, discriminant analysis can be "turned around" and used as a classification scheme, both as a predictive device (analogous to predicted scores in multiple regression) and as a means of determining the success of the initial discrimination. To illustrate, suppose a set of characteristics were chosen upon which a researcher hypothesized that compliant and noncompliant patients would be most likely to differ. Once this hypothesis had been tested and the appropriate discriminant function calculated, predicted group classifications could be determined for another sample of patients (or the present one recognizing the need for ultimate cross-validation) based only upon their possession of the relevant characteristics identified by the earlier function loadings. The fit between predicted and actual group membership (that is, whether patients complied or refused to comply with their treatment regimens) would determine the utility of the original set of characteristics chosen to discriminate said groups. SPSS even allows the researcher to set an a priori probability level that any given S would be likely to belong to any given group by chance alone.

Depending upon the researcher's objectives, other variations of discriminant analysis exist as well. As with factors in factor analysis, for example, functions can be rotated in various ways to improve their interpretability. Similarly, if the study contains a large number of potentially discriminating variables, a stepwise procedure (analogous to stepwise multiple regression) can be employed in which only those variables capable of yielding significantly unique discriminations between groups will be used to define the functions. Example 11-2 presents a more conventional use of the procedure.

EXAMPLE 11-2. Published Example of a Study Employing Discriminant Analysis

Title:	*One integrated cirriculum: An empirical evaluation.*
Source:	Richards, Nursing Research, vol. 26, March–April, 1977, pp. 90–95.
Purpose:	Although a relatively comprehensive study, the purpose for which discriminant analysis was used involved seeing if students completing a college of nursing program could be differentiated from those failing to complete same.

---

*These coefficients are analogous to beta weights in multiple regression in which the size of the coefficient is indicative of a particular item's importance in the construction of a discriminant function.

EXAMPLE 11-2. *Continued*

Procedure: 114 students (42 who either failed or withdrew, 72 who completed the program) were tested upon entry with respect to verbal and quantitative SATs, IQ, Gordon Personality Profile, a critical thinking test, and Kalisch's Empathy Scale.

Analysis: A discriminant analysis was performed using those who completed the program versus those who did not as the groups, the above mentioned tests as the discriminating variables.

Results: Graduating students were differentiated significantly from nongraduating students by the fact that the former scored higher on IQ, SAT scores, the ascendancy-leadership scale of the Gordon Personality Profile, the critical thinking test, and the Kalisch Empathy Scale.

Interpretation: The author concluded that it is possible to predict success, at least in general terms, based on the above test results. It was further concluded that the study possessed implications for predicting students who might benefit from special remedial and counseling services.

As a further example, suppose a nurse educator wished to see how three groups of graduate students — those graduating in the upper half of their class (Hi-GPA), those graduating in the lower half (Low-GPA), and those dropping out before graduation (Dropouts) — differed with respect to several professional and academic measures (GRE scores, SAT scores, undergraduate GPA, highest nursing position held, and years of nursing experience). Table 11-4 illustrates some of the information that a typical SPSS discriminant analysis might yield.

This completely hypothetical example illustrates both the discriminatory and classificational aspects of discriminant analysis. Sections a and b of the table are primarily concerned with the former, c with the latter.

To begin with, the information in section a tells the researcher that two significant discriminant functions resulted of moderate size and strength (37 percent of the variation in the first, 23 percent of the second, could be explained by group membership). The standardized discriminant coefficients indicate that the academic measures are the primary means by which the groups are differentiated on the first function and the professional variables are most important for the second function. Examination of the group centroids tells the researcher *how* the three groups differed on the five variables with (1) the first function primarily indicating a contrast between high achieving students at the positive end of the continuum versus low achievers *and* dropouts at the negative end, and (2) the second function differentiating dropouts from the other two groups (which are not really that different from one another according to their respective centroids, 0.767 versus 0.614). Examination of the standardized coefficients and the centroids simultaneously indicates that high achieving students tended to have higher GRE and SAT scores as well as higher undergraduate GPAs than both low achievers *and* dropouts. The second set of coefficients and centroids indicates that, after the relationship described by the first function had been partialled out, dropouts tended to have less (because of their group's negative centroid position) work experience and were less likely to have func-

TABLE 11-4. Hypothetical Discriminant Analysis Output

(a)

Discriminant Function	Relative Percent	Canonical Correlation . . . . Significance	
1	59.6	0.610	0.000
2	40.4	0.482	0.000

(b)

Standardized Discriminant Function Coefficients			Centroids of Groups in Reduced Space		
	Function I	Function II			
GRE	0.629	0.111	Hi-GPA	0.859	0.767
SAT	0.584	0.040	Low-GPA	−0.234	0.614
GPA	0.821	−0.089	Dropouts	−0.214	−0.914
Highest Position	0.012	0.698			
Yrs. Experience	−0.124	0.741			

(c)

	No. of Cases	Predicted Group Membership		
		Gp. 1	Gp. 2	Gp. 3
Group 1 Hi-GPA	50	30	17	3
Group 2 Low-GPA	50	10	28	12
Group 3 Dropouts	50	8	10	32

Percent of "known" groups correctly classified: 60%

tioned in a supervisory position than students completing the program (that is, those with both high and low GPAs).

The final section of Table 11-4 illustrates the classificational capabilities of discriminant analysis. This information indicates that when group membership is predicted for each student based upon the student's score on the five discriminatory variables alone a 60 percent degree of accuracy would be obtained. Although not particularly impressive, this figure does represent a significant improvement over chance alone (which would result in 33 percent accuracy). Obviously, as with other predictive studies, cross-validation would probably result in some shrinkage of this accuracy figure.

Although this cursory introduction to discriminant analysis can do little more than give the reader a general overview, it is hoped that some of the advantages of a multivariate procedure such as this can at least begin to be appreciated. Without the availability of such a tool, the researcher could have done little more than perform five separate one-way ANOVAs using each dependent variable in turn. Not only would this strategy have resulted in redundant information, it would have resulted in less power and presented far less information in the sense that the differences between groups with respect to the second function may not have even been ascertained. These advantages are equally operative in the final multivariate procedure to be discussed in this chapter, canonical correlation.

Canonical Correlation

Suppose that instead of wishing to differentiate among several groups with respect to several variables, a researcher was faced with the task of predicting a set of criteria on the basis of a set of predictor variables. To this point, none of the statistical procedures that have been discussed would provide a viable option.

Multiple regression, the closest alternative, could only be used on one criterion at a time and thus would result in redundant, hard to digest information. Factorial discriminant analysis (that is, using more than one independent variable) would only be possible if each predictor were dichotomized or trichotomized to yield grouped data, a strategy that would not only result in a great deal of lost precision but would also produce a bewildering array of interactions between independent variables (see Chapter 9). Factor analysis, while having the data reduction capabilities needed in this situation, does not allow independent/dependent variable distinctions.

What is obviously needed, therefore, is a technique that combines both the predictive capabilities of multiple regression with the data reduction ones of factor analysis to reduce *both* independent and dependent variable sets to manageable size and then to predict the former from the latter. Canonical correlation is precisely that technique.

Canonical correlation is basically a procedure that factor analyzes both independent and dependent variable sets to produce clusters of items that measure similar things, then assesses the relationship between these resulting *independent and dependent variable clusters*. The factoring process itself, however, is accomplished in a unique way. The two sets are not factor analyzed independently of one another; they are in effect accomplished *simultaneously* with the single objective of arriving at factors (called *canonical variates*) that share maximal variation *between sets*.

In other words, this procedure sifts through both independent and dependent variables and identifies a group of variables (or pieces thereof) that share the greatest amount of variance. These two "lumps" of variance, one from each set, then become the first canonical variate. The degree of relationship between the two factors or variates is given by the canonical R, which can be interpreted in much the same way a simple Pearson r is interpreted except that it is a correlation between two constructs (or linear combinations of independent and dependent variables). Each canonical variate, like discriminant functions and factors, possesses item (or variable) loadings that again are interpreted as simple correlations between each item and the appropriate canonical variate.

Interpretation of the canonical R itself should be tempered, however, by the fact that it is by definition the highest possible measure of relationship that can be empirically generated in a given situation. This means of course that a good deal of what is actually error gets treated as systematic variance, which leads to the fact that upon cross-validation both the canonical R and the individual item loadings are likely to change considerably. For this reason, canonical correlation should probably not be performed at all for studies involving fewer than 200 Ss, especially if a considerable number of variables is involved.

As an example of the type of information that might be generated from a canonical correlation program, suppose a researcher had interviewed both treatment staff and their respective patients in several drug abuse treatment facilities. Suppose further that the researcher wished to ascertain whether or not therapists' attitudes and demographics influenced their individual patients' perceptions of treatment efficacy. Designating the former independent (or predictor) and the latter dependent variables, the researcher might find the results in Table 11-5 accruing from an SPSS canonical correlation analysis.

TABLE 11-5. Hypothetical Canonical Correlation Output

(a)

(Canonical Variate)

Number	Eigenvalue	Canonical Correlation	Significance
1	0.615	0.784	0.000
2	0.411	0.641	0.000

(b) Coefficients for Canonical Variates of First Set

	Canvar 1	Canvar 2
Age	0.002	0.685
Educ. Level	−0.102	0.211
Attitudes toward Patients	0.681	−0.006
Sex	0.100	0.688

Coefficients for Canonical Variates of Second Set

Program's long term effectiveness	0.102	0.488
Program's short term effectiveness	0.062	0.562
Likelihood of pers. rehabilitation	0.624	0.614

Section a of this table indicates the presence of two highly significant canonical functions, one in which the shared variance between the sets is 62 percent, the other with 41 percent shared variance. Other programs such as Cooley and Lohnes'[7] CANON and BIOMED supply additional useful information such as the size of each function (variate) with respect to the total variance in each set, the redundancy (which is really nothing more than this figure multiplied by the eigenvalue), and correlations between each variable and each canonical variate. (SPSS does not print out actual loadings for each variable. Rather, it prints out what are really regression coefficients for each variable on the canonical variate.) Special heed should be paid to the relative size of a canonical function. One that accounts for very little of the total instrument variance should be interpreted with extreme caution regardless of the size of the canonical R simply because chances are good that it may not replicate in a different setting.

Section b basically tells the researcher which variables are related to which other variables across sets. Canvar 1 of the first set, for example, is correlated 0.784 with Canvar 1 of the second set and this relationship describes a situation in which therapists with positive attitudes toward their patients (that is, the 0.681 coefficient) are likely to have patients who believe they have a high chance of treatment success.

The second function is independent of the first and describes a situation in which older females (the negative coefficient must be interpreted with respect to how sex was coded; in this case it will be assumed that female = 1, male = 2) are associated with patients believing in the efficacy of both their programs' long and short term goals, but who are pessimistic about their own futures. This latter, completely hypothetical function, was included because it is unfortunately often typical of the smaller canonical variates that often do not make a great deal of conceptual or theoretical sense and often disappear in cross-validations unless a very large sample is used in the first place. This is because canonical correlation is the most powerful tool available to the researcher, more powerful in fact than many circumstances warrant. An example of a study employing canonical correlation is presented in Example 11-3.

EXAMPLE 11-3. Published Example of a Study Employing Canonical Correlation

Title:	*The relationship between treatment modality, demographic characteristics, and staff perceptions concerning their jobs in 26 Philadelphia drug treatment centers.*
Source:	Bausell, Rinkus, and Watson, International Journal of the Addictions (in press)
Purpose:	To ascertain how staff in different drug treatment modalities differ with respect to satisfaction with their jobs, the adequacy and organizational climate of their facilities, and their professional effectiveness.
Procedure:	198 staff members were interviewed in 26 drug treatment centers to ascertain their job satisfaction, perceived organizational climate, and professional effectiveness.
Analysis:	Both a set of predictors (type of treatment modality, institutional size, whether or not the respondent's position and training was primarily medical or nonmedical, his age, sex, race, and educational level) and a set of criteria (attitudes toward treatment and toward patients, perceptions of program effectiveness, overall satisfaction with the job, and organizational climate) were identified and subjected to a canonical correlation.
Results:	Four significant canonical functions were identified. The first indicated a relationship between nonmedical personnel in smaller therapeutic communities and positive attitudes toward treatment, clients, and the effectiveness of treatment. They also found their organizational climate less restrictive and were more satisfied with

EXAMPLE 11-3. *Continued*

their jobs. (The opposite relationship held for medical staff in methadone maintenance centers.) The second significant function of primary interest and relevance to the avowed purpose of the study concerned a relationship between positive attitudes and perceptions of outpatient drug free staff.

Interpretation: Treatment staff working in different treatment modalities do tend to view their jobs, facilities, and relative effectivenesses differently. Until more data are available concerning differential outcomes of treatment, policymakers would do well to consider these informed opinions.

BAYESIAN ANALYSIS

Descriptive studies employ summary statistics in an attempt to organize, describe, and communicate what exists in a situation. Experimental studies employ inferential statistics to make statements about an entire population on the basis of limited information regarding a small subset or sample of the population.

In Bayesian studies, which utilize statistical decision-making theory, a formal attempt is made to incorporate all that is known about a research question in order to reduce the amount of uncertainty in using the research results in real-life situations. During the conduct of the study, when new information about the research question is obtained, for example, from the literature or as a result of day-to-day experiences, it is combined with any previous information to form the basis for statistical procedures. The formal mechanism used to combine the new information with the previously available information is known as Bayes' Theorem, hence the term Bayesian is used to describe this type of analysis.

Bayesian studies use probabilities. At any given point in time, the researcher's state of information about some question can be represented by a set of probabilities. When new information is obtained, these probabilities are revised in order that they may represent all of the available information.

Examples of the types of research questions answered by Bayesian studies are:

1. A person chosen at random from the population of a certain city is given a tuberculin skin test and the reading is positive. Given the results of the skin test, one asks: what is the probability that this person has tuberculosis?
2. A nurse administrator must decide whether or not to establish ambulatory care services staffed by primary care nurses. This is the first time such a service will be made available to the community and her decision depends on the reaction of consumers and the payoff in terms of dollars saved. What should she do?

Questions of primary concern to nurse clinicians characteristically stem from their need to determine the probability of the occurrence of *unique events,* that is, events that occur in exactly the *same manner* only once. The traditional null hypothesis testing model, which forms the basis for inferential statistics, involves a relative frequency interpretation of probability that is based on the repetition of experiments under *identical* conditions. Although nurses may have some information regarding past occurrences in similar situations, they are usually without information in the form of observed frequencies of repeated trials under identical conditions. Thus, results from the null hypothesis testing approach generally lead to findings and conclusions that do not appear directly applicable to the work of the nurse clinician.

Bayesian analysis has a great deal of potential for nurses conducting clinical nursing research for the following reasons:

1. It allows for the consideration of the probability of the occurrence of unique events.
2. It provides a formal mechanism for including all information relevant to a given problem, including that resulting from day-to-day clinical experiences, during the ongoing conduct of the study.
3. It uses decision-making theory to choose from among a number of alternative actions, that is, results in a decision based on all available information in the unique situation.

Bayesian studies facilitate the incorporation of research results into ongoing practice because the actions to be taken in the clinical setting flow directly from the analysis. Unfortunately, published examples of nursing research employing Bayesian analysis are virtually nonexistent. Similarly, most nursing research textbooks in current use do not include content on Bayesian analysis. These factors suggest that Bayesian analysis is sorely underutilized in nursing research largely because it simply is not part of most nurse researchers' repertoires. In an attempt to correct this situation so that nurses, particularly those conducting clinical research, may begin to maximize the potential Bayesian analysis has for nursing, this section presents an elementary discussion of Bayesian analysis and provides examples of its use in the simplest cases of probability and decision-making. The intent here is to familiarize the reader with some of the concepts and terms employed in Bayesian studies. It is expected that the reader will be able to actually perform Bayesian analysis only after additional study.

Probability

A key concept in Bayesian analysis is *uncertainty*. The uncertainty in a situation is reflected by statements such as "it is probable," "the chances are," and "it is likely." When such statements are quantified, they are then translated into probability statements.

An elementary knowledge of probability is essential to the understanding of

Bayesian analysis. Thus, it is necessary to briefly consider the basic axioms of probability theory. In any problem involving uncertainty, the true situation is not known for certain. However, if the problem is well defined, it should be possible to anticipate the various possible outcomes. Any set or class of possible outcomes is referred to as an *event*. If an event cannot be broken down into a number of smaller events, it is called an *elementary event*; if it can be, it is called a *compound event*. For example, if the interest is in the cost of staffing an ambulatory setting with primary care nurses one year from now, the event "cost is $50,000" is an elementary event, whereas the event "cost is in excess of $50,000" is a compound event because it can be broken down into "cost is $51,000," "cost is $52,000," and many other elementary events. Similarly, if one is interested in the number of patients entering an emergency room during a particular hour, the event "50 patients enter the emergency room" is an elementary event whereas "at least 50 patients enter the emergency room" is a compound event.

In any problem involving uncertainty, one is interested in the *sample space* or *event space*, defined as the set of all possible elementary events that can be represented by zero and the positive integers. In any application of probability theory, it is important to define the sample space precisely. Events are *sets* of possible outcomes. A *set* is a well defined collection of objects, that is, given any object, one can tell whether or not it is a member of the set in question. Events can be illustrated by Venn diagrams. For example, in Figure 11-1, the rectangle (S) represents the sample space and the circle (E) represents the event.

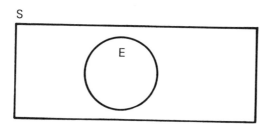

FIGURE 11-1. Venn diagram in which S = sample space and E = event.

A set may also be represented by a listing, enclosed in brackets, of the members of the set. For example, the compound event "fewer than six patients entering the emergency room" may be represented by the set {0, 1, 2, 3, 4, 5} or the elementary event "six patients enter the emergency room" by the set {6}.

Once the sample space is carefully defined, the next step is to consider the probabilities associated with the various events comprising the sample space. Winkler[26] presents the basic axioms of probability informally as:

1. The probability of an event E, written P(E), is non-negative.
2. If S denotes the set of all possible events (the sample space), then the probability of S, written P(S), is equal to one.

3. If two events, E_1 and E_2, are mutually exclusive (that is, they cannot both occur), then the probability that at least one of the two events will occur is the sum of the individual probabilities, that is, $P(E_1) + P(E_2)$.

In set theory, the event "E_1 or E_2 or both will occur" is called the *union* of E_1 and E_2. The event "both E_1 and E_2 will occur" is referred to as the *intersection* of E_1 and E_2 and is symbolized as $E_1 \cap E_2$. If E_1 and E_2 are mutually exclusive than $P(E_1 \cap E_2) = P(E_1) + P(E_2)$. If two events, E_1 and E_2, are not necessarily mutually exclusive, then the probability that at least one of them will occur is $P(E_1 \cup E_2)$ $= P(E_1) + P(E_2) - P(E_1 \cap E_2)$.

Another important concept in the theory of probability is that of *conditional probability*, that is, the probability that one event will occur, given that a particular second event has occurred or will occur. The conditional probability of event E_2, given event E_1, is written $P(E_2|E_1)$. *The joint probability* of two events, for example, 50 patients today and 50 patients tomorrow, is represented as $P(E_1, E_2)$. In general, for any two events, E_1 and E_2,

$$P(E_1, E_2) = P(E_1)\, P(E_2|E_1)$$

where the joint probability of the two events $P(E_1, E_2)$ is simply the probability of the intersection of E_1 and E_2 or $P(E_1 \cap E_2)$.

Bayes' Theorem

Bayes' Theorem is a convenient formula that gives the relationship among various conditional probabilities. It is useful when it is not easy to compute conditional probabilities directly from the probability formulas presented in the preceding section. The simpliest version of Bayes' Theorem is:[26]

$$P(E_1|E_2) = \frac{P(E_2|E_1)\, P(E_1)}{P(E_2|E_1)\, P(E) + P(E_2|\bar{E}_1)\, P(\bar{E}_1)}$$

where:
$\bar{E}_1$ = the complement of the event E_1, that is, "not E_1"

The application of Bayes' Theorem is best illustrated by example. Suppose that the probability that an adolescent's diabetes will be controlled is 0.90 if he complies with his treatment regimen and 0.40 if he does not. Furthermore, suppose that 70 percent of the adolescents in a particular diabetic clinic comply with their treatment regimens. If a patient is selected at random from the clinic, and is well controlled, what is the probability that he has complied with his treatment regimen? Let E_2 stand for the event, "diabetes is controlled" and let E_1 stand for the event, "complied with treatment regimen." $\bar{E}_1$ then stands for the event "did not comply with treatment regimen." The probability that is wanted is the probability that a patient complied with his treatment regimen, given that his diabetes was controlled. This is $P(E_1|E_2)$. Since 70 percent of the clinic patients complied and the adolescent patient of interest has been randomly chosen from the clinic population, the unconditional probability that he complied with his treatment regimen $P(E_1)$, is 0.70.

Bayes' Theorem can be used to determine the conditional probability that he complied, given that his diabetes was controlled:

$$P(E_1|E_2) = \frac{P(E_2|E_1)\,P(E_1)}{P(E_2|E_1)\,P(E_1) + P(E_2|\bar{E}_1)\,P(\bar{E}_1)}$$
$$= \frac{(0.90)\,(0.70)}{(0.90)\,(0.70) + (0.40)\,(0.30)}$$
$$= \frac{0.63}{0.63 + 0.12}$$
$$= \frac{0.63}{0.75}$$
$$= 0.84$$

In Bayesian analysis, the following terms are used to describe the various probabilities appearing in Bayes' Theorem:

$P(E_1)$ represents *a prior probability*

$P(E_2|E_1)$ represents *a likelihood* that involves the additional information E_2. The likelihood can be interpreted as the probability of the observed information E_2, given a particular event, E_1.

$P(E_1|E_2)$ represents *a posteriori probability*.

In the example, the prior probability of compliance with the treatment regimen was 0.70. After seeing some additional information, the likelihood of control with and without compliance, the a posteriori probability determined by Bayes' Theorem was 0.84. Because Bayes' Theorem provides a means of revising probabilities as new information is obtained, it is an extremely valuable tool in decision theory.

Prior probabilities should reflect the decision-maker's prior information about the uncertainty in question. This information may be obtained from the person's own prior study results, or observed relative frequencies from the literature, or whatever other relevant information is available. The choice of a prior probability is a subjective one so it is assumed that the prior probabilities are subjective probabilities. A subjective probability reflects the degree of belief of the researcher about a given proposition. If, however, probabilities are based on the judgments of an individual, what is needed is a way for the person to quantify those judgments (that is, to express them in probabilistic terms). Numerous objective techniques are available for the quantification of judgment, for example, lotteries, betting odds, reference contracts, insurance premiums, and so forth, or a researcher who understands the concept of probability might simply assign probabilities directly to the various values of the uncertain quantity of interest.

Since a likelihood is proportional to a conditional probability, many of the techniques used for the assessment of prior probabilities are relevant. That is, likelihoods can be assessed directly using conditional bets, lotteries, and so forth.

The simple case of Bayes' Theorem discussed here has been extended to allow the researcher to employ discrete and continuous probability models. These more sophisticated applications of Bayesian analysis are beyond the scope of this book. The reader who is interested in pursuing Bayesian analysis in more depth will find Winkler[26] and Mann and colleagues[16] useful references.

Decision-Making

Many decisions are made under the condition of uncertainty, that is uncertainty about the actual state of the world. For example, consider a major decision, such as the decision whether or not to employ a particular nursing plan or a decision to introduce primary care services in a particular ambulatory clinic. In such decisions, one evaluates such factors as the condition of the present plan or service and the cost of the new plan or service, the potential satisfaction or success of employing the new plan or service, and so forth. These are the types of decisions, those in which the consequence of making a wrong decision could be quite serious, for which formal decision theory employing Bayesian analysis may be useful. Formally, a consequence of a decision, which may be expressed in terms of a payoff or a loss to the decision-maker, is the result of the interaction of two factors: (1) the *decision* or the *action* selected by the decision-maker; and (2) the *event* or *state of the world* that actually occurs.

The problem of making decisions under uncertainty is complex and difficult. Hence, it is important when formally specifying a decision problem to keep it as simple as possible, including only the most relevant variables. The consequences of a decision can be expressed in terms of either payoffs or losses. A *payoff*, or *reward*, if expressed in monetary units, represents the net change in one's total wealth as a result of the decision and the actual state of the world. This can be either positive or negative. Payoffs are always expressed in net terms rather than gross terms so that all relevant factors can be taken into consideration. A *payoff table* consists of the set of payoffs for all possible combinations of actions and states of the world. All payoffs in the table are expressed in terms of dollars, even though the potential consequences include nonmonetary considerations, that is, the possible consequences are converted into cash equivalents. Figure 11-2 presents a payoff table for the decision-making regarding whether or not to change to primary care services discussed earlier. For simplicity, only the four variables change, not change, services improved, and not improved are illustrated.

In this example, it is assumed that the decision-maker feels the cost of changing to primary care in terms of actual dollars, time, effort expenditure, and the like is equivalent to $100,000 whether or not services are improved. Thus, −$100,000 is a cash equivalent for the consequences of "change to primary care" whether or not it improves services. Similarly, the consequences corresponding to "not change" when primary care does in fact improve services in-

STATE OF THE WORLD

	SERVICES IMPROVED	SERVICES NOT IMPROVED
CHANGE TO PC	− $100,000	− $100,000
ACTION		
DO NOT CHANGE TO PC	− $150,000	− $0

FIGURE 11-2. Example of a payoff table.

cludes the possible loss of clients, personnel dissatisfaction, danger to patients' health because of discontinuous care, and so forth. The cash equivalent of this consequence is −$150,000.

Loss refers to opportunity loss. For any combination of an action and a state of the world, the question is: could the decision-maker have obtained a higher payoff, given that particular state of the world? If the answer is no, then the loss is zero. If the answer is yes, then the loss is the positive difference between the given payoff and the highest possible payoff under that state of the world. Negative values in a payoff table are regarded as negative payoffs, negative rewards, or costs, in terms of opportunity loss; they may correspond to losses of zero. Figure 11-3 illustrates how the payoff table in Figure 11-2 can be converted to a loss table.

STATE OF THE WORLD

	SERVICES IMPROVED	SERVICES NOT IMPROVED
CHANGE TO PC	$0	$100,000
ACTION		
DO NOT CHANGE TO PC	$50,000	$0

FIGURE 11-3. Conversion of Table 11-2 into a loss table.

Consider the first entry in the first column of the payoff table (Fig. 11-2); it is higher than the other entry in that column, so it is the best the decision-maker could do given that services are improved and the loss is zero. For the second entry in column 1, the payoff is $50,000 lower than the first entry, so the loss is $50,000. Similarly, in the second column, the first entry is lower than the second, so the corresponding losses are $100,000 and 0. Figure 11-3 is also referred to as a *regret table*, since the entries reflect the decision-maker's regret at not having made the decision that turns out to be optimal under the actual state of the world.

An alternative way to present payoffs and losses in a decision-making problem is in terms of a *tree diagram* (Fig. 11-4).

In the diagram, the first fork corresponds to the action chosen by the

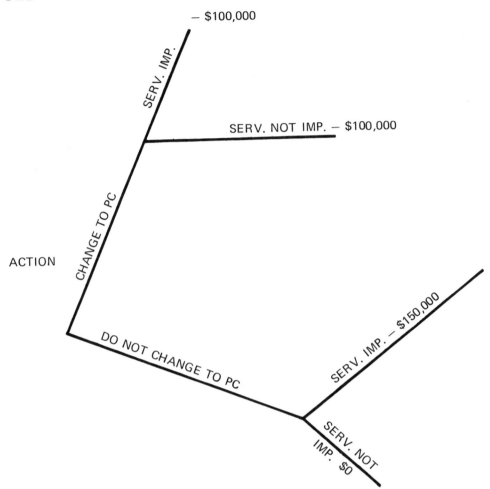

FIGURE 11-4. Example of a tree diagram.

decision-maker and the second fork corresponds to the state of the world. Thus, each terminal branch at the right-hand side corresponds to a combination of a particular action and a particular state of the world. The numbers at the end of the terminal branches are the corresponding payoffs. Tree diagrams are especially useful in representing complex decision-making problems with sequences of actions and events over time.

In making decisions, it is necessary to consider only *admissible acts*, acts that are not dominated by any other act. An action dominates a second action if, for each possible state of the world, the first action leads to at least as high a payoff as the second action and, for at least one state of the world, the first action leads to a higher payoff than the second action. If one action dominates another, then it would not make sense to choose the second action, thus the second action is said to be inadmissible. By confining attention to admissible acts, the decision-maker can greatly reduce the magnitude of the problem.

Decision-making rules that are based solely on the payoff loss table have been developed. One of these, the *maximum rule* states: find the smallest possible payoff for each action and choose the action for which this smallest payoff is largest. In Figure 11-2, the smallest payoffs for the two actions are −$100,000 and −$150,000. According to the rule, the decision-maker would choose the first, "change to primary care."

The *maximax rule* states: find the largest possible payoff for each action and then choose the action for which this largest payoff is largest. In Figure 11-2, the maximum payoff is $100,000.

The *minimax loss rule* states: find the largest possible loss for each action and choose the action for which this largest loss is smallest. In Figure 11-3, the losses are $100,000 and $50,000. The smallest of these is $50,000 and thus the action "do not change to primary care" would be chosen by the rule.

These rules have all been criticized for ignoring how likely the various states of the world are. Thus, two alternative decision-making criteria, expected payoff and expected loss, have been derived to allow the decision-maker to express uncertainty about the various states of the world in terms of probabilities that can be used as input to the decision-making process.

The *expected payoff* (ER) rule states: choose the action with the highest payoff. The *expected loss* (EL) rule states: choose the action with the smallest expected loss. For any decision-making problem, the ER and EL rules will yield identical decisions. In the primary care (PC) example, suppose that P(services improved) = 0.80 and P(services not improved) = 0.20 on the basis of research reports and an assessment of the present services. Then the expected payoffs for the two acts are:

$$ER(\text{change to PC}) = (0.80) (-100,000) + (0.20) (-100,000)$$
$$= \$100,000$$

$$ER(\text{do not change to PC}) = (0.80) (-\$150,000) + (0.20) (0)$$
$$= -\$120,000$$

$$EL(\text{change to PC}) = (0.80) (0) + (0.20) (100,000)$$
$$= \$20,000$$

$$EL(\text{do not change to PC}) = (0.80) (50,000) + (0.20) (0)$$
$$= \$40,000$$

The actual change to primary care has the larger expected payoff and the smaller expected loss.

It should be noted that the ER and EL depend on the values of the probabilities. Different sets of probabilities correspond to different information about the state of the world, and hence different information may lead to a different decision. Probabilities regarding the state of the world are best determined as a posteriori probabilities resulting from the application of Bayes' Theorem as discussed earlier. When determined in this manner, they represent all relevant information.

Example

The following discussion illustrates by example the relative utility of the null hypothesis testing decision model (NHTDM) and Bayesian analysis when the two alternative approaches were employed by one of the authors to analyze a common set of nursing data. Throughout this discussion, utility will be defined pragmatically as the expected net gain of doing the analysis to the clinical nurse whose concern is with the usefulness of research results for incorporation into ongoing practice.

Nurses are often interested in describing the characteristics of those who utilize their services in order to make inferences regarding the accessibility of nursing care to certain populations of patients. A central question in nursing at present relates to the utilization of health services by women over age 15 who have family incomes under $3,000 per year. Evidence has been presented in the literature that supports both the under- and overutilization of physician services by this low income group.[18] Since the accessibility of publically financed health care has been found to be associated with the use of physician services, one index by which nurses might assess the availability of health care to their clients is by estimating the proportion of low income women in a given population who have had three or more visits to a physician within a specified time.

In the classical null hypothesis testing approach to making inferences about p, the population proportion, the concern is with the proportion of units (women over age 15 with family incomes under $3,000 per year) in a population (all women in a small northeastern state) who possess some characteristic (have had three or more visits to a physician during the past year). The proportion of the women in the population who possess the characteristic will be denoted by p, which is equal to the number of units possessing the characteristic divided by the total number of units in the population. The hypothesis to be tested is that the proportion, p, who have had three or more physician visits within a 1-year period is equal to a value, a, that lies between 0 and 1.0 inclusive. The nurse's estimate of p most frequently is based on an idealized state of affairs in which the nurse feels that it is equally likely or similarly equally probable that a woman picked at random from the population of women with under $3,000 per year family income will have had three or more visits to a physician within the past year as it is that a woman picked at random will not have the characteristic of interest. It should be noted that the researcher's strategy in establishing the null hypothesis in this instance is a conceptual one and does not provide for the inclusion of evidence available on the basis of past clinical experience with similar clients nor does it provide for the incorporation of the nurse's degree of belief regarding the true value of the parameter, which might be the nurse's prior knowledge and/or available research findings. It appears, therefore, that a great deal of useful evidence that might be brought to bear on the statement of the research hypothesis is excluded by essence of the research strategy selected. That is to say that the NHTDM is an abstract model based on a theoretical sampling distribution that does not provide a formal mechanism for incorporating all sources of available information into the research process.

In the NHTDM then, it is conceivable that a nurse researcher, once the problem has been defined in conjunction with the clinical nurse, could carry out the investigation independent of further input or participation by the nurse clinician. Consequently, a major shortcoming of this approach would seem to be its tendency to perpetuate the gap between nursing research and nursing service rather than to lessen it, whereas, on the other hand, a research strategy that allowed for the formal incorporation of all information that might bear on the research problem would probably encourage the researcher to seek further input from the nurse clinician and thus facilitate collaboration between the two.

Returning to the data example, the nurse's null hypothesis is stated: "H_0: The proportion of women in the state over age 15, with family incomes under $3,000 per year who have had three or more visits to a physician during the year 1972 is 0.5." Similarly, her alternative hypothesis is: "H_1: p, the population proportion, is not equal to 0.5."

In classical hypothesis testing, the null hypothesis may be either true or false and the investigator decides on the basis of the sample data whether to reject or fail to reject the null hypothesis. That is, the parameter is viewed as fixed and the researcher is interested in the probability of the sample data, the random variable, given the fixed parameter. It becomes immediately evident that should the researcher reject the null hypothesis no direct statement can be made regarding the probable alternative value. This raises the general question of the utility of a point estimate of the parameter to the nurse clinician. That is, the clinician, in order to incorporate research findings into ongoing practice, would serve to gain more from information regarding the probability of observing a particular sample result given a number of alternative values of the population proportion.

The null hypothesis in the data example is to be tested at the 0.05 level of significance. This means that the researcher is willing to assume a certain degree of risk of incorrectly concluding on the basis of sample evidence that the null hypothesis is false when in fact it is true. This risk, alpha, stated as a probability is denoted by α and is called the level of significance of the hypothesis test. From the risk adopted, a set of values of the sample statistic is determined that will lead one to decide H_0 is false if the sample yields such a value. This set of values is called the critical region or region of rejection because the occurrence of a sample value that lies in the critical region leads one to reject the null hypothesis.

The next concern of the nurse investigator is the identification of assumptions necessary for determining the theoretical sampling distribution of the statistic that estimates the parameter about which the hypothesis is stated. Again, the concern is solely theoretical or conceptual and no provision is made for comparing the sample results to a prior distribution that reflects the researcher's degree of belief regarding the true value of the population proportion.

For purposes of testing H_0 against H_1 in the data example, the nurse need only assume that a random sample of size n is drawn from the population. From the population of women in the state, a random household sample of 92 women (n) with less than $3,000 per year family income was drawn. Upon questioning, 16 of these women indicated they had seen a physician three or more times within the past year. The number of successes or the number having the characteristic of interest, denoted r, is 16. The sample proportion p is the ratio of r to n or 0.1739. To test H_0 against H_1 at the 0.05 level of significance, the p value is transformed to a Z score. This Z of -6.2591 is then compared with the 100 $(\alpha/2)$ and 100 $1-(\alpha/2)$ percentiles in the unit normal distribution. The critical values of Z are ± 1.64 and evidence therefore exists for rejecting the null hypothesis that p = 0.5 at the 0.05 level of significance.

On the basis of this finding, however, the nurse can say only that the proportion of women with three or more visits to a physician is probably not 0.50; there is no basis for talking about the probability of an alternative value or the direction of the difference (that is, whether the true parameter is less than or greater than 0.50). Likewise, the nurse's prior beliefs regarding the true parameter have neither increased in precision as a result of this analysis nor have they necessarily been modified in anyway as a direct result of the research outcomes.

On the basis of these findings, the probabilities of the possible alternative values of the parameter are unknown, and the appropriate inferences to be made regarding the accessibility of physician services to low income women in the state remain unclear both to the nurse investigator and the nurse clinician.

The establishment of confidence intervals for the data example provides an opportunity to discuss in greater detail the relative frequency interpretation of probability upon which the NHTDM is based. The 95 percent confidence interval on P is found to extend from approximately 0.1562 to 0.1916. This confidence interval is viewed as a random variable and maybe interpreted to mean that in the long run or, similarly, over an infinite number of samples, the nurse is 95 percent confident that the intervals so constructed will contain the parameter. That is to say that the endpoints of the intervals will vary across samples and any particular interval may or may not contain the true parameter. The law of large numbers, which forms the basis for the relative frequency interpretation of probability, states, however, that if an experiment is repeated an infinite number of times under *identical* conditions (a situation that does not occur in most nursing research), the relative frequency of occurrence of any event is likely to be close to the probability of that event. Furthermore, the theorem states that the relative frequency and the probability are more likely to be close as the number of repetitions of the experiment increases. In the example, the uniqueness of the data, or inability to replicate the data under identical conditions, is illustrated by factors such as geographic mobility, economic mobility, and modifications in personal and community attitudes that would change conditions from the time of the first experiment to the time of the second or subsequent experiments.

A limited, yet useful, way to conceptualize the overall utility of the NHTDM to the study of clinical nursing problems might be found in terms analogous to the expected net gains of sampling (ENGS). ENGS is equal to the value of sample information (VSI) minus the cost of sampling (CS). It should be noted that sample information is the sum total of input into the NHTDM and, therefore, experimental outcomes depend solely on sample data. Since the clinical nurse practitioner in the data example gained no practical information from the outcomes of the research, on an arbitrary 10-point scale, the VSI might be estimated to be around 0 or 1. One unit is given here to reflect the gains, if any, incurred by the exchange between the nurse investigator and the nurse clinician during the delineation of the problem to be studied.

The cost of sampling, on the other hand, would be estimated to be high relative to the VSI. That is, the staff time and effort, transportation costs to collect data by making home visits, the cost of printing questionnaires, and analyzing and reporting results were expensive. On the 10-point scale, then, one might arbitrarily assign a value of 5 to the CS. The ENGS in this instance, then, might be estimated to be −4, which would represent a total net loss to both the researcher and the clinician. If nurse clinicians are to willingly become either consumers of or participants in ongoing nursing research, then the expected net gains to them need to be increased. One vehicle for increasing gains might be found in an alternative to the NHTDM approach to the study of clinical nursing problems. Such an alternative, in order to be more viable for the nurse clinician, would need to: (1) allow for the consideration of the probability of occurrence of unique events, (2) provide a formal mechanism for including all information relevant to the problem, (3) facilitate the articulation between nurse researchers and nurse clinicians throughout the investigation, and (4) provide results that clearly convey some information regarding the probability of alternative values of the parameter of interest and, therefore, appear to flow directly from the analysis. Not only would such an alternative approach serve a more utilitarian function regarding the implementation of empirical evidence into ongoing nursing practice but it would also serve to upgrade the overall quality of nursing research by legitimizing the explicit incorporation of the researcher's prior beliefs. Bayesian analysis is an alternative research strategy that meets the above four requirements and appears, therefore, to have greater utility for the investigation of the same clinical nursing problem.

In a Bayesian approach to the subjective interpretation of probability, a probability is interpreted as the quantified judgment of a particular researcher. Since a probability, in this sense, is a measure of a degree of belief rather than a long-run frequency, it is reasonable to assign a probability to an event that involves a nonrepetitive situation. As a result, one can think of a probability as representing the researcher's judgment concerning what will happen in a single trial of the uncertain situation in question rather than a statement about what will happen in the long run. It should be noted at this point, however, that it is not necessary for an experiment to be nonrepetitive for the subjective interpretation of probability to be applicable, that is, the subjective interpretation of probability makes sense whether the experiments in question are repetitive or nonrepetitive. The pragmatic advantage in this respect, therefore, is that a Bayesian approach will have utility for investigating the gamut of nursing problems, while the NHTDM should be limited to those in which a relative frequency interpretation of probability is feasible.

The subjective interpretation of probability can be thought of as an extension of the frequency interpretation of probability. That is, in the discussion of the NHTDM, it was mentioned that assumptions are made by the researcher regarding the appropriate theoretical sampling distribution and that the justification of long-run frequency is based on certain assumptions that are necessary for the proof of the law of large numbers (for example, that the trials or experiments are conducted under identical conditions). The point being made is that the researcher's decision as to whether these assumptions seem reasonable in any given situation is ultimately a subjective decision and, therefore, there is an element of subjectivity in the relative frequency interpretation of probability.

To illustrate the reanalysis of the same research question utilizing a Bayesian approach, suppose the nurse researcher is interested in assessing a probability distribution for p, the proportion of low income women who have had three or more visits to a physician in the past year. In this approach, probability can be thought of as a measure of uncertainty. The researcher does, however, have some subjective beliefs about the proportion. More specifically, the nurse investigator is aware of a body of research findings that suggests the lower the social status of the person, the less likely that person is to utilize medical facilities.[17] The nurse researcher's inclination, therefore, is to believe that the poor underutilize health services. The nurse clinician who brought the problem to the researcher's attention, however, has observed in the U.S. Health, Education and Welfare statistics[25] over the years 1963 to 1969 a trend that suggests to her that those with under $3,000 per year incomes are visiting physicians frequently. Combining this information with her knowledge of the characteristics of the clients for whom she provides care, the nurse clinician believes that the low income women in the state may, in fact, overutilize physician services. In attempting to reckon their disparate subjective judgments of what the population proportion might be, the two engage cooperatively in a literature search and a series of discussions which lead to the decision to obtain additional information in the form of a sample survey. It is important to note here that, unlike the NHTDM example in which the nurse clinician's involvement was limited to the problem identification stage, in the Bayesian approach, articulation between the nurse researcher and nurse clinician has evolved and will continue jointly as a natural result of the analysis.

Before collecting sample data, a second search of the literature reveals additional support for the clinician's belief regarding a trend reversal in the utilization of health services.[18] The nurse researcher is therefore willing to accept the prior beliefs of the clinician in the face of a variety of supporting sources for the clinician's view, that is, clinical experience, the literature, and discussions with knowledgeable others. The two agree to assume, therefore, that the low income women in the state probably overutilize physician services. In order to assess their belief further, it is now necessary for them to attempt to operationalize it. To accomplish this, they decide to use odds in a betting situation as a procedure, which forces them to state what action they would take in a particular decision-making situation rather than just to state directly what they think the probability is. They decide that the odds are 4 to 10 that a woman picked at random from the population of women over age 15 with less than $3,000 per year family income will have visited a physician three or more times in the past year. Their resulting estimate of pi, the population proportion, is 0.285.

The researchers are willing to assume that their data-generating process behaves like a Bernoulli process with two possible outcomes on each trial, such that the probabilities for these outcomes remain constant from trial to trial and the outcomes are independent. That is, the investigators view the population of women over age 15 with family incomes less than \$3,000 as a dichotomous one consisting of women who had three or more visits to a physician during the past year and those who had fewer than three visits. Furthermore, they believe p, the probability of success on a Bernoulli trial, conceptually can assume any real value from 0 to 1, so their prior distribution should be continuous rather than discrete (that is, they believe it is unrealistic to limit p to a finite number of values). They assume the probability distribution of p is a beta distribution with parameters r and n, the number of successes and sample size, respectively. The form of the function in which $n > r > 0$ then is:

$$f(p) = \frac{(n - 1)!}{(r - 1)! \, (n - r - 1)!} \, p^{r-1}(1 - p)^{n-r-1}$$
$$\text{if } 0 \leq p = 1,$$
$$0 \text{ elsewhere}$$

In the beta distribution, the uncertain quantity is p, which in terms of a Bernoulli process is the probability of success on any single Bernoulli trial. The shape of the beta distribution depends on r and n. The mean and variance of a beta distribution with parameters r and n are:

$$\text{mean} = E(p/r,n) = r/n$$
$$\text{variance} = V(p/r,n) = \frac{r(n - r)}{n^2(n + 1)}$$

A prior distribution is chosen from the beta class since it is usually possible, due to the variety of beta distributions, to choose a beta distribution that will approximate one's prior knowledge of the population. Let pi be the true proportion of the population with three or more visits to a physician. The first step in the specification of the prior distribution is to ask what is the most likely value for pi (0.285). The second step involves evaluating the amount of prior information available relative to sample information (denoted $m = 41$). Utilizing a B6700 Data Interactive Computer Program for calculating the Prior and Posterior Beta Binomial Models (BETAB), the researchers are able to express their prior beliefs in the form of a prior beta binomial distribution. The mode of the prior beta density is 0.258. Their selection of an m value of 41 implies that the researchers are willing to give even odds that the true value of pi will lie in the credibility interval that extends from 0.238 to 0.334. The mean of the prior distribution for pi is 0.295 and the SD is 0.07. The parameters of the distribution are 12.115 and 28.885. It should be noted that the prior distribution is a true probability distribution in that it meets the basic axioms of probability. That is, p cannot be negative and the total area under the curve must equal one. A credibility interval, then, is simply an interval of values with some given probability under a prior or a posteriori distribution. This is in contrast to the relative frequency interpretation of probability in the NHTDM, which does not obey the syntax of true probability.

From the population of women in the state with under $3,000 per year of family income, a random sample of 92 (n) women was collected. Randomization was ensured by utilization of a random household sampling procedure. The number of women who had three or more visits to a physician in the past year, or the number of successes, (r) was found to be 16.

Bayes' Theorem for continuous random variables is the mechanism for combining the prior probabilities and sample information represented by the likelihood function to determine the posterior distribution of the parameter of interest given this sample data. This is in contrast to the NHTDM, which is based solely on sample data and seeks the probability (relative frequency) of specific sample information given a fixed value of the parameter. The posterior distribution for pi is a beta distribution with a mode of 0.206, mean of 0.211 and a SD of 0.03. It has parameters 28.115 and 104.885. A 50 percent HDR credibility interval extends from 0.183 to 0.231. (Table 11-6).

TABLE 11-6. Summary of Prior and a Posteriori Results

	Mode	50% HDR	SD	Mean
Prior distribution	0.285	(0.238 − 0.334)	0.07	0.295
A posteriori distribution	0.206	(0.183 − 0.231)	0.03	0.211

It can be seen from Table 11-6 that both the mode and the mean have decreased somewhat from the prior estimate. Neither the prior mode nor mean lies in the a posteriori 50 percent HDR credibility interval. (This interval extends from 0.183 to 0.231.) The reduction in the a posteriori variance reflects the increased precision of the a posteriori estimate relative to the prior estimate. Because the 50 percent HDR credibility interval represents a true probability function, it may be interpreted to mean that the researcher is 50 percent sure that the parameter is between the values 0.183 and 0.231. The endpoints of this credibility interval are assumed to be fixed. In a Bayesian analysis, the credibility interval represents the researcher's degree of belief that the parameter is in the fixed interval. This differs from the confidence interval in the NHTDM, which is assumed to be a random variable whose endpoints are not fixed but vary over trials.

Since the a posteriori distribution in a Bayesian analysis is a true probability distribution, it is possible to talk more directly about the probability of alternative values of the population proportion. That is, given that the a posteriori probability that pi is less than 0.285 is 0.975, it would appear that the true value of pi is less than 0.285 and more likely closer to 0.206. Furthermore, assessing the probability that pi is greater than 0.137, the mode that the researchers believe would indicate underutilization of physician services, one finds the probability 0.989 that pi is greater than 0.137. In addition, the probability that pi is greater than 0.137 but less than 0.285 is 0.964.

The nurse researchers conclude on the basis of this analysis that their prior beliefs about pi that assume that low income women in the state overutilize physician services should be modified and consideration given to the probability that the true proportion is closer to 0.206. In fact, should the investigators decide to do another analysis, this a posteriori distribution of pi might become their subsequent prior distribution. In addition, one would expect the investigators' degree of belief regarding the population proportion to become more precise with each subsequent analysis. An important advantage of the Bayesian approach, then, is the ability it affords the researchers to increase the precision of their belief with subsequent analysis. It is evident then that the results of the Bayesian analysis provide the nurse researchers with information that allows them to talk directly about their concerns, that is, the probability of the value of the proportion comes in a straightforward manner from the analysis. Because there is a direct link between the inferential procedure and the belief that governs the researchers' actions, one would also expect the reporting of the research results to be improved in clarity, and the operational utility of the results to be greater for the nurse clinician. If this is so, it should follow that nurse clinicians will be more likely to accept Bayesian inferences as useful for consideration in their ongoing practice.

Using again the notion of the expected net gain of sampling (ENGS) to conceptualize the utility of the Bayesian approach, it is obvious that the value of sample information (VSI) is greater than in the NHTDM in that the researchers, as a result of their analysis, can make statements regarding the probability of alternative values of the population parameter given this sample information. Furthermore, the outcome of their analysis can be utilized in conjunction with another sample so that the utility of this sample outcome extends beyond this particular analysis. Therefore, the VSI in the Bayesian analysis might be arbitrarily assigned a value of 8 on a 10-point scale. The cost of sampling (CS) can be viewed as essentially the same as in the NHTDM, therefore, ENGS = VSI − CS = 3.

Table 11-7 summarizes the comparison of the ENGS for the NHTDM and the Bayesian analysis.

TABLE 11-7. Comparative ENGS in Two Alternative Approaches to Clinical Nursing Research

	NHTDM	Bayesian
VSI	1	8
CS	5	5
ENGS	−4	3

Summary

Questions of primary concern to nursing clinicians characteristically stem from a concern with the probability of the occurrence of unique events. The advantages of a Bayesian analysis may be realized in four areas of importance to nursing investigators:

1. Consideration of the probability of the occurrence of unique events.
2. Provision of a formal mechanism for the inclusion of all information relevant to a given problem.
3. Facilitation of the lessening of the gap that exists between nursing research and the incorporation and utilization of research results into ongoing nursing practice.
4. Provision of results that present information regarding the probability of alternative values of the parameter and, therefore, appear to flow directly from the analysis.

PRIMARY, SECONDARY, AND META-ANALYSIS OF NURSING RESEARCH DATA

The nurse researcher should be aware of and involved in three levels of research data analysis: primary, secondary, and meta-analysis.

Primary Analysis

Primary analysis is the original analysis of data in a research study. This form of analysis has been the subject of the discussions in this book and is by far the most popular type of analysis undertaken by researchers in nursing.

Secondary Analysis

Secondary analysis is the reanalysis of data for the purpose of answering the original research question with better statistical techniques, or answering new questions with old data.[6, 10] Secondary analysis may serve as a means for validating the results from primary analysis and is thus an especially important activity subsequent to large scale studies with potential for far-reaching consequences. Examples of this type of analysis are scant in the nursing literature, where the focus has been on the conduct of original investigations. Perhaps this reluctance on the part of editors to publish other than original research results from the early stage of development of nursing as a profession and reflects the same phenomenon observed in other developing fields during their early stages of research involvement. Hopefully, as nurse researchers recognize the need for secondary analysis and become involved in it, those responsible for the publication of research efforts will be forced to recognize secondary analysis not only as legitimate, but necessary for the development and testing of nursing theory and practice. A number of outstanding examples of secondary analysis are available in the field of education, including the Mosteller-Moynihan[19] secondary analysis of the Coleman study, Campbell-Erlebacher[5] secondary analysis of the Ohio-Westinghouse Headstart evaluation, and the Elashoff-Snow[9] secondary analysis of Pygmalion in the Classroom.

Secondary analysis can contribute to the advancement of nursing knowledge because it has the potential to consider important questions without some of the limitations, or with a different set of limitations, than those encountered in primary research. More specifically, Burstein[4] suggests the following merits of secondary analysis in the field of education, which hold for nursing as well:

1. Secondary analysis may determine whether or not persons from potentially different perspectives can arrive at similar conclusions if the same questions are investigated and whether or not different questions can be answered from the same data. It is virtually impossible for any primary nursing research investigation to incorporate all potentially relevant viewpoints. If the conclusions of primary and secondary analysis vary or are in conflict, the audience for the results of the original study has obtained interpretations from alternative points of view that can then clarify the difficulties encountered in implementing research findings in nursing settings.

2. Secondary analysis may not suffer from the closeness to the data that may affect the conclusions of primary research. They may reveal evidence that substantiates, elaborates, or refutes the interpretations of the original report. The nature of the research process seems to dictate that persons developing and testing a nursing theory tend to become very close to their problem and may overlook what seem to be peripheral questions. Investigation of these peripheral questions, however, may lead to important information that provides the critical test of a theory's worth. Hence, secondary analysis may lead to more objective consideration of the theoretical premises underlying nursing practice as well as provide for multiple perspectives to clarify the original findings.

3. Primary analysis may fail to focus on issues that become salient after the data are collected. Similarly, in longitudinal studies, the theory and practice that guided the original investigation may be obsolete when applied to prevailing nursing practice. Secondary analysis allows nurse researchers to test their ideas in the context of existing data sets before resources are allocated to support massive new data collection with the possibility of repeating the cycle of obsolescence.

4. Secondary analysis may alleviate some of the constraints operating in large scale studies by providing a fresh influx of capital for further data examination when money allocated for the primary investigation diminishes or by extending the time for research in large scale studies that have time deadlines to be met. Similarly, the psychologic letdown often experienced in the later stages of long term projects may be rejuvenated by the initiation of secondary analysis that brings fresh human resources to the study.

At this point, a word of caution seems in order: primary and secondary analysis should not be viewed as separate and distinct entities. Cooperation and collaboration between the primary and secondary researchers may afford opportunities for collegial exchange of ideas on topics of common interest and can also help to cultivate individuals to carry on the thrust of the original research. Several authors[4, 12, 21] have suggested ways in which collaboration between primary and secondary investigators may be fostered: (1) primary investigators should anticipate and invite secondary analysis of their study, (2) primary researchers should plan and budget for data archiving to ensure that access to data for secondary analysis is not problematic, (3) primary research contracts and consent forms should clearly indicate that the data may be used for multiple research purposes and if so used the secondary researchers are subject to the same legal and ethical obligations regarding confidentiality and privacy as the original researchers, (4) the rights to first access to data reporting by the primary investigators should be respected by secondary analysts, and (5) secondary analysts should avoid placing excessive or added work demands on the primary investigators.

The specific techniques employed in conducting a secondary analysis will be as varied as the research questions and hypotheses being investigated. In general, the secondary analyst should aim to select an approach that will improve upon the precision and hence the quality of the primary investigation. The reader who desires a more in-depth discussion of secondary analysis as well as more specifics regarding its employment will find Cook's[6] presentation of the potential and limitations of secondary evaluations particularly useful.

Meta-analysis

Meta-analysis involves the statistical analysis of a large collection of results from individual studies for the purpose of integrating the findings.[10] This approach represents a rigorous attempt to make sense of the often confusing and conflicting findings resulting from studies of the same variables across different contexts, subjects, and numerous other factors. For example, hundreds of studies on appraisal of faculty performance by nursing students exist, but the patterns of results across studies defy simple summary. Meta-analysis provides methods and techniques for organizing, depicting, and interrelating data from such studies so that knowledge can be aggregated and extracted from the myriad of individual investigations. Several problems in nursing warrant meta-analysis. For example, findings from studies of the expanded nursing role, prediction of success in baccalaureate, associate, and higher degree nursing programs, socialization of nursing students, care of decubitus ulcers, nurse-patient relationships, evaluation of clinical performance, and patient compliance, to name a few, could benefit from meta-analysis. Although the nursing research literature has been systematically reviewed and abstracted for a number of years, the reporting of the integration of the findings from this huge literature via meta-analysis is virtually nonexistent.

Essentially two major approaches exist for conducting a meta-analysis. The first focuses on the reanalysis of original raw data combined from studies that can meet criteria for comparison. Light and Smith[15] are advocates of this strategy, which they refer to as the *cluster approach*. The advantage of this approach is that it is precise and rigorous. An obvious limitation rests with its reliance upon the availability and accessibility of original data that are comparable. The second approach to meta-analysis centers on the results or outcomes of a number of studies rather than relying on original data. This strategy is more practical and less expensive than the first, but it lacks the degree of precision and rigor inherent in the first approach. A primary advocate of this approach is Glass,[10] who refers to it as the *effect size technique*.

The *cluster approach* to meta-analysis derives from cluster sampling originally developed in the field of sampling theory. It is based on the belief that many populations can be broken down into small identifiable subpopulations, which are called clusters. These clusters are natural aggregations within the population and they usually differ in broad and systematic ways. For example, suppose a community health nurse wanted to estimate mean income of the clients in her health district. She could assume in advance that incomes of clients living on the same neighborhood block would tend to be more similar than would incomes of two clients selected at random from the district population as a whole. A cluster sampling design would thus define a neighborhood block as a cluster and would allow for systematic differences in mean income among neighborhoods. A primary advantage of cluster sampling is that it allows data collection to be concentrated in a few conveniently compact areas, such as neighborhoods, and thus substantially reduces the cost of data collection. Another feature of cluster sampling is that clusters are assumed to differ from one another in ways that are not reflected in the variations within any one cluster. On the other hand, variations within clusters need not be reflected in variations among them.

Given a set of nursing studies, how does one identify the clusters? The smallest natural unit of the process under investigation that is available in the data should be taken as the cluster. The choice of a natural unit will then depend upon the research question at issue. Broad studies of patient compliance might focus on an entire hospital ambulatory service as their clustering unit, while other studies might require specific clinics, services, or even patient groups within services to be taken as clusters. For example, when research questions are directed toward the effects of the diabetic treatment regimen on compliance, each individual diabetic ambulatory service can be taken as an independent cluster. Conversely, when the effect of exit interviews on compliance in general is at issue, an entire hospital ambulatory service is a logical choice for a clustering unit. The point is that whatever unit is chosen to be a cluster, it should be the natural focal point or molar unit of whatever question one is investigating.

Hence, a cluster usually is not a complete study. That is, each study in a set to be combined will contain several individual clusters. When there is more than one treatment per study, the set of treatments comprises the set of clusters. Thus, a study will often contain several clusters and the cluster is the unit of analysis. Example 11-4 is a hypothetical example used to present a simplified view of the cluster approach to meta-analysis.

EXAMPLE 11-4. Hypothetical Example of Meta-Analysis Using the Cluster Approach

Purpose: To study the effects on patient compliance of four different kinds of programs:
1. Hospital-based ambulatory care centers.
2. HMOs.
3. Health department clinics.
4. Privately operated group practices comprised of teams of primary care practitioners.

Analysis: 1. Literature is reviewed to identify available studies. To ensure the quality of the meta-analysis, the studies must meet three standards in order to be selected for further analysis:
   a. All subjects in the study must have been selected from a known and precisely defined population.
   b. A study's dependent and independent variables must be measured in the same way as, or in a way subject to a conversion into, those employed in the rest of the studies.
   c. Overall, the instrumentation and quality of the experimental work in a study must be generally comparable to that in all the rest of the studies.[15]
2. In the literature, six studies are found to meet these standards. The six studies contain 14 sites:

| | Study Number | | | | | |
Program Type	1	2	3	4	5	6
Hospital	X	X	X		X	X
HMO	X	X				
Health Dept.			X	XX		X
Private			X		X	X

3. In this study, a cluster is defined as an individual site. Thus, the cluster approach focuses attention on the 14 sites rather than the six studies. Each of the 14 sites contains a group of patients. For each patient at each site, the researcher has a measurement on the dependent variable, compliance. In addition, for each client, the researcher has data on two continuous independent variables, a count of clinic attendance and a knowledge pretest score. Each patient's sex is also known. The researcher therefore has data on four variables.
4. The cluster approach requires access to the original data from these studies. Assuming the data are available, the first step is to group this information into 14 clusters. Thus, at the beginning of the analysis, there would be four measures on each patient assembled into 14 separate groups. It should be noted that one cannot assume that the data being analyzed came from a true experiment. In a true experiment, all patients would have been assembled into a single large group, pretested, and then randomly assigned among the 14 sites. In a meta-analysis, when the results of separate studies are to be combined, it needs to be known that no such group was assembled in advance and no such randomization took place.

EXAMPLE 11-4. *Continued*

5. The research question to be addressed in this meta-analysis is: which of the four types of programs offers the highest level of compliance? Fourteen clusters have been identified. These 14 clusters can differ in a variety of ways; thus, it is necessary to rephrase the research question to ask: in what ways do these 14 clusters differ from one another and, of the ways in which they differ, which can be identified with differences among the four types of programs?

6. A group of clusters can differ in at least five ways:[15]
   a. The means of their variables.
   b. Variances of their variables.
   c. Relations between the independent and dependent variables.
   d. Patient by treatment interactions.
   e. The complex manner in which each patient is affected by the composition of his group.

   If any of these types of differences is found, it follows that the clusters are not all alike and therefore cannot be directly combined. On the other hand, finding that clusters do not differ in any one respect does not lead to the conclusion that they are alike until all five ways have been examined. Even if clusters are found to differ, for example, in means, one must still search out other possible differences if only to explain the variation among means. (For a detailed discussion regarding how clusters can differ, why such differences are important and the implications of such differences for how data are analyzed and combined, the reader is referred to Light and Smith,[15] who present specific techniques and the like.)

7. When no differences in the five areas are found, data from the several clusters can be combined. When one or more differences are found, the differences must be explained and then data can still be combined after the differences are adjusted away (see Light and Smith[15] for specific ways in which this may be accomplished). When differences exist but no explanation is found, the data cannot be combined.

8. Once the problem of combining studies is resolved, cluster analysis may lead to varied and numerous insights into nursing concerns. Two frequently encountered uses of cluster analysis that would probably result from the findings of this hypothetical meta-analysis example are to: (a) resolve a contradiction that arises from two different analyses of the same data and (b) identify a fundamental relationship among several different ways in which a given program or programs can operate.

The *effect size technique* of meta-analysis, which is rapidly gaining favor, addresses the question(s): how large an effect does a particular treatment produce, or among several effective treatments which is the most effective? *Effect size* is the mean difference on the dependent variable between experimental and control subjects divided by the within-group standard deviation.[10] Since some studies may have more than one dependent variable and/or variables measured at more than one point in time, within any given meta-analysis there may be far more effect sizes than the actual number of studies. After the findings from each study are thus quantified, aggregate meanings can be summarized by (1) determining the average of the effect sizes across studies and (2) comparing the average effect size for experimental and control groups for each variable. A published example of meta-analysis using the effect size technique is presented in Example 11-5.

EXAMPLE 11-5. Published Example of Meta-Analysis Using the Effect Size Technique

Title: *Primary, secondary, and meta-analysis of research.*

Source: Glass, Educational Researcher, vol. 5, November, 1976, pp. 3 – 8.

Purpose: To integrate the outcome evaluation literature in psychotherapy and counseling.

Analysis:
1. An extensive literature search produced 375 controlled evaluations of the effects of psychotherapy.
2. In excess of 800 measures of effect size were determined from the 375 studies.
3. Additional factors described included, but were not limited to:
   a. Duration of therapy in hours.
   b. Years of experience.
   c. Subject's diagnosis.
   d. Type of therapy.
4. Aggregate meanings were summarized utilizing a variety of statistical analyses. For example:
   a. The average effect size over the 800 measures was found to be 0.68 standard deviations, indicating on the average the therapy group mean was found to be two thirds of a standard deviation above the control group mean on the outcome variable.
   b. Effect sizes of four different types of therapy were compared in relation to untreated control groups and it was found that the effect sizes for the four types of therapy were not greatly different in their average impact.
   c. To further control for differences among therapies in the types of problems dealt with, experience of therapists, duration, and so forth, all studies in which the conditions were strictly comparable for the different therapies were sorted out for special analysis.

Summary

In summary, primary analysis of data in nursing is not sufficient. Extracting knowledge from accumulated studies via secondary and meta-analysis is a complex endeavor that is important to a developing profession. Thus, both secondary and meta-analysis of nursing research data should become legitimate and inherent components of nursing research activity.

REFERENCES

1. Bausell, R. B., Rinkus, A., and Watson, D.: *The relationship between treatment modality, demographic characteristics, and staff perceptions concerning their jobs in*

26 *Philadelphia drug treatment centers.* International Journal of the Addictions (in press).

2. Bracht, G. H.: Experimental factors related to aptitude treatment interactions. Rev. Ed. Res. 40:627, 1970.

3. Brewer, J. K. and Knowles, R. D.: *Some statistical considerations in nursing research.* Nurs. Res. 23:68, 1974.

4. Burstein, L.: *Secondary analysis: An important resource for educational research and evaluation.* Ed. Res. 7(5):9, May, 1978.

5. Campbell, D. T. and Erebacher, A. E.: *How regression artifacts in quasi-experimental evaluations can mistakenly make compensatory education look harmful.* In Compensatory Education: A National Debate. Hellmuth, J. (ed.): The Disadvantaged Child, vol. 3. Brunner/Mazel, New York, 1970.

6. Cook, T. D.: *The potential and limitations of secondary evaluations.* In Apple, M. W., Subkoviak, H. S., and Lufler, J. R. (eds.): Educational Evaluation: Analysis and Responsibility. McCutchan, Berkeley, 1974, pp. 155–234.

7. Cooley, W. W. and Lohnes, P. R.: *Multivariate Data Analysis.* John Wiley and Sons, New York, 1971.

8. Dunkin, M. and Biddle, B.: *The Study of Teaching.* Holt, Rinehart and Winston, New York, 1974.

9. Elashoff, J. D. and Snow, R. E. (ed.): *Pygmalion Reconsidered.* Charles A. Jones, Worthington, Ohio, 1971.

10. Glass, G. V.: *Primary, secondary, and meta-analysis of research.* Ed. Res. 5(11):3, November, 1976.

11. Glass, G. V. and Stanley, J. C.: *Statistical Methods in Education and Psychology.* Prentice-Hall, Englewood Cliffs, New Jersey, 1970.

12. Hedrick, T. E., Boruch, R. F. and Ross, J.: *Policy and regulation for ensuring the availability of evaluation data for secondary analysis.* Paper presented at the Annual Meeting of the American Psychological Association, San Francisco, September, 1977.

13. Hutcenson, J. D., LaRetta, M. G., and Lowe, L. S.: *Antecedents of nursing school attrition: Attitudinal dimensions.* Nurs. Res. 28:57, 1979.

14. Jamison, D., Suppes, P., and Wells, S.: *The effectiveness of alternative instructional media: A survey.* Rev. Ed. Res. 44:1, 1974.

15. Light, R. J. and Smith, P. V.: *Accumulating evidence: Procedures for resolving contradictions among different research studies.* Harvard Ed. Rev. 41(4):429, November, 1971.

16. Mann, N. R., Schafer, R. E., and Singpurevalla, N. D.: *Methods for Statistical Analysis of Reliability and Life Data.* John Wiley and Sons, New York, 1974.

17. Mechanic, D.: *Medical Sociology.* Free Press, New York, 1968.

18. Monteiro, L. A.: *Expense is no object . . . Income and physician visits reconsidered.* J. Health Soc. Behav. 14:25, 1973.

19. Mosteller, F. M. and Moynihan, D. P. (eds.): *On Equality of Educational Opportunity.* Vintage Books, New York, 1972.

20. Nie, N. H., et al.: *Statistical Package for the Social Sciences,* ed. 2. McGraw-Hill, New York, 1975.

21. Powell, M.: *Necessary steps to insure availability of data for secondary analysis.* Paper presented at the Annual Meeting of the American Educational Research Association, New York, April, 1977.

22. Richards, M. A.: *One integrated curriculum: An empirical evaluation.* Nurs. Res. 26:90, 1977.

23. Schramm, W.: *Learning from instructional television.* Rev. Ed. Res. 32:156, 1962.

24. Tatsuoka, M. M.: *Multivariate Analysis.* John Wiley and Sons, New York, 1971.
25. U. S. Department of Health, Education and Welfare: *Health Statistics.* Volume of Physician Visits. Series 10, Number 75, U.S. Public Health Service, Washington, D.C., 1969.
26. Winkler, R. L.: *An Introduction to Bayesian Inference and Decision.* Holt, Rinehart and Winston, New York, 1972, p. 7.

APPENDIX. Statistical Tables

TABLE 1. Areas of the Unit Normal Distribution*

z	Area	z	Area	z	Area
−3.00	.0013	−2.28	.0113	−1.58	.0571
−2.98	.0014	−2.26	.0019	−1.56	.0594
−2.96	.0015	−2.24	.0125	−1.54	.0618
−2.94	.0016	−2.22	.0132	−1.52	.0643
−2.92	.0018	−2.20	.0139	−1.50	.0668
−2.90	.0019				
−2.88	.0020	−2.18	.0146	−1.48	.0694
−2.86	.0021	−2.16	.0154	−1.46	.0721
−2.84	.0023	−2.14	.0162	−1.44	.0749
−2.82	.0024	−2.12	.0170	−1.42	.0778
−2.80	.0026	−2.10	.0179	−1.40	.0808
−2.78	.0027	−2.08	.0188	−1.38	.0838
−2.76	.0029	−2.06	.0197	−1.36	.0869
−2.74	.0031	−2.04	.0207	−1.34	.0901
−2.72	.0033	−2.02	.0217	−1.32	.0934
−2.70	.0035	−2.00	.0228	−1.30	.0968
−2.68	.0037	−1.98	.0239	−1.28	.1003
−2.66	.0039	−1.96	.0250	−1.26	.1038
−2.64	.0041	−1.94	.0262	−1.24	.1075
−2.62	.0044	−1.92	.0274	−1.22	.1112
−2.60	.0047	−1.90	.0287	−1.20	.1151
−2.58	.0049	−1.88	.0301	−1.18	.1190
−2.56	.0052	−1.86	.0314	−1.16	.1230
−2.54	.0055	−1.84	.0329	−1.14	.1271
−2.52	.0059	−1.82	.0344	−1.12	.1314
−2.50	.0062	−1.80	.0359	−1.10	.1357
−2.48	.0066	−1.78	.0375	−1.08	.1401
−2.46	.0069	−1.76	.0392	−1.06	.1446
−2.44	.0073	−1.74	.0409	−1.04	.1492
−2.42	.0078	−1.72	.0427	−1.02	.1539
−2.40	.0082	−1.70	.0446	−1.00	.1587
−2.38	.0087	−1.68	.0465	−0.98	.1635
−2.36	.0091	−1.66	.0485	−0.96	.1685
−2.34	.0096	−1.64	.0505	−0.94	.1736
−2.32	.0102	−1.62	.0526	−0.92	.1788
−2.30	.0107	−1.60	.0548	−0.90	.1841

*Adapted from Tables I and II of Fisher and Yates: *Statistical Tables for Biological, Agricultural and Medical Research,* published by Longman Group Ltd., London, (previously published by Oliver and Boyd, Edinburgh), with permission.

TABLE 1. *Continued*

z	Area	z	Area	z	Area
−0.88	.1894	−0.08	.4681	0.72	.7642
−0.86	.1949	−0.06	.4761	0.74	.7704
−0.84	.2005	−0.04	.4840	0.76	.7764
−0.82	.2061	−0.02	.4920	0.78	.7823
−0.80	.2119	0.00	.5000	0.80	.7881
−0.78	.2177	0.02	.5080	0.82	.7939
−0.76	.2236	0.04	.5160	0.84	.7995
−0.74	.2296	0.06	.5239	0.86	.8051
−0.72	.2358	0.08	.5319	0.88	.8106
−0.70	.2420	0.10	.5398	0.90	.8159
−0.68	.2483	0.12	.5478	1.00	.8413
−0.66	.2546	0.14	.5557	1.02	.8461
−0.64	.2611	0.16	.5636	1.04	.8508
−0.62	.2676	0.18	.5714	1.06	.8554
−0.60	.2743	0.20	.5793	1.08	.8599
−0.58	.2810	0.22	.5871	1.10	.8643
−0.56	.2877	0.24	.5948	1.12	.8686
−0.54	.2946	0.26	.6026	1.14	.8729
−0.52	.3015	0.28	.6103	1.16	.8770
−0.50	.3085	0.30	.6179	1.18	.8810
−0.48	.3156	0.32	.6255	1.20	.8849
−0.46	.3228	0.34	.6231	1.22	.8888
−0.44	.3300	0.36	.6406	1.24	.8925
−0.42	.3372	0.38	.6480	1.26	.8962
−0.40	.3446	0.40	.6554	1.28	.8997
−0.38	.3520	0.42	.6628	1.30	.9032
−0.36	.3594	0.44	.6700	1.32	.9066
−0.34	.3669	0.46	.6772	1.34	.9099
−0.32	.3745	0.48	.6844	1.36	.9131
−0.30	.3821	0.50	.6915	1.38	.9162
−0.28	.3897	0.52	.6985	1.40	.9192
−0.26	.3974	0.54	.7054	1.42	.9222
−0.24	.4052	0.56	.7123	1.44	.9251
−0.22	.4129	0.58	.7190	1.46	.9279
−0.20	.4207	0.60	.7257	1.48	.9309
−0.18	.4286	0.62	.7324	1.50	.9332
−0.16	.4364	0.64	.7389	1.52	.9357
−0.14	.4443	0.66	.7454	1.54	.9382
−0.12	.4522	0.68	.7517	1.56	.9406
−0.10	.4602	0.70	.7580	1.58	.9429

TABLE 1. Continued

z	Area	z	Area
1.60	.9452	2.52	.9941
1.62	.9474	2.54	.9945
1.64	.9495	2.56	.9948
1.66	.9515	2.58	.9951
1.68	.9535	2.60	.9953
1.70	.9554		
1.72	.9573	2.62	.9956
1.74	.9591	2.64	.9959
1.76	.9608	2.66	.9961
1.78	.9625	2.68	.9963
1.80	.9641	2.70	.9965
1.90	.9733	2.72	.9967
1.92	.9726	2.74	.9969
1.94	.9738	2.76	.9971
1.96	.9750	2.78	.9973
1.98	.9761	2.80	.9974
2.00	.9772		
2.02	.9783	2.82	.9976
2.04	.9793	2.84	.9977
2.06	.9803	2.86	.9979
2.08	.9812	2.88	.9980
2.10	.9821	2.90	.9981
2.12	.9830	2.92	.9982
2.14	.9838	2.94	.9984
2.16	.9846	2.96	.9985
2.18	.9854	2.98	.9986
2.20	.9861	3.00	.9987
2.22	.9868		
2.24	.9875		
2.26	.9881		
2.28	.9887		
2.30	.9893		
2.32	.9898		
2.34	.9904		
2.36	.9909		
2.38	.9913		
2.40	.9918		
2.42	.9922		
2.44	.9927		
2.46	.9931		
2.48	.9934		
2.50	.9938		

TABLE 2. Critical Values of Chi-Square*

df	Probability under the Null Hypothesis that $X^2 \geq$ Chi-Square													
	.99	.98	.95	.90	.80	.70	.50	.30	.20	.10	.05	.02	.01	.001
1	.00016	.00063	.0039	.016	.064	.15	.46	1.07	1.64	2.71	3.84	5.41	6.64	10.83
2	.02	.04	.10	.21	.45	.71	1.39	2.41	3.22	4.60	5.99	7.82	9.21	13.82
3	.12	.18	.35	.58	1.00	1.42	2.37	3.66	4.64	6.25	7.82	9.84	11.34	16.27
4	.30	.43	.71	1.06	1.65	2.20	3.36	4.88	5.99	7.78	9.49	11.67	13.28	18.46
5	.55	.75	1.14	1.61	2.34	3.00	4.35	6.06	7.29	9.24	11.07	13.39	15.09	20.52
6	.87	1.13	1.64	2.20	3.07	3.83	5.35	7.23	8.56	10.64	12.59	15.03	16.81	22.46
7	1.24	1.56	2.17	2.83	3.82	4.67	6.35	8.38	9.80	12.02	14.07	16.62	18.48	24.32
8	1.65	2.03	2.73	3.49	4.59	5.53	7.34	9.52	11.03	13.36	15.51	18.17	20.09	26.12
9	2.09	2.53	3.32	4.17	5.38	6.39	8.34	10.66	12.24	14.68	16.92	19.68	21.67	27.88
10	2.56	3.06	3.94	4.86	6.18	7.27	9.34	11.78	13.44	15.99	18.31	21.16	23.21	29.59
11	3.05	3.61	4.58	5.58	6.99	8.15	10.34	12.90	14.63	17.28	19.68	22.62	24.72	31.26
12	3.57	4.18	5.23	6.30	7.81	9.03	11.34	14.01	15.81	18.55	21.03	24.05	26.22	32.91
13	4.11	4.76	5.89	7.04	8.63	9.93	12.34	15.12	16.98	19.81	22.36	25.47	27.69	34.53
14	4.66	5.37	6.57	7.79	9.47	10.82	13.34	16.22	18.15	21.06	23.68	26.87	29.14	36.12
15	5.23	5.98	7.26	8.55	10.31	11.72	14.34	17.32	19.31	22.31	25.00	28.26	30.58	37.70
16	5.81	6.61	7.96	9.31	11.15	12.62	15.34	18.42	20.46	23.54	26.30	29.63	32.00	39.29
17	6.41	7.26	8.67	10.08	12.00	13.53	16.34	19.51	21.62	24.77	27.59	31.00	33.41	40.75
18	7.02	7.91	9.39	10.86	12.86	14.44	17.34	20.60	22.76	25.99	28.87	32.35	34.80	42.31
19	7.63	8.57	10.12	11.65	13.72	15.35	18.34	21.69	23.90	27.20	30.14	33.69	36.19	43.82
20	8.26	9.24	10.85	12.44	14.58	16.27	19.34	22.78	25.04	28.41	31.41	35.02	37.57	45.32
21	8.90	9.92	11.59	13.24	15.44	17.18	20.34	23.86	26.17	29.62	32.67	36.34	38.93	46.80
22	9.54	10.60	12.34	14.04	16.31	18.10	21.24	24.94	27.30	30.81	33.92	37.66	40.29	48.27
23	10.20	11.29	13.09	14.85	17.19	19.02	22.34	26.02	28.43	32.01	35.17	38.97	41.64	49.73
24	10.86	11.99	13.85	15.66	18.06	19.94	23.34	27.10	29.55	33.20	36.42	40.27	42.98	51.18
25	11.52	12.70	14.61	16.47	18.94	20.87	24.34	28.17	30.68	34.38	37.65	41.57	44.31	52.62
26	12.20	13.41	15.38	17.29	19.82	21.79	25.34	29.25	31.80	35.56	38.88	42.86	45.64	54.05
27	12.88	14.12	16.15	18.11	20.70	22.72	26.34	30.32	32.91	36.74	40.11	44.14	46.96	55.48
28	13.56	14.85	16.93	18.94	21.59	23.65	27.34	31.39	34.03	37.92	41.34	45.42	48.28	56.89
29	14.26	15.57	17.71	19.77	22.48	24.58	28.34	32.46	35.14	39.09	42.56	46.69	49.59	58.30
30	14.95	16.31	18.49	20.60	23.36	25.51	29.34	33.53	36.25	40.26	43.77	47.96	50.89	59.70

*Abridged from Table IV of Fisher and Yates: *Statistical Tables for Biological, Agricultural and Medical Research,* published by Longman Group Ltd., London (previously published by Oliver and Boyd, Edinburgh), with permission.

TABLE 3. Percentile Points of F Distributions

75th percentiles

n_2 \ n_1	1	2	3	4	5	6	7	8	9	10	12	15	20	24	30	40	60	120	∞
1	5.83	7.50	8.20	8.58	8.82	8.98	9.10	9.19	9.26	9.32	9.41	9.49	9.58	9.63	9.67	9.71	9.76	9.80	9.85
2	2.57	3.00	3.15	3.23	3.28	3.31	3.34	3.35	3.37	3.38	3.39	3.41	3.43	3.43	3.44	3.45	3.46	3.47	3.48
3	2.02	2.28	2.36	2.39	2.41	2.42	2.43	2.44	2.44	2.44	2.45	2.46	2.46	2.46	2.47	2.47	2.47	2.47	2.47
4	1.81	2.00	2.05	2.06	2.07	2.08	2.08	2.08	2.08	2.08	2.08	2.08	2.08	2.08	2.08	2.08	2.08	2.08	2.08
5	1.69	1.85	1.88	1.89	1.89	1.89	1.89	1.89	1.89	1.89	1.89	1.89	1.88	1.88	1.88	1.88	1.87	1.87	1.87
6	1.62	1.76	1.78	1.79	1.79	1.78	1.78	1.78	1.77	1.77	1.77	1.76	1.76	1.75	1.75	1.75	1.74	1.74	1.74
7	1.57	1.70	1.72	1.72	1.71	1.71	1.70	1.70	1.69	1.69	1.68	1.68	1.67	1.67	1.66	1.66	1.65	1.65	1.65
8	1.54	1.66	1.67	1.66	1.66	1.65	1.64	1.64	1.63	1.63	1.62	1.62	1.61	1.60	1.60	1.59	1.59	1.58	1.58
9	1.51	1.62	1.63	1.63	1.62	1.61	1.60	1.60	1.59	1.59	1.58	1.57	1.56	1.56	1.55	1.54	1.54	1.53	1.53
10	1.49	1.60	1.60	1.59	1.59	1.58	1.57	1.56	1.56	1.55	1.54	1.53	1.52	1.52	1.51	1.51	1.50	1.49	1.48
11	1.47	1.58	1.58	1.57	1.56	1.55	1.54	1.53	1.53	1.52	1.51	1.50	1.49	1.49	1.48	1.47	1.47	1.46	1.45
12	1.46	1.56	1.56	1.55	1.54	1.53	1.52	1.51	1.51	1.50	1.49	1.48	1.47	1.46	1.45	1.45	1.44	1.43	1.42
13	1.45	1.55	1.55	1.53	1.52	1.51	1.50	1.49	1.49	1.48	1.47	1.46	1.45	1.44	1.43	1.42	1.42	1.41	1.40
14	1.44	1.53	1.53	1.52	1.51	1.50	1.49	1.48	1.47	1.46	1.45	1.44	1.43	1.42	1.41	1.41	1.40	1.39	1.38
15	1.43	1.52	1.52	1.51	1.49	1.48	1.47	1.46	1.46	1.45	1.44	1.43	1.41	1.41	1.40	1.39	1.38	1.37	1.36
16	1.42	1.51	1.51	1.50	1.48	1.47	1.46	1.45	1.44	1.44	1.43	1.41	1.40	1.39	1.38	1.37	1.36	1.35	1.34
17	1.42	1.51	1.50	1.49	1.47	1.46	1.45	1.44	1.43	1.43	1.41	1.40	1.39	1.38	1.37	1.36	1.35	1.34	1.33
18	1.41	1.50	1.49	1.48	1.46	1.45	1.44	1.43	1.42	1.42	1.40	1.39	1.38	1.37	1.36	1.35	1.34	1.33	1.32
19	1.41	1.49	1.49	1.47	1.46	1.44	1.43	1.42	1.41	1.41	1.40	1.38	1.37	1.36	1.35	1.34	1.33	1.32	1.30
20	1.40	1.49	1.48	1.47	1.45	1.44	1.43	1.42	1.41	1.40	1.39	1.37	1.36	1.35	1.34	1.33	1.32	1.31	1.29
21	1.40	1.48	1.48	1.46	1.44	1.43	1.42	1.41	1.40	1.39	1.38	1.37	1.35	1.34	1.33	1.32	1.31	1.30	1.28
22	1.40	1.48	1.47	1.45	1.44	1.42	1.41	1.40	1.39	1.39	1.37	1.36	1.34	1.33	1.32	1.31	1.30	1.29	1.28
23	1.39	1.47	1.47	1.45	1.43	1.41	1.41	1.40	1.39	1.38	1.37	1.35	1.34	1.33	1.32	1.31	1.30	1.28	1.27
24	1.39	1.47	1.46	1.44	1.43	1.41	1.40	1.39	1.38	1.38	1.36	1.35	1.33	1.32	1.31	1.30	1.29	1.28	1.26
25	1.39	1.47	1.46	1.44	1.42	1.41	1.40	1.39	1.38	1.37	1.36	1.34	1.33	1.32	1.31	1.29	1.28	1.27	1.25
26	1.38	1.46	1.45	1.44	1.42	1.41	1.39	1.38	1.37	1.36	1.35	1.34	1.32	1.31	1.30	1.29	1.28	1.26	1.25
27	1.38	1.46	1.45	1.43	1.42	1.40	1.39	1.38	1.37	1.36	1.35	1.33	1.32	1.31	1.30	1.28	1.27	1.25	1.24
28	1.38	1.46	1.45	1.43	1.41	1.40	1.39	1.38	1.37	1.36	1.34	1.33	1.31	1.30	1.29	1.28	1.26	1.25	1.24
29	1.38	1.45	1.45	1.43	1.41	1.40	1.38	1.37	1.36	1.35	1.34	1.32	1.31	1.30	1.29	1.27	1.26	1.25	1.23
30	1.38	1.45	1.44	1.42	1.41	1.39	1.38	1.37	1.36	1.35	1.34	1.32	1.30	1.29	1.28	1.27	1.26	1.24	1.23
40	1.36	1.44	1.42	1.40	1.39	1.37	1.36	1.35	1.34	1.33	1.31	1.30	1.28	1.26	1.25	1.24	1.22	1.21	1.19
60	1.35	1.42	1.41	1.38	1.37	1.35	1.33	1.32	1.31	1.30	1.29	1.27	1.25	1.24	1.22	1.21	1.19	1.17	1.15
120	1.34	1.40	1.39	1.37	1.35	1.33	1.31	1.30	1.29	1.28	1.26	1.24	1.22	1.21	1.19	1.18	1.16	1.13	1.10
∞	1.32	1.39	1.37	1.35	1.33	1.31	1.29	1.28	1.27	1.25	1.24	1.22	1.19	1.18	1.16	1.14	1.12	1.08	1.00

Reprinted from *Biometrika Tables for Statisticians* (2nd ed., 1962), eds. E. S. Pearson and H. O. Hartley, by permission of the *Biometrika* Trustees and the publisher, Cambridge University Press.

90th percentiles

n_2 \ n_1	1	2	3	4	5	6	7	8	9	10	12	15	20	24	30	40	60	120	∞
1	39.86	49.50	53.59	55.83	57.24	58.20	58.91	59.44	59.86	60.19	60.71	61.22	61.74	62.00	62.26	62.53	62.79	63.06	63.33
2	8.53	9.00	9.16	9.24	9.29	9.33	9.35	9.37	9.38	9.39	9.41	9.42	9.44	9.45	9.46	9.47	9.47	9.48	9.49
3	5.54	5.46	5.39	5.34	5.31	5.28	5.27	5.25	5.24	5.23	5.22	5.20	5.18	5.18	5.17	5.16	5.15	5.14	5.13
4	4.54	4.32	4.19	4.11	4.05	4.01	3.98	3.95	3.94	3.92	3.90	3.87	3.84	3.83	3.82	3.80	3.79	3.78	3.76
5	4.06	3.78	3.62	3.52	3.45	3.40	3.37	3.34	3.32	3.30	3.27	3.24	3.21	3.19	3.17	3.16	3.14	3.12	3.10
6	3.78	3.46	3.29	3.18	3.11	3.05	3.01	2.98	2.96	2.94	2.90	2.87	2.84	2.82	2.80	2.78	2.76	2.74	2.72
7	3.59	3.26	3.07	2.96	2.88	2.83	2.78	2.75	2.72	2.70	2.67	2.63	2.59	2.58	2.56	2.54	2.51	2.49	2.47
8	3.46	3.11	2.92	2.81	2.73	2.67	2.62	2.59	2.56	2.54	2.50	2.46	2.42	2.40	2.38	2.36	2.34	2.32	2.29
9	3.36	3.01	2.81	2.69	2.61	2.55	2.51	2.47	2.44	2.42	2.38	2.34	2.30	2.28	2.25	2.23	2.21	2.18	2.16
10	3.29	2.92	2.73	2.61	2.52	2.46	2.41	2.38	2.35	2.32	2.28	2.24	2.20	2.18	2.16	2.13	2.11	2.08	2.06
11	3.23	2.86	2.66	2.54	2.45	2.39	2.34	2.30	2.27	2.25	2.21	2.17	2.12	2.10	2.08	2.05	2.03	2.00	1.97
12	3.18	2.81	2.61	2.48	2.39	2.33	2.28	2.24	2.21	2.19	2.15	2.10	2.06	2.04	2.01	1.99	1.96	1.93	1.90
13	3.14	2.76	2.56	2.43	2.35	2.28	2.23	2.20	2.16	2.14	2.10	2.05	2.01	1.98	1.96	1.93	1.90	1.88	1.85
14	3.10	2.73	2.52	2.39	2.31	2.24	2.19	2.15	2.12	2.10	2.05	2.01	1.96	1.94	1.91	1.89	1.86	1.83	1.80
15	3.07	2.70	2.49	2.36	2.27	2.21	2.16	2.12	2.09	2.06	2.02	1.97	1.92	1.90	1.87	1.85	1.82	1.79	1.76
16	3.05	2.67	2.46	2.33	2.24	2.18	2.13	2.09	2.06	2.03	1.99	1.94	1.89	1.87	1.84	1.81	1.78	1.75	1.72
17	3.03	2.64	2.44	2.31	2.22	2.15	2.10	2.06	2.03	2.00	1.96	1.91	1.86	1.84	1.81	1.78	1.75	1.72	1.69
18	3.01	2.62	2.42	2.29	2.20	2.13	2.08	2.04	2.00	1.98	1.93	1.89	1.84	1.81	1.78	1.75	1.72	1.69	1.66
19	2.99	2.61	2.40	2.27	2.18	2.11	2.06	2.02	1.98	1.96	1.91	1.86	1.81	1.79	1.76	1.73	1.70	1.67	1.63
20	2.97	2.59	2.38	2.25	2.16	2.09	2.04	2.00	1.96	1.94	1.89	1.84	1.79	1.77	1.74	1.71	1.68	1.64	1.61
21	2.96	2.57	2.36	2.23	2.14	2.08	2.02	1.98	1.95	1.92	1.87	1.83	1.78	1.75	1.72	1.69	1.66	1.62	1.59
22	2.95	2.56	2.35	2.22	2.13	2.06	2.01	1.97	1.93	1.90	1.86	1.81	1.76	1.73	1.70	1.67	1.64	1.60	1.57
23	2.94	2.55	2.34	2.21	2.11	2.05	1.99	1.95	1.92	1.89	1.84	1.80	1.74	1.72	1.69	1.66	1.62	1.59	1.55
24	2.93	2.54	2.33	2.19	2.10	2.04	1.98	1.94	1.91	1.88	1.83	1.78	1.73	1.70	1.67	1.64	1.61	1.57	1.53
25	2.92	2.53	2.32	2.18	2.09	2.02	1.97	1.93	1.89	1.87	1.82	1.77	1.72	1.69	1.66	1.63	1.59	1.56	1.52
26	2.91	2.52	2.31	2.17	2.08	2.01	1.96	1.92	1.88	1.86	1.81	1.76	1.71	1.68	1.65	1.61	1.58	1.54	1.50
27	2.90	2.51	2.30	2.17	2.07	2.00	1.95	1.91	1.87	1.85	1.80	1.75	1.70	1.67	1.64	1.60	1.57	1.53	1.49
28	2.89	2.50	2.29	2.16	2.06	2.00	1.94	1.90	1.87	1.84	1.79	1.74	1.69	1.66	1.63	1.59	1.56	1.52	1.48
29	2.89	2.50	2.28	2.15	2.06	1.99	1.93	1.89	1.86	1.83	1.78	1.73	1.68	1.65	1.62	1.58	1.55	1.51	1.47
30	2.88	2.49	2.28	2.14	2.05	1.98	1.93	1.88	1.85	1.82	1.77	1.72	1.67	1.64	1.61	1.57	1.54	1.50	1.46
40	2.84	2.44	2.23	2.09	2.00	1.93	1.87	1.83	1.79	1.76	1.71	1.66	1.61	1.57	1.54	1.51	1.47	1.42	1.38
60	2.79	2.39	2.18	2.04	1.95	1.87	1.82	1.77	1.74	1.71	1.66	1.60	1.54	1.51	1.48	1.44	1.40	1.35	1.29
120	2.75	2.35	2.13	1.99	1.90	1.82	1.77	1.72	1.68	1.65	1.60	1.55	1.48	1.45	1.41	1.37	1.32	1.26	1.19
∞	2.71	2.30	2.08	1.94	1.85	1.77	1.72	1.67	1.63	1.60	1.55	1.49	1.42	1.38	1.34	1.30	1.24	1.17	1.00

TABLE 3. Continued

95th percentiles

n_2 \ n_1	1	2	3	4	5	6	7	8	9	10	12	15	20	24	30	40	60	120	∞
1	161.4	199.5	215.7	224.6	230.2	234.0	236.8	238.9	240.5	241.9	243.9	245.9	248.0	249.1	250.1	251.1	252.2	253.3	254.3
2	18.51	19.00	19.16	19.25	19.30	19.33	19.35	19.37	19.38	19.40	19.41	19.43	19.45	19.45	19.46	19.47	19.48	19.49	19.50
3	10.13	9.55	9.28	9.12	9.01	8.94	8.89	8.85	8.81	8.79	8.74	8.70	8.66	8.64	8.62	8.59	8.57	8.55	8.53
4	7.71	6.94	6.59	6.39	6.26	6.16	6.09	6.04	6.00	5.96	5.91	5.86	5.80	5.77	5.75	5.72	5.69	5.66	5.63
5	6.61	5.79	5.41	5.19	5.05	4.95	4.88	4.82	4.77	4.74	4.68	4.62	4.56	4.53	4.50	4.46	4.43	4.40	4.36
6	5.99	5.14	4.76	4.53	4.39	4.28	4.21	4.15	4.10	4.06	4.00	3.94	3.87	3.84	3.81	3.77	3.74	3.70	3.67
7	5.59	4.74	4.35	4.12	3.97	3.87	3.79	3.73	3.68	3.64	3.57	3.51	3.44	3.41	3.38	3.34	3.30	3.27	3.23
8	5.32	4.46	4.07	3.84	3.69	3.58	3.50	3.44	3.39	3.35	3.28	3.22	3.15	3.12	3.08	3.04	3.01	2.97	2.93
9	5.12	4.26	3.86	3.63	3.48	3.37	3.29	3.23	3.18	3.14	3.07	3.01	2.94	2.90	2.86	2.83	2.79	2.75	2.71
10	4.96	4.10	3.71	3.48	3.33	3.22	3.14	3.07	3.02	2.98	2.91	2.85	2.77	2.74	2.70	2.66	2.62	2.58	2.54
11	4.84	3.98	3.59	3.36	3.20	3.09	3.01	2.95	2.90	2.85	2.79	2.72	2.65	2.61	2.57	2.53	2.49	2.45	2.40
12	4.75	3.89	3.49	3.26	3.11	3.00	2.91	2.85	2.80	2.75	2.69	2.62	2.54	2.51	2.47	2.43	2.38	2.34	2.30
13	4.67	3.81	3.41	3.18	3.03	2.92	2.83	2.77	2.71	2.67	2.60	2.53	2.46	2.42	2.38	2.34	2.30	2.25	2.21
14	4.60	3.74	3.34	3.11	2.96	2.85	2.76	2.70	2.65	2.60	2.53	2.46	2.39	2.35	2.31	2.27	2.22	2.18	2.13
15	4.54	3.68	3.29	3.06	2.90	2.79	2.71	2.64	2.59	2.54	2.48	2.40	2.33	2.29	2.25	2.20	2.16	2.11	2.07
16	4.49	3.63	3.24	3.01	2.85	2.74	2.66	2.59	2.54	2.49	2.42	2.35	2.28	2.24	2.19	2.15	2.11	2.06	2.01
17	4.45	3.59	3.20	2.96	2.81	2.70	2.61	2.55	2.49	2.45	2.38	2.31	2.23	2.19	2.15	2.10	2.06	2.01	1.96
18	4.41	3.55	3.16	2.93	2.77	2.66	2.58	2.51	2.46	2.41	2.34	2.27	2.19	2.15	2.11	2.06	2.02	1.97	1.92
19	4.38	3.52	3.13	2.90	2.74	2.63	2.54	2.48	2.42	2.38	2.31	2.23	2.16	2.11	2.07	2.03	1.98	1.93	1.88
20	4.35	3.49	3.10	2.87	2.71	2.60	2.51	2.45	2.39	2.35	2.28	2.20	2.12	2.08	2.04	1.99	1.95	1.90	1.84
21	4.32	3.47	3.07	2.84	2.68	2.57	2.49	2.42	2.37	2.32	2.25	2.18	2.10	2.05	2.01	1.96	1.92	1.87	1.81
22	4.30	3.44	3.05	2.82	2.66	2.55	2.46	2.40	2.34	2.30	2.23	2.15	2.07	2.03	1.98	1.94	1.89	1.84	1.78
23	4.28	3.42	3.03	2.80	2.64	2.53	2.44	2.37	2.32	2.27	2.20	2.13	2.05	2.01	1.96	1.91	1.86	1.81	1.76
24	4.26	3.40	3.01	2.78	2.62	2.51	2.42	2.36	2.30	2.25	2.18	2.11	2.03	1.98	1.94	1.89	1.84	1.79	1.73
25	4.24	3.39	2.99	2.76	2.60	2.49	2.40	2.34	2.28	2.24	2.16	2.09	2.01	1.96	1.92	1.87	1.82	1.77	1.71
26	4.23	3.37	2.98	2.74	2.59	2.47	2.39	2.32	2.27	2.22	2.15	2.07	1.99	1.95	1.90	1.85	1.80	1.75	1.69
27	4.21	3.35	2.96	2.73	2.57	2.46	2.37	2.31	2.25	2.20	2.13	2.06	1.97	1.93	1.88	1.84	1.79	1.73	1.67
28	4.20	3.34	2.95	2.71	2.56	2.45	2.36	2.29	2.24	2.19	2.12	2.04	1.96	1.91	1.87	1.82	1.77	1.71	1.65
29	4.18	3.33	2.93	2.70	2.55	2.43	2.35	2.28	2.22	2.18	2.10	2.03	1.94	1.90	1.85	1.81	1.75	1.70	1.64
30	4.17	3.32	2.92	2.69	2.53	2.42	2.33	2.27	2.21	2.16	2.09	2.01	1.93	1.89	1.84	1.79	1.74	1.68	1.62
40	4.08	3.23	2.84	2.61	2.45	2.34	2.25	2.18	2.12	2.08	2.00	1.92	1.84	1.79	1.74	1.69	1.64	1.58	1.51
60	4.00	3.15	2.76	2.53	2.37	2.25	2.17	2.10	2.04	1.99	1.92	1.84	1.75	1.70	1.65	1.59	1.53	1.47	1.39
120	3.92	3.07	2.68	2.45	2.29	2.17	2.09	2.02	1.96	1.91	1.83	1.75	1.66	1.61	1.55	1.50	1.43	1.35	1.25
∞	3.84	3.00	2.60	2.37	2.21	2.10	2.01	1.94	1.88	1.83	1.75	1.67	1.57	1.52	1.46	1.39	1.32	1.22	1.00

97.5th percentiles

n_2 \ n_1	1	2	3	4	5	6	7	8	9	10	12	15	20	24	30	40	60	120	∞
1	647.8	799.5	864.2	899.6	921.8	937.1	948.2	956.7	963.3	968.6	976.7	984.9	993.1	997.2	1001	1006	1010	1014	1018
2	38.51	39.00	39.17	39.25	39.30	39.33	39.36	39.37	39.39	39.40	39.41	39.43	39.45	39.46	39.46	39.47	39.48	39.49	39.50
3	17.44	16.04	15.44	15.10	14.88	14.73	14.62	14.54	14.47	14.42	14.34	14.25	14.17	14.12	14.08	14.04	13.99	13.95	13.90
4	12.22	10.65	9.98	9.60	9.36	9.20	9.07	8.98	8.90	8.84	8.75	8.66	8.56	8.51	8.46	8.41	8.36	8.31	8.26
5	10.01	8.43	7.76	7.39	7.15	6.98	6.85	6.76	6.68	6.62	6.52	6.43	6.33	6.28	6.23	6.18	6.12	6.07	6.02
6	8.81	7.26	6.60	6.23	5.99	5.82	5.70	5.60	5.52	5.46	5.37	5.27	5.17	5.12	5.07	5.01	4.96	4.90	4.85
7	8.07	6.54	5.89	5.52	5.29	5.12	4.99	4.90	4.82	4.76	4.67	4.57	4.47	4.42	4.36	4.31	4.25	4.20	4.14
8	7.57	6.06	5.42	5.05	4.82	4.65	4.53	4.43	4.36	4.30	4.20	4.10	4.00	3.95	3.89	3.84	3.78	3.73	3.67
9	7.21	5.71	5.08	4.72	4.48	4.32	4.20	4.10	4.03	3.96	3.87	3.77	3.67	3.61	3.56	3.51	3.45	3.39	3.33
10	6.94	5.46	4.83	4.47	4.24	4.07	3.95	3.85	3.78	3.72	3.62	3.52	3.42	3.37	3.31	3.26	3.20	3.14	3.08
11	6.72	5.26	4.63	4.28	4.04	3.88	3.76	3.66	3.59	3.53	3.43	3.33	3.23	3.17	3.12	3.06	3.00	2.94	2.88
12	6.55	5.10	4.47	4.12	3.89	3.73	3.61	3.51	3.44	3.37	3.28	3.18	3.07	3.02	2.96	2.91	2.85	2.79	2.72
13	6.41	4.97	4.35	4.00	3.77	3.60	3.48	3.39	3.31	3.25	3.15	3.05	2.95	2.89	2.84	2.78	2.72	2.66	2.60
14	6.30	4.86	4.24	3.89	3.66	3.50	3.38	3.29	3.21	3.15	3.05	2.95	2.84	2.79	2.73	2.67	2.61	2.55	2.49
15	6.20	4.77	4.15	3.80	3.58	3.41	3.29	3.20	3.12	3.06	2.96	2.86	2.76	2.70	2.64	2.59	2.52	2.46	2.40
16	6.12	4.69	4.08	3.73	3.50	3.34	3.22	3.12	3.05	2.99	2.89	2.79	2.68	2.63	2.57	2.51	2.45	2.38	2.32
17	6.04	4.62	4.01	3.66	3.44	3.28	3.16	3.06	2.98	2.92	2.82	2.72	2.62	2.56	2.50	2.44	2.38	2.32	2.25
18	5.98	4.56	3.95	3.61	3.38	3.22	3.10	3.01	2.93	2.87	2.77	2.67	2.56	2.50	2.44	2.38	2.32	2.26	2.19
19	5.92	4.51	3.90	3.56	3.33	3.17	3.05	2.96	2.88	2.82	2.72	2.62	2.51	2.45	2.39	2.33	2.27	2.20	2.13
20	5.87	4.46	3.86	3.51	3.29	3.13	3.01	2.91	2.84	2.77	2.68	2.57	2.46	2.41	2.35	2.29	2.22	2.16	2.09
21	5.83	4.42	3.82	3.48	3.25	3.09	2.97	2.87	2.80	2.73	2.64	2.53	2.42	2.37	2.31	2.25	2.18	2.11	2.04
22	5.79	4.38	3.78	3.44	3.22	3.05	2.93	2.84	2.76	2.70	2.60	2.50	2.39	2.33	2.27	2.21	2.14	2.08	2.00
23	5.75	4.35	3.75	3.41	3.18	3.02	2.90	2.81	2.73	2.67	2.57	2.47	2.36	2.30	2.24	2.18	2.11	2.04	1.97
24	5.72	4.32	3.72	3.38	3.15	2.99	2.87	2.78	2.70	2.64	2.54	2.44	2.33	2.27	2.21	2.15	2.08	2.01	1.94
25	5.69	4.29	3.69	3.35	3.13	2.97	2.85	2.75	2.68	2.61	2.51	2.41	2.30	2.24	2.18	2.12	2.05	1.98	1.91
26	5.66	4.27	3.67	3.33	3.10	2.94	2.82	2.73	2.65	2.59	2.49	2.39	2.28	2.22	2.16	2.09	2.03	1.95	1.88
27	5.63	4.24	3.65	3.31	3.08	2.92	2.80	2.71	2.63	2.57	2.47	2.36	2.25	2.19	2.13	2.07	2.00	1.93	1.85
28	5.61	4.22	3.63	3.29	3.06	2.90	2.78	2.69	2.61	2.55	2.45	2.34	2.23	2.17	2.11	2.05	1.98	1.91	1.83
29	5.59	4.20	3.61	3.27	3.04	2.88	2.76	2.67	2.59	2.53	2.43	2.32	2.21	2.15	2.09	2.03	1.96	1.89	1.81
30	5.57	4.18	3.59	3.25	3.03	2.87	2.75	2.65	2.57	2.51	2.41	2.31	2.20	2.14	2.07	2.01	1.94	1.87	1.79
40	5.42	4.05	3.46	3.13	2.90	2.74	2.62	2.53	2.45	2.39	2.29	2.18	2.07	2.01	1.94	1.88	1.80	1.72	1.64
60	5.29	3.93	3.34	3.01	2.79	2.63	2.51	2.41	2.33	2.27	2.17	2.06	1.94	1.88	1.82	1.74	1.67	1.58	1.48
120	5.15	3.80	3.23	2.89	2.67	2.52	2.39	2.30	2.22	2.16	2.05	1.94	1.82	1.76	1.69	1.61	1.53	1.43	1.31
∞	5.02	3.69	3.12	2.79	2.57	2.41	2.29	2.19	2.11	2.05	1.94	1.83	1.71	1.64	1.57	1.48	1.39	1.27	1.00

TABLE 3. Continued

99th percentiles

n_2 \ n_1	1	2	3	4	5	6	7	8	9	10	12	15	20	24	30	40	60	120	∞
1	4052	4999.5	5403	5625	5764	5859	5928	5982	6022	6056	6106	6157	6209	6235	6261	6287	6313	6339	6366
2	98.50	99.00	99.17	99.25	99.30	99.33	99.36	99.37	99.39	99.40	99.42	99.43	99.45	99.46	99.47	99.47	99.48	99.49	99.50
3	34.12	30.82	29.46	28.71	28.24	27.91	27.67	27.49	27.35	27.23	27.05	26.87	26.69	26.60	26.50	26.41	26.32	26.22	26.13
4	21.20	18.00	16.69	15.98	15.52	15.21	14.98	14.80	14.66	14.55	14.37	14.20	14.02	13.93	13.84	13.75	13.65	13.56	13.46
5	16.26	13.27	12.06	11.39	10.97	10.67	10.46	10.29	10.16	10.05	9.89	9.72	9.55	9.47	9.38	9.29	9.20	9.11	9.02
6	13.75	10.92	9.78	9.15	8.75	8.47	8.26	8.10	7.98	7.87	7.72	7.56	7.40	7.31	7.23	7.14	7.06	6.97	6.88
7	12.25	9.55	8.45	7.85	7.46	7.19	6.99	6.84	6.72	6.62	6.47	6.31	6.16	6.07	5.99	5.91	5.82	5.74	5.65
8	11.26	8.65	7.59	7.01	6.63	6.37	6.18	6.03	5.91	5.81	5.67	5.52	5.36	5.28	5.20	5.12	5.03	4.95	4.86
9	10.56	8.02	6.99	6.42	6.06	5.80	5.61	5.47	5.35	5.26	5.11	4.96	4.81	4.73	4.65	4.57	4.48	4.40	4.31
10	10.04	7.56	6.55	5.99	5.64	5.39	5.20	5.06	4.94	4.85	4.71	4.56	4.41	4.33	4.25	4.17	4.08	4.00	3.91
11	9.65	7.21	6.22	5.67	5.32	5.07	4.89	4.74	4.63	4.54	4.40	4.25	4.10	4.02	3.94	3.86	3.78	3.69	3.60
12	9.33	6.93	5.95	5.41	5.06	4.82	4.64	4.50	4.39	4.30	4.16	4.01	3.86	3.78	3.70	3.62	3.54	3.45	3.36
13	9.07	6.70	5.74	5.21	4.86	4.62	4.44	4.30	4.19	4.10	3.96	3.82	3.66	3.59	3.51	3.43	3.34	3.25	3.17
14	8.86	6.51	5.56	5.04	4.69	4.46	4.28	4.14	4.03	3.94	3.80	3.66	3.51	3.43	3.35	3.27	3.18	3.09	3.00
15	8.68	6.36	5.42	4.89	4.56	4.32	4.14	4.00	3.89	3.80	3.67	3.52	3.37	3.29	3.21	3.13	3.05	2.96	2.87
16	8.53	6.23	5.29	4.77	4.44	4.20	4.03	3.89	3.78	3.69	3.55	3.41	3.26	3.18	3.10	3.02	2.93	2.84	2.75
17	8.40	6.11	5.18	4.67	4.34	4.10	3.93	3.79	3.68	3.59	3.46	3.31	3.16	3.08	3.00	2.92	2.83	2.75	2.65
18	8.29	6.01	5.09	4.58	4.25	4.01	3.84	3.71	3.60	3.51	3.37	3.23	3.08	3.00	2.92	2.84	2.75	2.66	2.57
19	8.18	5.93	5.01	4.50	4.17	3.94	3.77	3.63	3.52	3.43	3.30	3.15	3.00	2.92	2.84	2.76	2.67	2.58	2.49
20	8.10	5.85	4.94	4.43	4.10	3.87	3.70	3.56	3.46	3.37	3.23	3.09	2.94	2.86	2.78	2.69	2.61	2.52	2.42
21	8.02	5.78	4.87	4.37	4.04	3.81	3.64	3.51	3.40	3.31	3.17	3.03	2.88	2.80	2.72	2.64	2.55	2.46	2.36
22	7.95	5.72	4.82	4.31	3.99	3.76	3.59	3.45	3.35	3.26	3.12	2.98	2.83	2.75	2.67	2.58	2.50	2.40	2.31
23	7.88	5.66	4.76	4.26	3.94	3.71	3.54	3.41	3.30	3.21	3.07	2.93	2.78	2.70	2.62	2.54	2.45	2.35	2.26
24	7.82	5.61	4.72	4.22	3.90	3.67	3.50	3.36	3.26	3.17	3.03	2.89	2.74	2.66	2.58	2.49	2.40	2.31	2.21
25	7.77	5.57	4.68	4.18	3.85	3.63	3.46	3.32	3.22	3.13	2.99	2.85	2.70	2.62	2.54	2.45	2.36	2.27	2.17
26	7.72	5.53	4.64	4.14	3.82	3.59	3.42	3.29	3.18	3.09	2.96	2.81	2.66	2.58	2.50	2.42	2.33	2.23	2.13
27	7.68	5.49	4.60	4.11	3.78	3.56	3.39	3.26	3.15	3.06	2.93	2.78	2.63	2.55	2.47	2.38	2.29	2.20	2.10
28	7.64	5.45	4.57	4.07	3.75	3.53	3.36	3.23	3.12	3.03	2.90	2.75	2.60	2.52	2.44	2.35	2.26	2.17	2.06
29	7.60	5.42	4.54	4.04	3.73	3.50	3.33	3.20	3.09	3.00	2.87	2.73	2.57	2.49	2.41	2.33	2.23	2.14	2.03
30	7.56	5.39	4.51	4.02	3.70	3.47	3.30	3.17	3.07	2.98	2.84	2.70	2.55	2.47	2.39	2.30	2.21	2.11	2.01
40	7.31	5.18	4.31	3.83	3.51	3.29	3.12	2.99	2.89	2.80	2.66	2.52	2.37	2.29	2.20	2.11	2.02	1.92	1.80
60	7.08	4.98	4.13	3.65	3.34	3.12	2.95	2.82	2.72	2.63	2.50	2.35	2.20	2.12	2.03	1.94	1.84	1.73	1.60
120	6.85	4.79	3.95	3.48	3.17	2.96	2.79	2.66	2.56	2.47	2.34	2.19	2.03	1.95	1.86	1.76	1.66	1.53	1.38
∞	6.63	4.61	3.78	3.32	3.02	2.80	2.64	2.51	2.41	2.32	2.18	2.04	1.88	1.79	1.70	1.59	1.47	1.32	1.00

99.5th percentiles

n_2 \ n_1	1	2	3	4	5	6	7	8	9	10	12	15	20	24	30	40	60	120	∞
1	16211	20000	21615	22500	23056	23437	23715	23925	24091	24224	24426	24630	24836	24940	25044	25148	25253	25359	25465
2	198.5	199.0	199.2	199.2	199.3	199.3	199.4	199.4	199.4	199.4	199.4	199.4	199.4	199.5	199.5	199.5	199.5	199.5	199.5
3	55.55	49.80	47.47	46.19	45.39	44.84	44.43	44.13	43.88	43.69	43.39	43.08	42.78	42.62	42.47	42.31	42.15	41.99	41.83
4	31.33	26.28	24.26	23.15	22.46	21.97	21.62	21.35	21.14	20.97	20.70	20.44	20.17	20.03	19.89	19.75	19.61	19.47	19.32
5	22.78	18.31	16.53	15.56	14.94	14.51	14.20	13.96	13.77	13.62	13.38	13.15	12.90	12.78	12.66	12.53	12.40	12.27	12.14
6	18.63	14.54	12.92	12.03	11.46	11.07	10.79	10.57	10.39	10.25	10.03	9.81	9.59	9.47	9.36	9.24	9.12	9.00	8.88
7	16.24	12.40	10.88	10.05	9.52	9.16	8.89	8.68	8.51	8.38	8.18	7.97	7.75	7.65	7.53	7.42	7.31	7.19	7.08
8	14.69	11.04	9.60	8.81	8.30	7.95	7.69	7.50	7.34	7.21	7.01	6.81	6.61	6.50	6.40	6.29	6.18	6.06	5.95
9	13.61	10.11	8.72	7.96	7.47	7.13	6.88	6.69	6.54	6.42	6.23	6.03	5.83	5.73	5.62	5.52	5.41	5.30	5.19
10	12.83	9.43	8.08	7.34	6.87	6.54	6.30	6.12	5.97	5.85	5.66	5.47	5.27	5.17	5.07	4.97	4.86	4.75	4.64
11	12.23	8.91	7.60	6.88	6.42	6.10	5.86	5.68	5.54	5.42	5.24	5.05	4.86	4.76	4.65	4.55	4.44	4.34	4.23
12	11.75	8.51	7.23	6.52	6.07	5.76	5.52	5.35	5.20	5.09	4.91	4.72	4.53	4.43	4.33	4.23	4.12	4.01	3.90
13	11.37	8.19	6.93	6.23	5.79	5.48	5.25	5.08	4.94	4.82	4.64	4.46	4.27	4.17	4.07	3.97	3.87	3.76	3.65
14	11.06	7.92	6.68	6.00	5.56	5.26	5.03	4.86	4.72	4.60	4.43	4.25	4.06	3.96	3.86	3.76	3.66	3.55	3.44
15	10.80	7.70	6.48	5.80	5.37	5.07	4.85	4.67	4.54	4.42	4.25	4.07	3.88	3.79	3.69	3.58	3.48	3.37	3.26
16	10.58	7.51	6.30	5.64	5.21	4.91	4.69	4.52	4.38	4.27	4.10	3.92	3.73	3.64	3.54	3.44	3.33	3.22	3.11
17	10.38	7.35	6.16	5.50	5.07	4.78	4.56	4.39	4.25	4.14	3.97	3.79	3.61	3.51	3.41	3.31	3.21	3.10	2.98
18	10.22	7.21	6.03	5.37	4.96	4.66	4.44	4.28	4.14	4.03	3.86	3.68	3.50	3.40	3.30	3.20	3.10	2.99	2.87
19	10.07	7.09	5.92	5.27	4.85	4.56	4.34	4.18	4.04	3.93	3.76	3.59	3.40	3.31	3.21	3.11	3.00	2.89	2.78
20	9.94	6.99	5.82	5.17	4.76	4.47	4.26	4.09	3.96	3.85	3.68	3.50	3.32	3.22	3.12	3.02	2.92	2.81	2.69
21	9.83	6.89	5.73	5.09	4.68	4.39	4.18	4.01	3.88	3.77	3.60	3.43	3.24	3.15	3.05	2.95	2.84	2.73	2.61
22	9.73	6.81	5.65	5.02	4.61	4.32	4.11	3.94	3.81	3.70	3.54	3.36	3.18	3.08	2.98	2.88	2.77	2.66	2.55
23	9.63	6.73	5.58	4.95	4.54	4.26	4.05	3.88	3.75	3.64	3.47	3.30	3.12	3.02	2.92	2.82	2.71	2.60	2.48
24	9.55	6.66	5.52	4.89	4.49	4.20	3.99	3.83	3.69	3.59	3.42	3.25	3.06	2.97	2.87	2.77	2.66	2.55	2.43
25	9.48	6.60	5.46	4.84	4.43	4.15	3.94	3.78	3.64	3.54	3.37	3.20	3.01	2.92	2.82	2.72	2.61	2.50	2.38
26	9.41	6.54	5.41	4.79	4.38	4.10	3.89	3.73	3.60	3.49	3.33	3.15	2.97	2.87	2.77	2.67	2.56	2.45	2.33
27	9.34	6.49	5.36	4.74	4.34	4.06	3.85	3.69	3.56	3.45	3.28	3.11	2.93	2.83	2.73	2.63	2.52	2.41	2.29
28	9.28	6.44	5.32	4.70	4.30	4.02	3.81	3.65	3.52	3.41	3.25	3.07	2.89	2.79	2.69	2.59	2.48	2.37	2.25
29	9.23	6.40	5.28	4.66	4.26	3.98	3.77	3.61	3.48	3.38	3.21	3.04	2.86	2.76	2.66	2.56	2.45	2.33	2.21
30	9.18	6.35	5.24	4.62	4.23	3.95	3.74	3.58	3.45	3.34	3.18	3.01	2.82	2.73	2.63	2.52	2.42	2.30	2.18
40	8.83	6.07	4.98	4.37	3.99	3.71	3.51	3.35	3.22	3.12	2.95	2.78	2.60	2.50	2.40	2.30	2.18	2.06	1.93
60	8.49	5.79	4.73	4.14	3.76	3.49	3.29	3.13	3.01	2.90	2.74	2.57	2.39	2.29	2.19	2.08	1.96	1.83	1.69
120	8.18	5.54	4.50	3.92	3.55	3.28	3.09	2.93	2.81	2.71	2.54	2.37	2.19	2.09	1.98	1.87	1.75	1.61	1.43
∞	7.88	5.30	4.28	3.72	3.35	3.09	2.90	2.74	2.62	2.52	2.36	2.19	2.00	1.90	1.79	1.67	1.53	1.36	1.00

TABLE 3. Continued

99.9th percentiles

n_2 \ n_1	1	2	3	4	5	6	7	8	9	10	12	15	20	24	30	40	60	120	∞
1	4053*	5000*	5404*	5625*	5764*	5859*	5929*	5981*	6023*	6056*	6107*	6158*	6209*	6235*	6261*	6287*	6313*	6340*	6366*
2	998.5	999.0	999.2	999.2	999.3	999.3	999.4	999.4	999.4	999.4	999.4	999.4	999.4	999.5	999.5	999.5	999.5	999.5	999.5
3	167.0	148.5	141.1	137.1	134.6	132.8	131.6	130.6	129.9	129.2	128.3	127.4	126.4	125.9	125.4	125.0	124.5	124.0	123.5
4	74.14	61.25	56.18	53.44	51.71	50.53	49.66	49.00	48.47	48.05	47.41	46.76	46.10	45.77	45.43	45.09	44.75	44.40	44.05
5	47.18	37.12	33.20	31.09	29.75	28.84	28.16	27.64	27.24	26.92	26.42	25.91	25.39	25.14	24.87	24.60	24.33	24.06	23.79
6	35.51	27.00	23.70	21.92	20.81	20.03	19.46	19.03	18.69	18.41	17.99	17.56	17.12	16.89	16.67	16.44	16.21	15.99	15.75
7	29.25	21.69	18.77	17.19	16.21	15.52	15.02	14.63	14.33	14.08	13.71	13.32	12.93	12.73	12.53	12.33	12.12	11.91	11.70
8	25.42	18.49	15.83	14.39	13.49	12.86	12.40	12.04	11.77	11.54	11.19	10.84	10.48	10.30	10.11	9.92	9.73	9.53	9.33
9	22.86	16.39	13.90	12.56	11.71	11.13	10.70	10.37	10.11	9.89	9.57	9.24	8.90	8.72	8.55	8.37	8.19	8.00	7.81
10	21.04	14.91	12.55	11.28	10.48	9.92	9.52	9.20	8.96	8.75	8.45	8.13	7.80	7.64	7.47	7.30	7.12	6.94	6.76
11	19.69	13.81	11.56	10.35	9.58	9.05	8.66	8.35	8.12	7.92	7.63	7.32	7.01	6.85	6.68	6.52	6.35	6.17	6.00
12	18.64	12.97	10.80	9.63	8.89	8.38	8.00	7.71	7.48	7.29	7.00	6.71	6.40	6.25	6.09	5.93	5.76	5.59	5.42
13	17.81	12.31	10.21	9.07	8.35	7.86	7.49	7.21	6.98	6.80	6.52	6.23	5.93	5.78	5.63	5.47	5.30	5.14	4.97
14	17.14	11.78	9.73	8.62	7.92	7.43	7.08	6.80	6.58	6.40	6.13	5.85	5.56	5.41	5.25	5.10	4.94	4.77	4.60
15	16.59	11.34	9.34	8.25	7.57	7.09	6.74	6.47	6.26	6.08	5.81	5.54	5.25	5.10	4.95	4.80	4.64	4.47	4.31
16	16.12	10.97	9.00	7.94	7.27	6.81	6.46	6.19	5.98	5.81	5.55	5.27	4.99	4.85	4.70	4.54	4.39	4.23	4.06
17	15.72	10.66	8.73	7.68	7.02	6.56	6.22	5.96	5.75	5.58	5.32	5.05	4.78	4.63	4.48	4.33	4.18	4.02	3.85
18	15.38	10.39	8.49	7.46	6.81	6.35	6.02	5.76	5.56	5.39	5.13	4.87	4.59	4.45	4.30	4.15	4.00	3.84	3.67
19	15.08	10.16	8.28	7.26	6.62	6.18	5.85	5.59	5.39	5.22	4.97	4.70	4.43	4.29	4.14	3.99	3.84	3.68	3.51
20	14.82	9.95	8.10	7.10	6.46	6.02	5.69	5.44	5.24	5.08	4.82	4.56	4.29	4.15	4.00	3.86	3.70	3.54	3.38
21	14.59	9.77	7.94	6.95	6.32	5.88	5.56	5.31	5.11	4.95	4.70	4.44	4.17	4.03	3.88	3.74	3.58	3.42	3.26
22	14.38	9.61	7.80	6.81	6.19	5.76	5.44	5.19	4.99	4.83	4.58	4.33	4.06	3.92	3.78	3.63	3.48	3.32	3.15
23	14.19	9.47	7.67	6.69	6.08	5.65	5.33	5.09	4.89	4.73	4.48	4.23	3.96	3.82	3.68	3.53	3.38	3.22	3.05
24	14.03	9.34	7.55	6.59	5.98	5.55	5.23	4.99	4.80	4.64	4.39	4.14	3.87	3.74	3.59	3.45	3.29	3.14	2.97
25	13.88	9.22	7.45	6.49	5.88	5.46	5.15	4.91	4.71	4.56	4.31	4.06	3.79	3.66	3.52	3.37	3.22	3.06	2.89
26	13.74	9.12	7.36	6.41	5.80	5.38	5.07	4.83	4.64	4.48	4.24	3.99	3.72	3.59	3.44	3.30	3.15	2.99	2.82
27	13.61	9.02	7.27	6.33	5.73	5.31	5.00	4.76	4.57	4.41	4.17	3.92	3.66	3.52	3.38	3.23	3.08	2.92	2.75
28	13.50	8.93	7.19	6.25	5.66	5.24	4.93	4.69	4.50	4.35	4.11	3.86	3.60	3.46	3.32	3.18	3.02	2.86	2.69
29	13.39	8.85	7.12	6.19	5.59	5.18	4.87	4.64	4.45	4.29	4.05	3.80	3.54	3.41	3.27	3.12	2.97	2.81	2.64
30	13.29	8.77	7.05	6.12	5.53	5.12	4.82	4.58	4.39	4.24	4.00	3.75	3.49	3.36	3.22	3.07	2.92	2.76	2.59
40	12.61	8.25	6.60	5.70	5.13	4.73	4.44	4.21	4.02	3.87	3.64	3.40	3.15	3.01	2.87	2.73	2.57	2.41	2.23
60	11.97	7.76	6.17	5.31	4.76	4.37	4.09	3.87	3.69	3.54	3.31	3.08	2.83	2.69	2.55	2.41	2.25	2.08	1.89
120	11.38	7.32	5.79	4.95	4.42	4.04	3.77	3.55	3.38	3.24	3.02	2.78	2.53	2.40	2.26	2.11	1.95	1.76	1.54
∞	10.83	6.91	5.42	4.62	4.10	3.74	3.47	3.27	3.10	2.96	2.74	2.51	2.27	2.13	1.99	1.84	1.66	1.45	1.00

* Multiply these entries by 100.

INDEX